D1583304

SYMPTOMS AND SIGNS IN CLINICAL MEDICINE

AN INTRODUCTION TO MEDICAL DIAGNOSIS

BY

E. NOBLE CHAMBERLAIN, M.D., M.Sc., F.R.C.P.

Lecturer in Medicine, University of Liverpool ; Physician to Out-patients, Royal Liverpool United Hospital, Royal Infirmary Branch ; Visiting Physician, Smithdown Road Hospital, Liverpool ; Formerly Beit Memorial Research Fellow

FOURTH EDITION

WITH 346 ILLUSTRATIONS, OF WHICH 19 ARE IN COLOUR

BRISTOL : JOHN WRIGHT AND SONS LTD.

LONDON : SIMPKIN MARSHALL (1941) LTD.

1947

TO MY WIFE

First Issued, April, 1936
Reprinted, November, 1936
Second Edition, September, 1938
Reprinted, February, 1940
Reprinted, November, 1941
Third Edition, June, 1943
Reprinted, May, 1944
Reprinted, May, 1945
Fourth Edition, June, 1947
Reprinted, October, 1948

PRINTED IN GREAT BRITAIN BY
JOHN WRIGHT AND SONS LTD., BRISTOL

PREFACE TO THE FOURTH EDITION

SYMPTOMS and physical signs do not change, but their interpretation must often be reconsidered in the light of advances in pathology and special methods of examination. This book has been thoroughly revised in the present edition and certain chapters have been largely rewritten, especially those dealing with the Nervous System. A number of additional sections have been added where there appeared to be omissions or changes in understanding as, for example, tracheal tug, d'Espine's sign, and the myotonic pupil. Descriptions have been given of paracentesis pericardii and sternal puncture, and the parts dealing with liver function and pancreatic insufficiency have been brought up to date. Dr. Whitaker has prefaced his chapter on Radiology by some introductory remarks which should be helpful to the student in the interpretation of the normal radiograph. Professor Capon has also made some minor modifications in his popular chapter.

It would be wearisome to give a full account of the many changes which have been made in the chapters on Examination of the Nervous System, but fuller details have been given of paralysis, epilepsy, muscle tone, and involuntary movements, and more attention has been devoted to the sensory neurones and to the effects of spinal cord compression and retention of urine.

Comparison with previous editions will emphasize that the main amplifications in the present edition have been made in essentially clinical problems, and the laboratory and mechanical methods of approach have not been expanded more than was necessary to bring them up to date. It is hoped that the new edition will help the student to maintain a proper sense of proportion between the older clinical methods of examination and the more modern scientific accessory methods which may tend to assume an undue position of importance in his knowledge of medicine.

E. NOBLE CHAMBERLAIN.

Liverpool,
May, 1947.

FROM THE PREFACE TO THE FIRST EDITION

WHEN the student first enters hospital he is initiated into the art of medicine, as distinct from the purer sciences of anatomy and physiology with which he has become familiar. He must learn to obtain from the patient an accurate history of his illness, and be able to appreciate the significance of his symptoms. He must master the technique of medical examination and of eliciting physical signs. The interpretation of these signs, and their co-relation with the symptoms, is the basis of diagnosis. It is the object of this book primarily to help the student in this difficult intermediary period in which he is first introduced to the practice of his art, and the practitioner who wishes to refresh his memory.

As the title implies, an account has been given of the common symptoms and physical signs of disease, but since his student days the author has felt that these are often wrongly described divorced from diagnosis. An attempt has been made, therefore, to take the student a stage further to the visualization of symptoms and signs as forming a clinical picture of some pathological process. In each chapter some of the commoner or more important diseases have been included to illustrate how symptoms and signs are pieced together in the jig-saw puzzle of diagnosis.

In most chapters brief mention has been made of those special methods of laboratory or instrumental investigations which in modern medicine are usually necessary for a full and accurate diagnosis. A rightful place of importance has been given to physical signs which are demonstrated by the use of the unaided senses, but when the special investigations, as occasionally happens, are of more value than the physical signs, this has been pointed out. The technique of these special investigations finds no place here, but those simple laboratory and instrumental procedures, such as lumbar punctures, blood-counts, urine examinations, and so forth, which are generally carried out in the ward or clinic room, have been gathered together in two separate chapters for ease of reference.

In writing this book many standard text-books and monographs have been consulted, and free acknowledgement is made to these sources, which are too numerous to be mentioned by name. In the hope of avoiding the undue influence of particular works, each chapter was written before any book was consulted. In the same way after each chapter had taken shape, certain of them were submitted to colleagues who had a special interest in the subject discussed.

E. NOBLE CHAMBERLAIN.

Liverpool,
March, 1936.

CONTENTS

CHAPTER XI

THE EXAMINATION OF SICK CHILDREN

CHAPTER XII

MEDICAL OPERATIONS AND INSTRUMENTAL INVESTIGATIONS

CHAPTER XIII

RADIOLOGY

CHAPTER XIV

CLINICAL PATHOLOGY AND BIOCHEMISTRY

SYMPTOMS AND SIGNS IN CLINICAL MEDICINE

CHAPTER I

THE ROUTINE OF INTERROGATION AND EXAMINATION

INTRODUCTION

FOR the investigation of a medical case the student must develop a definite system of interrogation and examination, which must be carried out in a routine fashion to save time and to ensure that no important data are omitted. In time this routine system becomes a habit in his professional life, a habit which must be cultivated assiduously. No book can do more than assist in this : the habit can only come by constant practice in dealing with sick persons.

The ultimate object of interrogation and examination is diagnosis. Without diagnosis there can be no satisfactory prognosis or treatment, and the diagnosis depends on a well-balanced judgment of all the facts relating to the case.

These facts fall into four groups : (1) The present symptoms ; (2) The antecedent history, personal and familial ; (3) The physical signs ; (4) The special investigations. Sometimes the diagnosis depends chiefly on one of these, but all must be considered in conjunction before a diagnosis is made.

The Symptoms.—These are *subjective* disturbances which cause dis-ease—that is, cause the patient to appreciate that he is not well. An account of them is obtained by taking a history of the present condition.

The Antecedent History.—This reveals facts in the patient's personal life or in those of his near relatives which may have a direct bearing on the problem under consideration.

The Physical Signs.—These are *objective* marks of disease appreciated by the trained observer by the use of his senses, generally unaided, though the aid of the stethoscope is usually allowed under this definition.

The Special Investigations.—This term is used in the present book to include various accessory methods of examination requiring special apparatus, e.g., radiography, microscopy, and electrocardiography. These special investigations are now an integral part of many medical examinations, and in some cases diagnosis is impossible without them. They are described in Chapters XII-XIV.

When the facts of the case have been gathered together, the final stage is reached, that of *diagnosis*, a word implying knowledge of the organs or tissues affected by disease, and of the pathological changes which have taken place in them.

A complete diagnosis includes an accurate idea of the anatomical localization of the disease, and an understanding of the type of pathological process which is at work. It should also give an impression of the activity of the disease, whether this is stationary as in old healed lesions, or progressing slowly or rapidly. These facts cannot always be elicited, but an attempt must be made to make the diagnosis as comprehensive as possible, both in anatomical and aetiological detail.

In a valvular lesion of the heart, for example, not only must the valve affected be known, but whether it is damaged by rheumatic, syphilitic, or other infection, and whether this infection is actively present, or past and healed. Similarly recognition of a lesion such as paraplegia must be amplified when possible by indicating the cause of the paraplegia, e.g., compression paraplegia due to tumour.

It is also important to recognize that structural changes may exist without functional derangement, and vice versa. Thus certain congenital abnormalities of the heart are consistent with normal function ; whilst in certain abnormal rhythms of the heart, function may be disturbed without any gross underlying structural change.

From the beginning it is essential for the student to train himself to piece together the evidence he has accumulated by taking the history and making a physical examination, with the object of establishing a diagnosis. Only in this way will he avoid that indecisive mental state in which the multiplicity of facts prevents him from appreciating their significance.

Errors will be many at first, and indeed for most of us continue to be made throughout our professional life, but they will become fewer as judgment matures and experience ripens.

Though the necessity for an early attempt at diagnosis has been emphasized here, it is equally important to stress the necessity for that receptivity of mind which allows the physician to reconsider his diagnosis, should fresh evidence be forthcoming.

In subsequent chapters of this book an attempt has been made to describe briefly the symptoms and physical signs of disease, with illustrative examples in each system of the way in which they are employed to make a diagnosis. Variations from this general scheme have been necessary occasionally, notably in Chapter II, dealing with the external manifestations of disease, and in the special chapter on pyrexia.

In the present chapter the important subjects of history-taking and the physical examination of the patient are discussed.

THE PATIENT'S SYMPTOMS AND HISTORY

To take a good history of a case requires as much or more skill than the subsequent physical examination, and accuracy and patience are usually well rewarded by the diagnostic value of the data obtained.

Difficulties arise when the patient's mental status is low and he is unable to grasp the meaning of the questions, but experience soon teaches the interrogator to formulate his questions in a manner suitable to each patient's intelligence.

Likewise it is necessary to learn how to appraise the value of the symptoms or details of personal or family life given by the patient, who on the one hand may wish to conceal or minimize the significance of these, or, on the other, to exaggerate them. We must always be tolerant towards the natural reserve which certain persons show when details of their personal or family life are required. To us these details may appear commonplace, but to the patient they are intimate and therefore not always given without reluctance to a stranger. It is wise to ask, firstly, questions which will cause no embarrassment, leaving questions of a more delicate nature until the patient's confidence has been secured.

The individual physician, in the course of practice, usually develops a particular scheme of interrogation and examination which to him seems most appropriate. Most schemes follow similar lines and the following embodies the general principles involved.

The Complaint : The Patient's Description of his Present Symptoms.—It is most advisable to allow the patient to *express his symptoms in his own words*. The intelligent patient may, in a few minutes, give a history pointing conclusively to the system or systems involved. Others, of less education, are unable to describe the nature of their complaint without help from the examiner in the form of simple questions.

One patient may complain that he gets a crushing pain in the upper part of the chest, which spreads to the left arm, and occurs after effort, thus establishing by the history alone strong diagnostic evidence of the cardiac origin of his pain. Another with " pain in the stomach " may be unable to describe its character until a choice of such terms as griping, cutting, burning, sharp, etc., is offered to him, and is uncertain as to its position until asked to point to any places where it has been felt. It is sometimes necessary to keep loquacious patients to the essential story by interruption with pertinent questions, but impatience on the part of the examiner may cause valuable information to be suppressed, and will certainly destroy the patient's confidence.

The *complaint* should be stated briefly on the case sheet, as it is to be amplified by the subsequent history of the present condition.

History of the Development of the Symptoms : Amplification of the Patient's Description of his Complaint.—Exceptionally, the patient gives an adequate account of his symptoms. More often they are poorly described owing chiefly to his natural lack of technical knowledge and inability to express himself adequately. It therefore becomes the duty of the examiner to put such questions as will bring out a fuller description of individual symptoms. In doing so care must be taken *not to put 'leading questions'*, questions which suggest the nature of the answer.

The following general points should be noted :—

1. *The Duration of the Symptom.*—If more than one, the duration of each should be recorded. Examples : Breathlessness, 6 months ; palpitation, 3 months ; swelling of the feet, 3 days.

It should also be recorded whether the symptoms have been present continuously since their onset ; or, if there have been *intervals of freedom*, the length of these.

2. *The Mode of Onset.*—Did the symptoms come on suddenly or gradually ? If the illness consists of a series of 'attacks', the mode of onset, course, duration, mode of decline, and after-effects of each should be compared.

3. *Modifications of Symptoms.*—The patient should be asked *whether any circumstances aggravate or relieve the symptoms.* Epigastric pain after food and relieved by alkalis or more food is suggestive evidence of pylorospasm, most commonly due to peptic ulcer, but sometimes to the reflex effects of cholecystitis, appendicitis, etc. Pain in the chest aggravated by breathing would point to affections of the pleura or chest wall, e.g., pleurisy or intercostal myositis. These examples could be multiplied indefinitely, and for a true appreciation of symptoms and the questions which should be asked about them, considerable knowledge of medicine is necessary.

4. *Associated Phenomena.*—Does the patient notice other phenomena accompanying the main symptom ? Attacks of pain in the right hypochondrium constantly followed by jaundice are suggestive of intermittent biliary obstruction. Paroxysmal cough followed by a crowing inspiration (the 'whoop') suggests whooping-cough. Pain in the loin followed by hæmaturia suggests renal lesions such as calculus. Again many similar examples could be chosen.

For the junior student a table has been inserted at the end of this chapter in which some of the commoner symptoms of disease are considered, with certain questions designed to amplify the patient's description of them. This table should be studied in conjunction with the present description of history taking.

Care must be taken to trace *any modification which has taken place in the symptoms since their onset.* Not infrequently the patient describes the existent symptoms accurately, but is confused about their character in the beginning. Sometimes, however, he is able to describe changes in their character which may be of diagnostic value.

The history of the development of the symptoms is the most important section of history taking. By close analysis of the patient's statements, the nature of his symptoms will be appreciated and their significance interpreted in the light of the physical examination.

Time spent in questioning the patient intelligently is never lost, but the types of questions to ask need experience. This experience is based on clinical practice, for which reading is a poor substitute. In the present chapter only a skeleton outline of history-taking and an elementary table of symptoms have been provided.

In later chapters the symptoms are discussed in more detail, in their relation to the different systems. When the student has read these accounts and had the opportunity of talking to patients, he will be able to formulate questions which he considers are suitable, for he will then understand what information he expects the question to provide.

Past History.—This should not be confused with the earlier symptoms of the present condition, but may reasonably include attacks of a similar nature when a long interval has elapsed. Thus an attack of pneumonia ten years previously in a patient now suffering from this disease should be included. On the other hand in a patient with a suspected gastric ulcer, attacks of epigastric pain six months previously would rightly be recorded in the present complaint.

The past history relates particularly to those circumstances or illnesses which may have caused or contributed towards the development of the present disease. A successful record of this history really demands considerable knowledge of pathology. *The junior student is well-advised to make a note of all previous illnesses and accidents,* but as his knowledge of the causation of disease increases he may justifiably discard irrelevant facts in the history. It is also important, quite apart from details of actual illnesses, to form some conception as to whether the patient was previously in robust health or has always ' ailed '.

In the case of women, the past history should include an account of the number of *children,* and of any *miscarriages* or *still-births,* and the period of gestation at which these took place. Any difficulties attendant on delivery, and abnormalities of the child or fœtus, should be recorded.

Personal Habits.—It is usually easier to consider the personal habits separately from the past illnesses. The following should be noted :—

1. The patient's *occupation* and any changes which have taken place in it throughout his life. It is necessary to know the conditions of his work, whether the hours are long, the work unduly fatiguing or tedious, whether the place of work is healthy or not, and, perhaps not least, whether the occupation is agreeable to him. The importance of occupation is well illustrated by the prevalence of silicosis (a lung disease) in stone-masons, of lead poisoning in plumbers, and of certain nervous symptoms in workers in manganese.

2. *Hours and regularity of meals.* Amount and variety of food and drink taken. Whether the food is chewed properly and adequate time is

taken over the meal. These points are of great importance in digestive disorders.

3. Amount of *alcohol* and *tobacco* (if any) per week.

4. Amount and quality of *sleep*.

5. *Exercise* and *holidays*.

6. *Menstrual cycle* in women.

7. *Sexual life*, if deemed relevant.

Family History.—Frequently this is irrelevant, but again the inexperienced student would do better to include irrelevant matter rather than to omit facts which might be of importance. In most cases it is sufficient to record any serious illnesses occurring in the immediate relatives (father, mother, sisters, and brothers), or the cause of death if any have died.

In the case of suspected disease of an hereditary or familial type (e.g., hæmophilia, deafness, myopathies, etc.) a more detailed analysis of the family history should be made. This applies also to diseases which, though not strictly hereditary, are commonly found in several members or generations of the same family, e.g., tuberculosis, rheumatic heart disease, etc.

When the history of the case is complete, the physician should have a mental picture not only of the patient's present symptoms, but of the manner in which these developed and of the type of background of personal and family life upon which they have been grafted. Too often we are rightly accused of studying the disease rather than the patient.

THE PHYSICAL EXAMINATION

In most cases the history gives a lead to the system or part of the body affected which should be examined first after a general inspection of the patient has been made (*see* Table, pp. 8–15).

Where no clue is provided by the history, examination must needs be systematic—for example, when the patient complains of vague symptoms such as fatigue, insomnia, or loss of appetite. Even when a particular system is suspected, examination should be made of other related systems, and more briefly of the whole body.

Shortly, systematic examination should comprise the following :—

1. *General inspection* of the whole body for external evidence of disease, in particular for such signs as jaundice, anæmia, cyanosis and rashes, abnormalities in stature and development, abnormal facial characteristics, pathological changes in the limbs, hands and feet, and joints, and pathological swellings (e.g., thyroid, lymphatic glands, and new growths).

2. *The respiratory system*, including the nose, nasal sinuses, throat, bronchi and lungs, and the character of the sputa.

3. *The cardio-vascular system*, including the heart, blood-vessels, and blood-pressure.

4. *The digestive system*, including the mouth, œsophagus, stomach, intestines, liver, gall-bladder, and other abdominal viscera. The fæces and any vomitus should also be inspected.

5. *The hæmopoietic system*, including the blood, lymphatic glands, spleen, and liver.

6. *The genito-urinary system*, including the kidneys, bladder, and genital organs, with an examination of the urine in every case.

7. *The nervous system*, including examination of the cranial nerves, brain functions, and motor and sensory systems in the brain, spinal cord, and peripheral nerves.

8. *The special senses*, when relevant—the eyes, ears, and nose.

The general inspection and the symptoms may make a diagnosis possible without further examination, though a complete examination should not be omitted, as facts supporting or modifying the diagnosis are usually discovered. Moreover, although an attempt should be made to explain all the symptoms and signs on the basis of one disease, the possibility of multiple diseases must not be overlooked. Thus tabes and aortic disease are not infrequently found in the same patient, both having a syphilitic basis, and even unrelated diseases such as pernicious anæmia and myxœdema may be found together.

Some of the diseases diagnosable chiefly by inspection are considered in the next chapter, and the subsequent sections deal with the routine methods of examination of each system in turn. It would be redundant to consider these methods of examination in the present chapter, but it is convenient to mention here certain general observations which are necessary in most medical cases. These include a record of the temperature, of the pulse and respiratory rates, of the frequency with which the bowels are opened, and of the amount of urine passed daily. These facts are generally recorded by the nurse on the temperature chart in all cases admitted to hospital, but a record of them should not be omitted in private practice.

It is usually sufficient to chart the temperature, pulse, and respiratory rate in the morning and evening, but in cases of pyrexia or when changes in the heart or respiratory rates are anticipated, more frequent observations are necessary (four-hourly or two-hourly). (*See also* FEVER, Chapter X.)

Further details relating to height, weight, and general appearance of the patient will be considered in the next chapter.

TABLE OF SYMPTOMS

(This table must not be regarded as complete, but it will serve as a skeleton outline to which the student can add after further reading, and experience in the wards. Fuller details of the *symptoms* of disease are given in each chapter and will suggest the type of question to be asked.)

SYMPTOM	QUESTIONS	EXAMINATION
ANÆMIA (*see* PALLOR)		
ANOREXIA (LOSS OF APPETITE)	1. Whether for all, or special foods 2. Duration 3. Degree	1. Digestive system 2. Respiratory system 3. Other systems if symptoms suggest involvement. Consider also psychological causes
BLOOD IN FÆCES	(*See* EXAMINATION OF FÆCES, pp. 202–204, 415)	
BLOOD IN URINE (HÆMATURIA)	1. Amount. Colour of urine (bright-red : smoky) 2. Relation to micturition (before, during, or after) 3. Pain (renal or bladder) 4. Other urinary symptoms	1. Urinary system 2. Hæmopoietic system 3. Cardio-vascular system
BREATHLESSNESS (DYSPNŒA) *A.* Dyspnœa on Effort	1. What grade of effort causes dyspnœa (e.g., walking, climbing)? 2. Did the dyspnœa appear suddenly or gradually in the first place? 3. Are there other cardiac or respiratory symptoms?	1. Cardio-vascular system 2. Respiratory system 3. Hæmopoietic system
B. Paroxysmal Dyspnœa	1. Circumstances under which attacks come on, e.g., in bed, with excitement 2. Character of breathing (rapid, wheezing, laboured, periodic) 3. Degree of distress (any collapse?) 4. Associated symptoms (cough, sweating, palpitation)	
COLLAPSE	1. Patient's description of what happened 2. Did he fall? Was he unconscious? 3. Associated symptoms (dizziness, sweating, pallor, pain, diarrhœa, fever, hæmorrhage) 4. Food or drugs taken 5. Previous health. Any similar collapse before	1. For evidence of poisoning, infections, intestinal derangement, and internal hæmorrhage 2. Cardio-vascular system 3. Central nervous system

Symptom	Questions	Examination
Constipation	1. Recent or long-standing 2. Normal habits 3. Partial or absolute 4. If partial, is it increasing? 5. Associated symptoms (pain, vomiting) 6. Any alternation with diarrhœa	1. Intestinal tract (abdominal and rectal examination) 2. Examine for general state of health 3. Character of stools
Cough	1. Frequency and severity 2. Duration 3. Whether present any special time of day or night 4. Whether dry or accompanied by expectoration 5. Is the cough brought on by special circumstances such as posture, effort? 6. Amount and character of sputum	1. Note character of cough and nature of sputum 2. Respiratory system, including upper respiratory passages 3. Cardio-vascular system 4. More rarely other systems for reflex causes (e.g., ear, stomach)
Coughing of Blood (Hæmoptysis)	1. Evidence that the blood was coughed (blood bright red, frothy, etc.) 2. Amount of blood. Was the sputum subsequently stained? 3. Previous symptoms of respiratory or heart disease	1. Respiratory system 2. Cardio-vascular system 3. Hæmopoietic system
Decreased Quantity of Urine (Oliguria, Anuria)	1. Amount passed and frequency 2. Duration of symptom 3. Appearance of urine 4. Other symptoms of renal or heart disease	1. Cardio-vascular system 2. Urinary system
Diarrhœa	1. Recent or of long duration 2. Frequency of motions and their character 3. Any fever or loss of weight 4. Food eaten. Other persons affected	1. Intestinal tract (abdominal and rectal examination) 2. Examination of fæces
Difficulty in Micturition (Dysuria)	1. Exact nature (e.g., in starting, in force of stream, in inhibition) 2. If accompanied by pain	1. Urinary system 2. Nervous system
Difficulty in Swallowing (Dysphagia)	1. Whether for fluids or only solids	1. Neck and chest—clinically

Continued on next page

Symptom	Questions	Examination
DIFFICULTY IN SWALLOWING (DYSPHAGIA)—continued.	2. Whether increasing 3. History of possible trauma to œsophagus (hot liquids ; corrosive poisons) 4. Loss of weight	2. Œsophagus—radiologically 3. Heart and great vessels —clinically and radiologically 4. Mouth, pharynx, and larynx
DIZZINESS (VERTIGO)	1. Continuous or paroxysmal 2. Does patient tend to fall in a particular direction? 3. Severity (does he fall ?) 4. Variation with posture 5. Associated phenomena, e.g., vomiting, deafness, tinnitus	1. Ears, including labyrinthine function 2. Nervous system (especially cerebellar tests) 3. Cardio-vascular system 4. Eyes 5. Evidence of toxæmia
DOUBLE VISION (DIPLOPIA)	1. Is the object seen double with one eye (monocular) or with both eyes (binocular)? (Test objectively) 2. Does the diplopia increase on looking to the right, left, upwards, or downwards ?	1. Close each eye in turn to see if diplopia is monocular or binocular 2. In monocular diplopia examine for local disease of the eye 3. In binocular diplopia test integrity of cranial nerves, especially external ocular muscles 4. Examine central nervous system
FAINTING	1. Is consciousness lost completely ? If so, duration 2. Are there any convulsive movements ? 3. Colour of patient 4. Associated phenomena (nausea, sweating, trembling) 5. Circumstances of onset (emotion, pain, prolonged standing) (Obtain history from observer)	1. Nervous system 2. Cardio-vascular system 3. Other systems if symptomatology suggests involvement 4. Evidence of vasomotor instability
FITS (CONVULSIONS)	1. Duration and frequency 2. Generalized or localized (if localized, obtain accurate description of point of origin and spread of fits) 3. Loss of consciousness 4. Injury or incontinence during attacks 5. Other neurological symptoms	1. Nervous system 2. Urinary system 3. Cardio-vascular system

Symptom	Questions	Examination
Flatulence	1. Relation to meals 2. Whether wind belched or passed per anum 3. Is the flatus offensive?	1. Observe for air-swallowing 2. Examine gastro-intestinal tract and associated viscera
Frequency of Micturition	1. Number of times urine is passed 2. Whether at night or in daytime or both 3. Amount of urine passed each time 4. If accompanied by pain	1. Urinary system 2. Nervous system
Headache	1. Situation 2. Character and severity 3. Time of occurrence 4. Aggravating factors (e.g., sneezing, posture) 5. Associated symptoms, especially vomiting, drowsiness, fits	(See Headache, p. 293)
Inability to pass Urine (Retention or Suppression)	1. Sudden onset or increasing difficulty 2. Any psychical trauma 3. Symptoms of cardiac or renal disease	1. Abdomen for distension of bladder 2. If distension, examine for surgical causes of retention (especially stricture and prostatic enlargement), and also nervous system. Catheterize if necessary 3. Cardio-vascular system and renal system for causes of anuria
Incontinence of Fæces	1. Is the symptom occasional or persistent? 2. Is there a call to stool? 3. Is the patient conscious of defæcation?	1. Anus, rectum, and colon 2. Nervous system
Incontinence of Urine	1. Does it occur only at night (in which case the term enuresis is used)? 2. Does the urine dribble away all the time or only periodically?	1. Urinary system 2. Central nervous system
Increased Quantity of Urine (Polyuria)	1. Approximate amount passed, and frequency 2. Appearance of urine 3. Whether continually or only occasionally present 4. Is there undue thirst?	1. Urinary system, including urine 2. Endocrine organs (especially for diabetes mellitus and insipidus)

Continued on next page

SYMPTOM	QUESTIONS	EXAMINATION
INDIGESTION	1. Exact definition, e.g., pain, flatulence, anorexia 2. Relation to food, and bowel movement 3. General health ; diet	1. Digestive system 2. Other systems for evidence of ill health and reflex causes, e.g., tuberculosis, tabes
INVOLUNTARY MOVEMENTS (TREMORS, CHOREIFORM MOVEMENTS, SPASMS, ETC.)	1. Parts of body affected 2. Effect of voluntary muscular action and sleep upon	1. Nervous system 2. Evidence of toxæmia
LOSS OF POWER (PARESIS, PARALYSIS)	1. Sudden or gradual 2. Portion of body involved. 3. Whether maximum at onset or increasing 4. Previous attacks 5. Other symptoms of nervous disease	1. Nervous system 2. Other systems which may give indications of the cause, e.g., sites of embolus formation, malignant disease, etc.
LOSS OF SPEECH (APHASIA AND DYSARTHRIA)	1. Mode of onset, sudden or gradual 2. Does patient understand speech, (e.g., execute a simple command, given without signs) ? 3. Does he understand written words, e.g., will he execute a command given in writing ? 4. Does the patient speak ? If so, is the speech intelligible 5. Can he write ?	1. Nervous system, especially :— a. Intellectual function b. For evidence of paralysis (hemiplegia) of limbs c. For evidence of paralysis of muscles of articulation (larynx, tongue, etc.)
LOSS OF WEIGHT	1. Rapid or gradual 2. Continuous or interrupted by periods of gain in weight 3. Total loss	1. Examine for wasting diseases (See p. 18)
NAUSEA	1. Whether related to food 2. Whether accompanied by vomiting	1. Gastro-intestinal tract and associated viscera 2. Nervous system
NEURALGIA	(See PAIN, p. 264)	(See PAIN, p. 264)
NOISES IN THE EARS OR HEAD	1. Type of noise, e.g., singing, buzzing, voices, etc. 2. Are the noises persistently or occasionally present ?	1. Ears 2. Cardio-vascular system, especially arteries and blood-pressure 3. Nervous system
NUMBNESS, TINGLING, PINS AND NEEDLES (DYSÆSTHESIÆ)	1. Extent and distribution 2. Sudden or gradual onset 3. Periodic or continuous	1. Nervous system, especially for involvement of sensory tracts 2. Cardio-vascular system, especially peripheral vessels

Symptom	Questions	Examination
Obesity	1. Family history 2. Sudden or gradual onset 3. Generalized or localized 4. Habits of diet and exercise 5. If associated with pain	1. Distribution of fat 2. Endocrine organs
Pain (see details under each system)	1. Position 2. Localized, or direction of spread, if any 3. Character and severity 4. Aggravating factors 5. Relieving factors 6. Associated phenomena	1. Tissues or organs over which the pain is experienced 2. Organs and tissues innervated from the same segments of the spinal cord as the area where the pain is felt 3. Nervous system, including structures surrounding or along the course of the nerve
Pallor (Anæmia)	1. The patient's usual colour 2. Whether of sudden or gradual appearance 3. Has there been any hæmorrhage? 4. Any symptoms of anæmia? (see p. 205)	1. Hæmopoietic system. Blood-count in all cases 2. Other systems or tissues, affections of which are known to produce anæmia
Palpitation	1. Whether in attacks. If so, mode of onset and offset, with particular reference to suddenness 2. Consciousness of irregularity 3. Whether the patient has been taking drugs 4. Association with emotion and exercise	1. Cardio-vascular system 2. Nervous system
Rashes	1. Duration and associated symptoms 2. Distribution (if not present now) 3. Is there (a) pain, (b) itching? 4. Is the patient taking drugs?	1. Distribution and character of rash 2. Presence of fever and signs of toxæmia
Sore Tongue and Mouth	1. Duration 2. Patchy (e.g., ulcers) or diffuse 3. Whether taking any medicines 4. Any dysphagia	1. Digestive system, especially tongue, teeth, and buccal mucosa 2. Hæmopoietic system

Continued on next page

SYMPTOM	QUESTIONS	EXAMINATION
SWELLING OF ABDOMEN	1. Sudden or gradual onset 2. Total duration 3. Whether the swelling varies in size 4. Whether body weight is increasing	For general obesity, tympanites, ascites, enlarged viscera, pregnancy, or abdominal tumours
SWELLING OF FEET (ŒDEMA)	1. Whether persistent or only after standing 2. Degree and duration 3. Other symptoms of cardiac and renal disease, anæmia, etc.	1. Cardio-vascular system 2. Urine 3. Blood
THIRST	1. Quantity of fluid taken 2. Is there polyuria ?	1. Examine urine (sugar and albumin) 2. Look for causes and evidence of dehydration
UNCONSCIOUSNESS	1. Is the patient aware of anything going on around him whilst 'unconscious' ? 2. Sensations, if any, immediately prior to attack 3. Duration of attacks 4. Whether accompanied by fits 5. Previous health and the history of any known disease or accident, e.g., diabetes and renal disease 6. Any symptoms immediately preceding coma 7. Possibility of poisoning	1. For patients who are in an unconscious state when seen, see COMA (p. 291) 2. If seen between attacks examine especially :— a. Central nervous system b. Cardio-vascular system c. Urinary system
UNSTEADINESS IN STANDING OR WALKING (ATAXIA)	1. Is it worse in the dark ? 2. Are these associated symptoms (e.g., motor or sensory disturbances, vertigo, etc.) ? 3. Does the patient tend to fall to one particular side ? 4. If of short duration, inquire as to possible poisoning, including alcohol and hypnotic drugs	1. Nervous system 2. Ears (labyrinthine function)
VOMITING	1. Frequency and forcibility 2. Relation to meals ; time of day	1. Digestive system 2. Nervous system

Symptom	Questions	Examination
Vomiting—*continued*	3. Whether preceded by nausea or pain 4. Quantity and nature of vomitus	3. Other systems if symptoms suggest involvement, e.g., renal disease
Vomiting of Blood (Hæmatemesis)	1. Amount and character of hæmorrhage 2. Signs indicating its origin (e.g., bleeding gums, dyspeptic history) 3. Appearance of stools (melæna)	1. Digestive system 2. Hæmopoietic system 3. Evidence of bleeding which might have led to swallowing of blood
Yellow Skin (Jaundice)	1. Is the skin yellow or only sallow? 2. Are the conjunctivæ yellow? 3. Are the attacks associated with (a) pain, (b) gastro-intestinal disturbance, (c) rigors? 4. What is the colour of the urine and stools? 5. Has the patient been taking drugs or having any injections (e.g., atophan, arsenicals)?	1. Skin and mucosæ for signs of present jaundice and anæmia 2. Abdomen (especially liver, gall-bladder, and spleen) 3. Urine and stools

CHAPTER II

EXTERNAL CHARACTERISTICS OF DISEASE

INSPECTION OF EXTERIOR OF BODY

IN the examination of every case it is well to inspect the whole body and to record the following details : (1) Height and weight ; (2) Bodily configuration ; (3) Posture and gait ; (4) Shape of head ; (5) Character of hair ; (6) Facial characteristics ; (7) Skin characters ; (8) Condition of genitalia ; (9) Condition of joints ; (10) Condition of extremities.

These observations are necessary in every medical case even when the symptoms point to an affection of some particular system, but may of themselves give sufficient data for a provisional diagnosis.

1. HEIGHT AND WEIGHT

Height.—The height should be taken in consideration with the age and build of the patient (*see also* EXAMINATION OF SICK CHILDREN, Chapter XI), but although tables of height and weight give a rough indication of the correct proportion between these, they must be interpreted with considerable latitude.

Excessive height, *gigantism*, is nearly always an expression of over-activity of the anterior lobe of the pituitary gland occurring before puberty, i.e., before the long bones have attained their full length. Other features of pituitary hyperfunction may also be present (*see* pp. 42-3).

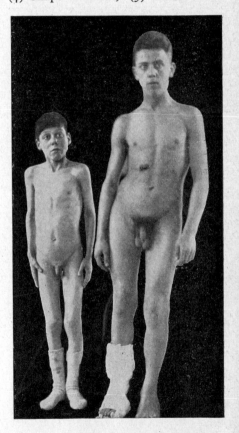

Fig. 1.—Infantilism. Due to congenital heart disease in a boy aged 17 years ; contrasted with a normal boy of the same age. Note also delayed sexual development.

Occasionally gigantism may occur in the rare disease leontiasis ossea.

Small stature, *dwarfism*, may exist physiologically in certain races such as the pygmies of Central Africa, but in this country is generally a symptom of various types of infantilism. A comprehensive list of these cannot be given here, but they may be associated with any serious disease in childhood (e.g., congenital syphilis, congenital or acquired heart disease),

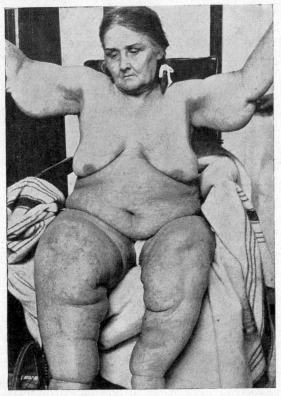

Fig. 2.—Lipomatosis (Dercum's adiposis dolorosa). The enormous deposits of fat have been present for many years. Some are painful to touch.

endocrine dyscrasias (e.g., pituitary and thyroid dystrophies), and metabolic disorders (e.g., cœliac disease and rickets). The term *infantilism* implies more than mere defective height, and includes genital hypoplasia, defective mental development, etc. (*Fig.* 1).

Weight.—The weight may be permanently below or above the average, but more significance attaches to a rapid change in weight.

Great *increase in weight* may be a familial characteristic, often occurring at the same age in different members. Although common in middle age, it may occur even in youth. This familial obesity may be aggravated by over-eating and lack of exercise. Extreme obesity is seen in childhood in hypofunction of the pituitary gland, and in adults from thyroid deficiency and eunuchoidism.

2

Irregular distribution of fat occurs in the rarer lipodystrophies, in some of which the lower part of the body is obese and the upper part emaciated (descending lipodystrophy). In Dercum's disease, adiposis dolorosa (*Fig.* 2), the masses of fat are painful to touch.

Decrease of weight is a feature of many diseases, and it is important to have *exact information* as to the amount of weight lost and the length of time during which it has been decreasing.

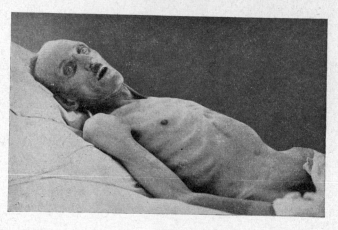

Fig. 3.—Cachexia. Note the extreme emaciation, sunken eyes, pigmented and dry skin. The patient is in the terminal stages of malignant disease.

Almost all serious diseases produce some loss of weight. Those of short duration, e.g., pneumonia, are generally accompanied by loss of weight which is restored partially or completely soon after the illness terminates. Continuous loss of weight is of graver omen, and may require thorough systematic examination for its elucidation. It is a common early symptom, for example, in all forms of tuberculosis, malignant disease, and diabetes, the other signs of which may only appear later. When no obvious cause is found for the loss of weight the urine should always be tested for *sugar*.

The term *cachexia* usually implies serious wasting, a greyish or 'earthy' pallor, and frequently an altered texture of the skin (dry and wrinkled). Although originally used for some conditions of which wasting was not essentially a part (e.g., cachexia thyreopriva in hypothyroidism), it is now commonly reserved for cases of malignant disease, of which wasting is an essential symptom (*Fig.* 3). This is accurately described as malignant cachexia. Occasionally the word is applied to the general condition in fatal diseases such as leukæmia, chronic Bright's disease, chronic tuberculosis, and so forth. A special type, described as pituitary cachexia, results from deficiency in the secretions of the anterior lobe of the pituitary (*see* SIMMOND'S DISEASE, p. 43).

2. BODILY CONFIGURATION

Apart from obesity or wasting, variations in physical type should be observed.

Asthenic Type.—The individual is tall, with a long neck, a tendency to a long flat chest, and a protuberant lower abdomen (*Fig.* 4). The

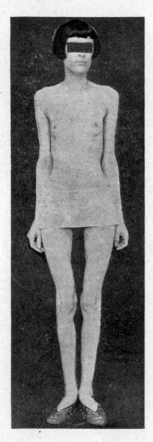

Fig. 4.—The asthenic type. The patient is long and thin but has no disease.

hands are slender and the fingers long. Neurasthenic individuals with visceroptosis are frequently found in this category.

Sthenic Type.—The sthenic type is short, with broad chest and short neck, and usually of considerable strength. The hands are broad and the fingers stumpy. This type may develop into the plethoric type.

Plethoric Type.—This is characterized by short stature, broad chest, short neck, disproportionately large abdominal girth, and florid complexion (*Fig.* 5). The eyes are suffused and watery. Cardio-vascular, renal, and respiratory troubles are common in such persons. It is sometimes called the apoplectic type owing to the frequency with which cerebral hæmorrhage is found.

Phthisical Type.—An exaggerated form of the asthenic in which chest deformities (*see* Chapter III) are more pronounced and nutrition is poor characterizes the phthisical type (*Figs.* 6, 7).

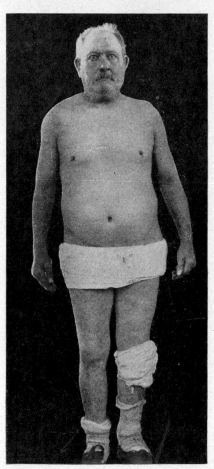

Fig. 5.—The plethoric type.

Endocrine Imbalance.—Endocrine imbalance is often exhibited in altered bodily configuration. Attention should be paid to the contour of the body, the sites of fat deposit, and the distribution of hair.

Deficiency of testicular or pituitary internal secretions results, in the male, in the preponderance of feminine characteristics. Fat is deposited in feminine sites, especially in the breasts and round the hips ; hair is scanty on the face, chest, abdomen, and legs, slight genu valgum is often present, and the skin is soft and delicate, the whole appearance of the individual being feminine (*See* EUNUCHOIDISM, p. 45, and HYPOPITUITARISM, p. 43).

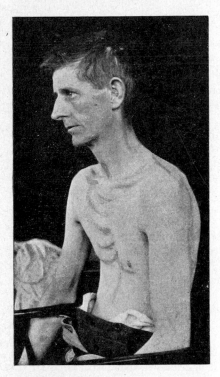

Fig. 6.—The phthisical type. Note the long, rather flat chest, with kyphosis and pronounced depression at the lower end of the sternum. The bony landmarks stand out prominently.

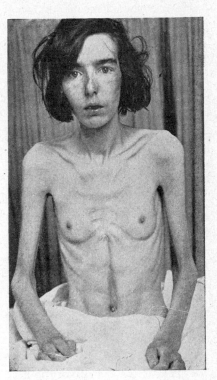

Fig. 7.—The phthisical type. The chest is long and flat, the ribs obliquely set. The emaciation is the result of advanced phthisis.

Conversely, in suprarenal cortical overactivity (tumours) the bodily contour, masculine distribution of hair, and other characteristics (*see* GENITALIA, p. 32) give an excessively virile appearance to the male and overshadow feminine characteristics in the female (*see Fig.* 40, p. 43). Basophil adenoma of the pituitary may result in somewhat similar hypertrichosis and obesity, but genital atrophy is commonly present. Minor degrees of femininity in the male and masculinity in the female are often to be noted without gross changes in the ductless glands.

3. POSTURE AND GAIT

Posture and gait will be considered more fully under the nervous system. In the ambulatory patient they play an important part in the diagnosis of nervous diseases.

Posture.—In conditions other than nervous diseases posture may also give information. Serious debilitating diseases and old age cause loss of muscular tone, which is shown by the drooping attitude and round shoulders of the patient. Pain may influence posture. Thus joint affections in one leg may cause the patient to lean heavily on the other. This becomes more obvious when the patient walks.

Posture in bed should also be noted carefully. In cardiac and respiratory diseases the patient frequently seeks comfort by sitting up, whilst in typhoidal states and coma he lies flat and log-like. In abdominal pain the knees are often drawn up. Pleural pain causes the individual to lie sometimes on the affected side, sometimes on the opposite.

In nervous diseases special postures may be almost pathognomonic, as in the opisthotonos and head retraction of meningeal irritation, but these will be considered more fully later.

Diseases of bones and joints not infrequently cause characteristic postures. Kyphosis in Pott's disease, emphysema, acromegaly, and Paget's disease (osteitis deformans), for example, gives a stooping appearance.

Gait.—The patient should be asked to walk first slowly, then more rapidly, if able. The gait revealed is often an important physical sign in neurological diagnosis, as described later. More rarely it may suggest affections of other systems. A limp, for example, apart from disturbances of the joints and their musculature, may be found in intra-abdominal lesions, such as appendicitis, which cause pain on movement of the hip-joint.

4. THE HEAD*

The shape and size of the head is sometimes of diagnostic importance. In *hydrocephalus* it is often immense in proportion to the rest of the body, and the forehead appears to overhang the orbits, giving a sunken effect to the eyes, which are directed downwards. In such cases the sutures are unduly separated and the fontanelles enlarged and bulging.

Frontal bossing occurs in rickets and in congenital syphilis. In rickets the forehead also overhangs to a slight extent. In congenital syphilis the bossing sometimes leads to the 'hot-cross-bun' appearance.

Generalized gradual enlargement of the head in adults, noticeable to the patient by the increase in the size of his hats, is almost a pathognomonic sign of osteitis deformans.

The great thickening and prominence of the supra-orbital ridges with the receding forehead above contribute much to the simian appearance of the acromegalic (*Fig.* 8).

---

* *See also* THE EXAMINATION OF SICK CHILDREN, Chapter XI.

Leontiasis ossea may produce changes in the shape of the skull, giving the characteristic leonine appearance.

Lastly, *nodular irregularities* should suggest the possibility of secondary growths or syphilitic tumours of the cranium.

5. THE NECK

Enlargement of the thyroid gland is known as a *goitre*. Note should be taken of the size, regularity or irregularity, and movements of the gland

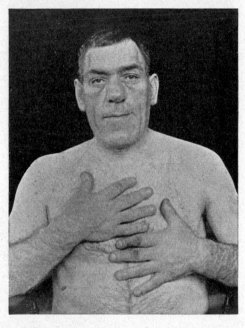

Fig. 8.—Acromegaly. Note especially the large nose, large and prominent lower jaw, and big hands (*see also* Figs. 36, 37). (*Professor Henry Cohen's case.*)

on swallowing. Free movement distinguishes the goitre from enlargement of lymphatic glands. When the latter are present their extent and physical characters (pp. 206, 224) should be observed.

The position of the trachea (p. 70) is of great importance in respiratory diseases.

Undue vascular pulsation and prominence of the jugular veins will be observed. Their significance is dealt with under THE CARDIO-VASCULAR SYSTEM (pp. 112, 113).

6. THE HAIR

The hair is often modified by disease. It is common knowledge that even trivial departures from normal health may be sufficient to cause the hair to lose its lustre and for natural waves or curls to disappear.

More serious illness results in dryness and loss of hair. In hypo-thyroidism these characters are especially noticeable, and the hair is thick, coarse, and scanty, falling out particularly over the frontal region. The outer third of the eyebrows is also sometimes lost in myxœdema (*Figs.* 9, 13, 18). Conversely, in hyperthyroidism the hair is often thin and softer

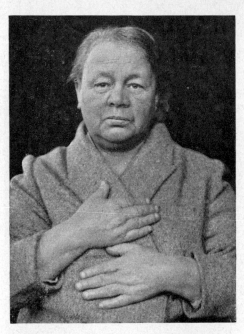

Fig. 9.—Myxœdema. The patient had had some treatment with thyroid, but the coarseness of the skin (especially the hands) and loss of eyebrows are still apparent.

than normal. In mongolism it is silky. Patchy loss of hair occurs in alopecia areata, a skin condition of nervous origin. Infections of the scalp must not be overlooked, especially when enlarged glands in the neck are otherwise unexplained.

7. THE FACE

The *temperament* rarely fails to leave an impression on the facial characteristics, and even the untrained observer is familiar with the facies of the anxious and placid types of individual. *Mental deficiency* may give the face a stupid expression, often with a fatuous grin. The woeful face of the melancholic, the agitated mien of the maniac, and the slanting eyes of the mongol, are other examples of the importance of a study of the face in mental disease. Changes in character due to alcohol, morphine, and cocaine are often suggested by the facies. The expression of the drug-taker is shifty ; that of the alcoholic self-satisfied and plausible.

It is none the less important not to jump to conclusions about such characteristics, which may merely indicate nervousness, shyness, or other evidence of psychological imbalance.

Physical diseases may also produce changes in the facies. In pneumonia the bright eyes, the flushed cheeks, and the presence of herpes labialis (*see* THE LIPS, p. 27) give a characteristic appearance. The patient with typhoid fever has a similar appearance at first, but the flushed cheeks and bright eyes give way to an apathetic heavy look as the disease progresses. The fixed grin in cases of tetanus has been given the name of risus sardonicus (*Fig.* 10).

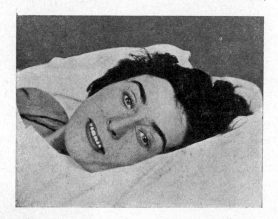

Fig. 10.—Risus sardonicus. From a case of tetanus.

Wasting and plumpness may be noticed first in the face, and many nervous diseases (e.g., Parkinsonism, myopathies, etc.), which will be described later, leave their mark on the countenance.

The condition of the face depends partly on the individual features, which will be discussed shortly, but changes in the bony prominences may be helpful diagnostic features in diseases such as acromegaly, leontiasis ossea, oxycephaly, achondroplasia, and congenital syphilis.

Other examples of the effect of physical disease on facial appearance are dealt with in subsequent chapters.

The individual features should be carefully inspected.

The Eyes.—The eyes may exhibit local disease, which sometimes has a bearing on general medical diagnosis. Cataract may call attention to diabetes, interstitial keratitis (*Fig.* 11) to congenital syphilis.

Exophthalmos is a notable feature of primary hyperthyroidism (*Fig.* 12), and may occur more rarely in brain tumours extending into the orbit, or in thrombosis of the lateral sinus (generally unilateral). Enophthalmos (recession of the eyes) may occur in serious wasting diseases and in dehydration (e.g., cholera). It is also a sign of sympathetic paralysis. Subconjunctival hæmorrhages may occur in high blood-pressure and chronic renal disease, in fractured skull, and in various forms of cerebral hæmorrhage. Squint, irregularity in the pupils, and other evidence of

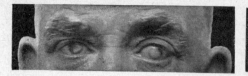

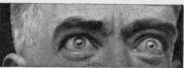

Fig. 11.—Interstitial keratitis. The corneæ have a 'ground glass' appearance.

Fig. 12.—Exophthalmos, due to hyperthyroidism. Greater in the left eye than the right. Such inequality in the degree of exophthalmos is not uncommon.

oculomotor paresis are of particular importance in the diagnosis of nervous diseases, and will be considered more fully in Chapter IX. Care should be taken not to 'lose face' by overlooking a glass eye, which is not always so easy to recognize as it sounds to be.

The eyes have been called "the windows of the soul", and apart from the grosser changes described above, the experienced observer will take into account the apathy portrayed in long illnesses or the anguish caused by pain or mental suffering. A common complaint of mothers is that their children have dark rings under the eyes. They can usually be reassured that these have little or no significance, though delicate persons, both children and adults, are liable to exhibit this evidence of loss of circulatory tone.

The Skin.—The colour and texture of the skin of the face must be observed. Anæmia causes pallor ; jaundice, yellow discoloration modified by the natural colour of the cheeks ; cyanosis, blueness. Polycythæmia causes a brick-red coloration, becoming purplish with cold or exercise. Pigmentation of the skin in Addison's disease is of brownish character, and slaty-grey in the now rare argyria. These changes will be considered in relation to the body as a whole. Certain rashes are most evident on the face—for example, those of measles and small-pox.

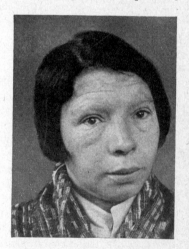

Fig. 13.—Myxœdema. Note especially the loss of hair on the forehead and outer parts of the eyebrows. The face is 'puffy', somewhat resembling a nephritic facies.

Thickening of the subcutaneous tissues may be seen in acromegaly and myxœdema, and the puffiness of the eyelids in the latter condition (*Fig.* 13) may simulate the true subcutaneous œdema of renal disease. In acute nephritis the puffy swollen face and closure of the eyelids by œdema often make a provisional diagnosis possible by inspection, though the possibility of urticaria should not be overlooked. In old age and dehydration (e.g., in diabetes and severe diarrhœa), the skin may be parched and wrinkled.

The condition of the blood-vessels should be recorded. Dilated vessels are often seen in mitral disease (*see Fig.* 90, p. 102) and prolonged dyspepsia : in the former especially on the cheeks ; in the latter on the nose. Spider-like venules (telangiectases) are common in cirrhosis of the liver.

The Lips.—Indications of ill health may be given by the lips. They are dry and cracked in most illnesses, even of a trivial nature, but *sordes*, a collection of epithelial debris, food, and bacteria, are present in serious diseases such as pneumonia, typhoid, etc.

Herpes labialis is recognized as an eruption of vesicles which soon burst and form scabs. It is seen not only on the lips but on other parts of the face (*Fig.* 14),

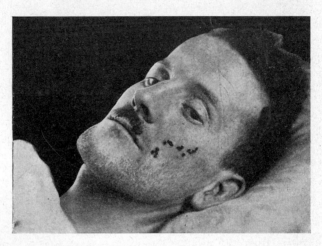
Fig. 14.—Herpes labialis et facialis. Case of pneumonia.

especially on the chin and nose, and is found frequently with the common cold, and more extensively distributed in pneumonia, cerebrospinal fever, and malaria.

Anæmia and cyanosis are particularly well seen in the lips, but are considered elsewhere. The lips are thick in myxœdema and acromegaly. In the myopathic facies the lower lip is pendulous, exhibiting part of the mucous membrane (*see Figs.* 197, 198, p. 257).

The Nose.—The nose is large in acromegaly, due partly to thickening of the subcutaneous tissues, and partly to bony overgrowth. In hypothyroidism it is also large and broad.

A sharp, peaky nose is characteristic of the Hippocratic facies seen in patients who are moribund, especially from peritonitis. In congenital syphilis the bridge of the nose is depressed, giving a *saddle-back* appearance (*Fig.* 15).

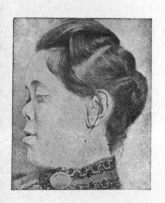
Fig. 15.—Congenital syphilis, showing prominent forehead and depressed nasal bridge. (*Professor Rendle Short's case.*) (*From French's 'Index of Diagnosis'.*)

Acne rosacea is characterized by a reddening of the nose and cheeks, giving the 'butterfly-wings' appearance. This appearance is also seen in lupus erythematosus. Acne rosacea occurs in dyspeptics and in alcoholics and heavy tea drinkers. In an exaggerated form it occurs as the 'strawberry nose'.

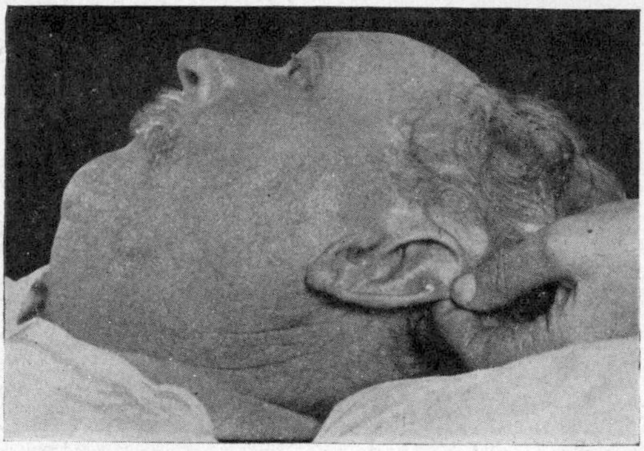

The Ears.—The ears may be deformed in degenerate types. The usual malformation is an absence of well-defined lobes and a fusion of the ear to the face where the lobe should normally be freely dependent. Ears of this type are common in mental deficients and in epileptics. In mongolian idiots the ears are usually large.

Fig. 16.—Gouty tophus in the ear.

Note should be taken of any cyanosis of the periphery of the ear, which may occur in all conditions causing cyanosis, and also in the rare disease ochronosis, which darkens the cartilages. Any *discharge* from the meatus should be recorded, as it may indicate middle-ear infection and have important bearings in suspected intracranial abscess.

Tophi ('chalk-stones') are collections of uric acid salts in the ears, and appear as whitish masses stretching the skin and sometimes protruding through it (*Fig.* 16). They are found in gout, and like this disease are now rarely seen. Similar tophaceous deposits may be seen in other parts of the body (*Fig.* 17).

The Salivary Glands.—The salivary glands may be enlarged. Parotid swellings are situated chiefly in front of the ear. The most important from the physician's point of view is the bilateral painful swelling of these glands caused by *mumps*.

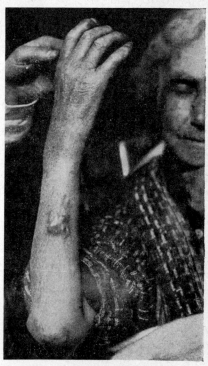

Fig. 17.—Gouty deposit in the arm.

In this disease there is pyrexia and constitutional disturbance. Unilateral parotitis is more often due to sepsis, but may complicate 'medical' illnesses such as typhoid. Swellings beneath the chin may be due to enlargement of the submaxillary or sublingual glands, but their diagnosis falls more within the scope of surgical practice.

Facial Movements.—These are considered under the nervous system. They give indications of lesions of the facial nerve, of hypertonicity or hypotonicity of the facial muscles, choreiform movements, and other signs of neurological importance.

8. THE SKIN

Some of the points to be observed have been mentioned in describing the skin of the face, but it is necessary to inspect the skin of the whole body.

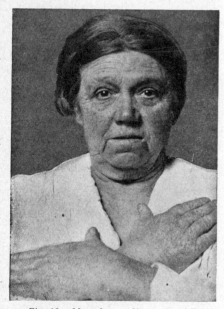

Fig. 18.—Myxœdema. Shows especially the coarse wrinkled skin of the face and hands. The hair is also coarse and tends to fall out—note the right eyebrow.

Undue *sweating* is common in certain fevers, especially rheumatic fever and tuberculosis, and is also usual during the subsidence of any pyrexia. The sweating of pulmonary tuberculosis occurs characteristically during sleep. Sweating is also common in hyperthyroidism and neurasthenia, and in most illnesses which cause exhaustion or sudden collapse.

Dryness of the skin is also common in fevers—for example, during the course of pneumonia, though sweating occurs at the crisis. It is a characteristic of myxœdema (*Fig.* 18) and some skin diseases, and also results from loss of body fluid by diarrhœa or polyuria, e.g., in cholera and diabetes.

The degree of *pigmentation* of the skin should next be noted. Increased pigmentation varying from light to dark shades of brown is a classical sign of Addison's disease (suprarenal insufficiency, usually due to tuberculosis), but should be sought also in the mucous membrane of the mouth. Similar pigmentation may be caused by arsenical poisoning but the mucous membranes are rarely affected. Patchy pigmentation may alternate with white patches in leucoderma, and 'café au lait' spots may be seen in von Recklinghausen's disease.

The dark skin of silver poisoning is now rarely seen. Blackness of the skin may occur in gangrene, commonly the result of arterial obstruction (*see Fig.* 30).

The *texture* of the skin may change. Apart from skin diseases, reference has already been made, in describing facial characteristics, to the increased thickness and coarse texture in myxœdema. This may affect the skin of other parts of the body.

Nævi may be important in neurological conditions, suggesting the possibility of meningeal nævi.

Rashes.—Rashes are of great clinical importance. Sometimes the rash is the principal physical sign, as in the exanthemata (measles, scarlet fever, etc.) ; sometimes it is only subsidiary—for example, the purpura of hæmorrhagic fevers and certain blood diseases. Its extent and exact distribution should be noted, the colour and type, the duration, and whether or not it is accompanied by distress (itching, burning).

The commoner types of skin eruption are :—

1. *Macular*, consisting of coloured spots, not raised above the surrounding skin. Examples are the roseolar rashes of syphilis and typhoid fever, and the more diffuse and densely distributed spots of scarlet fever. Hæmorrhagic rashes, *purpura*, also fall into this category.

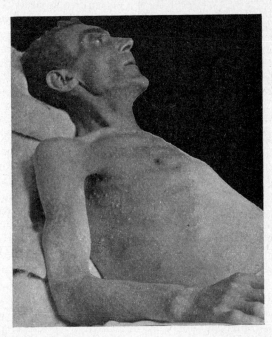

Fig. 19.—Secondary nodules. The nodules were widely distributed on the chest and abdominal wall. From a case of malignant disease of the stomach. Note also the cachectic appearance.

2. *Papular*, or rashes in which the elements are raised into tiny nodes. This type of rash occurs in certain stages of the exanthemata, e.g., chicken-pox and small-pox, and in essential diseases of the skin with which this book has no concern.

3. *Vesicular*, comprised of small blisters or papules, the tops of which are filled with a clear fluid. Good examples are seen in herpes labialis (*see* THE LIPS, p. 27), and herpes zoster, a vesicular rash due to an infection of the posterior root ganglia, and usually distributed in a girdle-like manner round one-half of the chest (to which the disease owes its popular name of 'shingles' (Lat. *cingulum*, a girdle).

4. *Bullous*, consisting of larger blisters generally containing clear fluid. They are well seen in burns and scalds and occasionally in erysipelas. Sometimes they occur in severe nervous lesions such as myelitis and syringomyelia. The various forms of pemphigus,

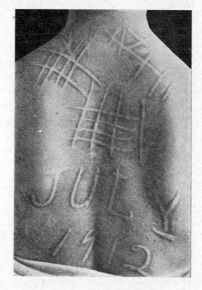

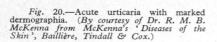

Fig. 20.—Acute urticaria with marked dermographia. (*By courtesy of Dr. R. M. B. McKenna from McKenna's 'Diseases of the Skin', Baillière, Tindall & Cox.*)

of which bullæ are the essential features, cannot be considered here.

5. *Pustular*, in many ways resembling a vesicular rash, but in which the little nodules are filled with turbid or purulent instead of clear fluid. Pustules are familiarly seen in acne vulgaris, and are a characteristic sign in small-pox and to a lesser extent in chicken-pox.

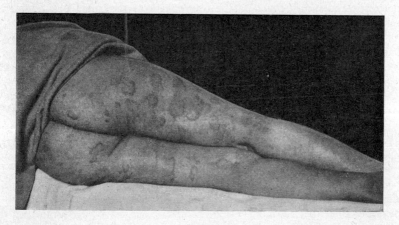

Fig. 21.—Giant urticaria following insulin injection.

They are the usual element found in the rashes of bromide and iodide overdosage.

6. *Nodular* rashes consist of swellings in the skin generally of greater size than the average vesicle or pustule (the pustules of small-pox are an exception in attaining large size by fusion). An important example of a nodular rash is found in *erythema nodosum*. This rash occurs on the legs and arms as painful reddish-blue nodules varying in size from a millimetre to several centimetres in diameter. It is thought by some to be of rheumatic origin. Other examples of a nodular rash are the secondary deposits in the skin of carcinoma or sarcoma (*Fig.* 19), and the deposition of syphilitic, tuberculous, and leprous granulation tissue in the form of gummata, tuberculomata, and leprous nodules.

7. *Weals.*—These are raised areas, sometimes pale, sometimes red, which are often seen in sensitive skins even after slight trauma (*Fig.* 20). They occur spontaneously in various forms of urticaria, and are often an expression of hypersensitivity to foreign proteins (*Fig.* 21). Thus they have an important connexion with allergic diseases such as asthma, hay fever, and angioneurotic œdema. Other essential features of a weal are its transient nature and irritable characteristics (itching, burning).

These essential elements of a rash may be accompanied by secondary changes. The area around pustules is usually reddened and swollen from inflammatory reaction. When the pustules burst *crusts* may form, e.g., in small-pox. *Desquamation* is the name given to shedding of the superficial layers of the epidermis which occurs after many fevers, but is particularly characteristic of scarlet fever. Erosion of the deeper layers of the skin and loss of tissue result in *ulcers*, and may occur from the breakdown of nodules such as gummata, sarcomata, tuberculomata, etc. *Scars* may be significant of old skin lesions, especially of old syphilitic infections such as a chancre on the penis or gummata on the legs. The pitting of small-pox is another example of scarring. The scars of operations and injury must not be overlooked, as they may bear upon the present illness.

In many rashes several elements are combined. Thus in small-pox, macules, papules, vesicles, and pustules are seen on the skin successively. In arthritic purpura the essential hæmorrhagic rash is frequently combined with the weals of urticaria.

9. THE GENITALIA

The size and form of the genitalia are of especial importance in endocrine disorders, for their normal development depends on a correct balance of the ductless glands.

The penis and testicles fail to reach adult proportions in several types of infantilism : hypopituitarism, hypothyroidism, and eunuchoidism are notable causes. In these cases the normal sexual functions are also in abeyance, and the secondary sex characters (in boys, deepening of the voice, growth of hair on the pubes and in masculine sites) do not develop at puberty. In females the main sign of genital infantilism is the failure to menstruate, though the pubic hair may be delayed in appearance, and the general bodily configuration remain sexless.

By contrast, sexual precocity is usually found in suprarenal tumours. Male children may develop genitalia of adult proportions at an early age (erection and ejaculation of spermatozoa may occur). In the female the genitalia have certain masculine attributes, notably the large clitoris. The secondary sex characters are also those of the male—hair on the face, chest, thighs, etc., and a masculine voice.

10. THE JOINTS

Most affections of joints fall more within the scope of a surgical than a medical text-book, and space only allows a brief description of the method of examination of the joints and of the commoner joint diseases found in the medical wards.

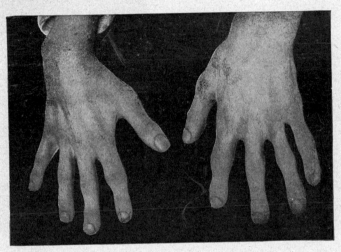

Fig. 22.—Rheumatoid arthritis. Moderate spindle-shaped swelling of joints.

The most important points to be recorded are : (1) The size ; (2) The shape ; (3) The mobility ; (4) The presence or absence of inflammation ; (5) The joints affected.

1. **Size.**—The joints are enlarged in most types of arthritis. Swelling is partly due to changes in the articulating bones and cartilages and their connecting structures, the synovial membranes and ligaments, and partly to effusion of fluid into the joint. These facts should be borne in mind whilst the joint is under examination. To assign the causes of the joint enlargement correctly requires considerable skill, and palpation must be employed in addition to inspection.

2. **Shape.**—In rheumatoid arthritis the small joints of the hands are

3

frequently involved, and the proximal phalangeal joints often assume the classical *spindle shape* (*Figs.* 22, 23). The larger joints show a uniform smooth enlargement in rheumatic fever, but in rheumatoid arthritis (*Fig.* 24), and even more in osteo-arthritis and gout, they are nodular owing to the changes in the bony and periarticular tissues. Similarly, great deformity and disorganization occur in the arthropathies of tabes and syringomyelia (*see Fig.* 49, p. 53, and *Fig.* 182, p. 238).

3. **Mobility.**—Limitation of movement is an important sign of articular disease, but may be caused by pain on movement of the periarticular tissues, especially the muscles, or by fear of movement. The range of movement in the suspected joint must be carefully compared with that in the corresponding unaffected one. Limitation may be caused by pain in acute lesions of the joints, or in chronic arthritis by destructive or proliferative changes resulting in partial or complete ankylosis.

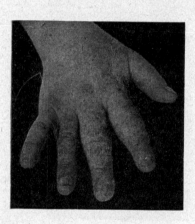

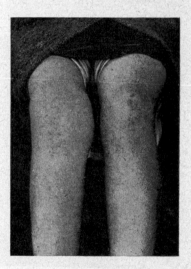

Fig. 23.—Rheumatoid arthritis. Extreme spindle-shaped swelling of fingers.

Fig. 24.—Rheumatoid arthritis. The right knee is irregularly swollen.

4. **Signs of Inflammation.**—The cardinal signs of inflammation—pain, heat, redness, swelling, and loss of function—are present in all forms of acute arthritis, e.g., acute rheumatism and acute rheumatoid arthritis. Heat is easily appreciated by placing the hand on an unaffected and the affected joint in turn.

The absence of important inflammatory signs is notably observed in subacute and chronic affections of the joints such as the later stages of rheumatoid arthritis, osteo-arthritis, and gout.

5. **Joints Involved.**—The distribution of the arthritis is of considerable diagnostic importance. Rheumatic fever generally involves the larger joints, e.g., the shoulders, elbows, wrists, knees, and ankles ; whilst

acute rheumatoid arthritis, though also frequently affecting these joints, generally involves the small joints of the hands, and sometimes the temporomaxillary, sternoclavicular, and spinal joints. Gout is classically seen in the great toe, and senile forms of osteo-arthritis in the hips. These

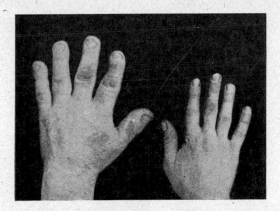

Fig. 25.—Acromegalic hand. The relatively enormous acromegalic hand is contrasted with an average normal hand.

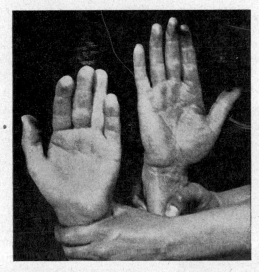

Fig. 26.—Acromegalic hand. Note the large palm, short fingers, and general ' paw-like' appearance. Contrasted with a normal hand.

special distributions are by no means pathognomonic, but are helpful when considered with other physical signs.

The length of time the joint remains inflamed is also important. In rheumatic fever, the arthritis is often fleeting, remaining in one joint only for a comparatively short time—one to three days—though several joints are not uncommonly affected in varying degrees at the same time. In rheumatoid arthritis several joints are almost invariably involved together,

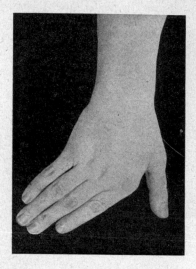

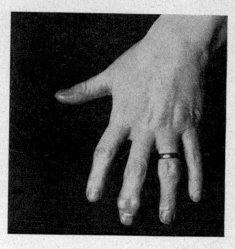

Fig. 27.—Ulnar deviation. Due to rheumatoid arthritis.

Fig. 28.—Heberden's nodes. Note the deformity of the ring finger also.

and the signs of inflammation may remain for days or weeks. Gonococcal arthritis, though affecting several joints, tends to be most pronounced and resistant to treatment in one or two. Similarly in senile forms of osteo-arthritis one joint is singled out.

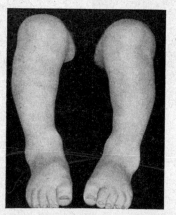

11. THE EXTREMITIES

The hands and feet should always be examined carefully.

The hands of the manual worker are rough, lined, red, and often engrimed in spite of personal cleanliness. The condition

Fig. 29.—Epiphysial enlargement. Marked enlargement of the epiphyses of the ankles in a case of rickets. Note also bow-legs.

of the feet may give some indication of the hygienic habits of the individual.

In certain diseases the shape of the hands may be modified. In myxœdema they are broad and the fingers appear short and stubby from thickening of the subcutaneous tissues (see Fig. 9). In acromegaly they are large, broad, and paw-like (Figs. 25, 26), but in hypopituitarism and hyperthyroidism they are often slender and feminine in type.

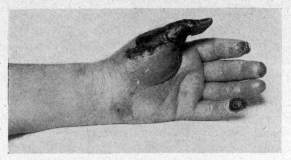

Fig. 30.—Embolic gangrene due to auricular fibrillation.
(*see p.* 29).

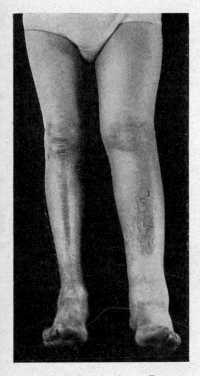

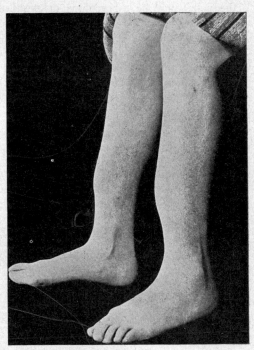

Fig. 31.—Unilateral œdema. Due to carcinoma of the rectum.

Fig. 32.—Sabre-shaped tibiæ. Due to syphilis.

The joint affections of the hands have already been considered. It remains to add that many types of crippling deformity may result from arthritis. Two are worthy of mention here : firstly, *ulnar deviation*, in which the whole hand, but especially the fingers from the metacarpophalangeal joints, is deflected to the ulnar side (*Fig.* 27) ; secondly, *Heberden's nodes* (*Fig.* 28), bony prominences at the distal phalangeal joints which occur in advanced and usually non-progressive osteo-arthritis.

Epiphysial enlargement is commonly found in rickets (*Fig.* 29); less frequently in congenital syphilis and infantile scurvy.

Arterial spasm in *Raynaud's disease* results in altered appearance of the fingers and toes. These are pallid in most cases when the extremities are exposed to cold, and the patient complains of the fingers " going dead ", but in more advanced cases cyanosis occurs and occasionally gangrene (*see Fig.* 125, p. 140). (*See also* pp. 139, 140.)

In respiratory and cardiac disease clubbing of the fingers and toes should be sought, but this and the abnormalities of the hands due to nervous diseases will be considered in later chapters.

Finally, the *nails* should be inspected. Pitting, ribbing, and brittleness are often seen after severe illnesses. The short irregular nails of the nail-biter may suggest some instability of the nervous system. Onychia (infection of the nails) may be tuberculous or syphilitic in origin, and other signs of these diseases should be looked for. Discoloration of the nails may be seen in silver and mercurial poisoning and also in Addison's disease. Hæmorrhages may appear beneath the nails in blood diseases.

The *legs* should be specially examined for œdema (*Fig.* 31), ulcers, and vascular disturbances such as phlebitis and gangrene. Bony deformities such as bow legs, knocked knees, and sabre tibiæ (*Fig.* 32) must also be noted.

SOME DISEASES DIAGNOSED CHIEFLY BY INSPECTION

Signs pointing to an affection of one particular system or even to one particular disease are commonly seen on inspection—for example, clubbing of the fingers in respiratory or cardiac disease, and jaundice in affections

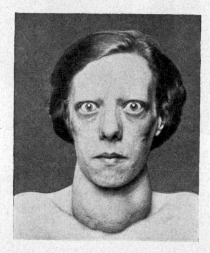

Fig. 33.—Hyperthyroidism. Note large goitre and marked exophthalmos, giving an expression of terror to the face. (*Dr. William Johnson's case.*)

of the biliary tract. These will be described in the chapters relating to the special systems. In the present chapter a few common diseases are described to illustrate those disorders which depend *chiefly on inspection* for their diagnosis. They may be grouped under three headings :—

1. Endocrine disorders.
2. Diseases characterized by a rash.
3. Bone and joint affections.

1. ENDOCRINE DISORDERS

Thyroid Diseases.—

Hyperthyroidism (Exophthalmic goitre ; Graves' disease ; Basedow's disease).—The facial expression of the patient often suggests the diagnosis immediately. It is one of fright or terror, due to the exophthalmos and retraction of the upper eyelid. Goitre of variable size is present in most cases, but is not always proportionate to the degree of hyperthyroidism (*Fig.* 33).

Confirmatory signs are the loss of weight, fine tremor of the hands, tachycardia, sweating, nervousness, and various eye signs. Most of the

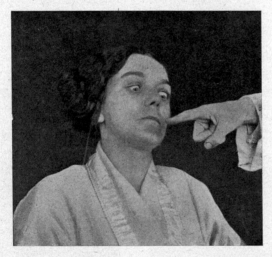

Fig. 34.—Von Graefe's sign. Although the lower margin of the iris is level with the lower eyelid, the upper eyelid has not moved downwards. The finger has been moved slowly from the level of the hair to its present position.

eye signs depend upon the primary sign, exophthalmos, but von Graefe's sign (*Fig.* 34) is of value and sometimes present without much exophthalmos. It consists in lagging of the upper eyelid when the patient is asked to follow the observer's finger downwards as it is slowly moved in front of the eyes from the level of the forehead to the level of the cheeks. Cases of 'toxic adenoma' or secondary Graves' disease present similar signs, but are distinguished by the *nodular* enlargement of the thyroid

(*Fig.* 35), by the absence of exophthalmos, and by the fact that some thyroid enlargement is often present before the signs of hyperthyroidism appear. Cardio-vascular symptoms and signs are also prominent in toxic adenoma. The heart is usually enlarged, the mitral first sound accentuated, and auricular fibrillation may follow.

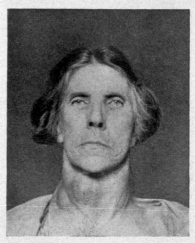

Fig. 35.—Adenoma of the thyroid. Note the lobular appearance of the right lobe of the gland.

Hypothyroidism (*Myxœdema* ; *Cretinism*).—Underactivity of the thyroid may occur in adult life (*myxœdema*), or in infancy (*cretinism*). Both diseases have similar symptoms and signs, modified by the age of the patient. The appearance of the patient suggests sluggish or defective

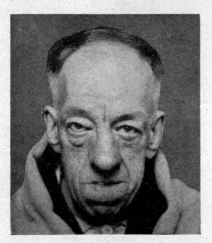 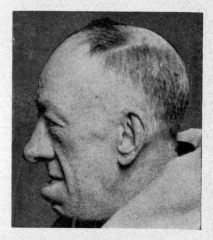

Figs. 36, 37.—Acromegaly. Note the large nose, thickened and pendulous lower lip, and prominent lower jaw. (*Prof. John Hay's case.*)

mentality, amounting to idiocy in untreated cretins. Lethargy is noticeable in adults, with impairment of mental activity. The face is puffy and pale, with coarse skin and broad nose. The hair falls out, especially

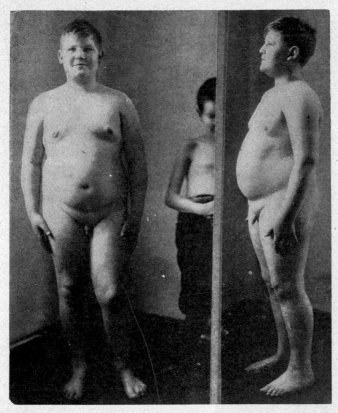

Fig. 38.—Dystrophia adiposo-genitalis due to dyspituitarism. Note the general fatness, the hypertrophy of the mammæ, and the smallness of the penis. A normal boy of the same age is partly in view in the left-hand illustration. (*From French's 'Index of Diagnosis'.*)

over the frontal region and outer third of the eyebrows ; the remainder is coarse in texture and dry. The lips and ears are thickened. Dryness, and a *solid thickening* of the skin of the whole body are also present, the latter leading to increase in the patient's weight. (*See Figs.* 9, 13, and 18.)

These signs contrast with those of hyperthyroidism. Further points of contrast are the slow pulse, absence of sweating, and constipation in hypothyroidism.

In the cretin the deficiency of thyroid secretion also causes stunted growth, late closure of the fontanelles, delayed dentition, and other signs of deficient development. (*See* p. 360 and *Figs.* 265, 266.)

Pituitary Diseases.—Tumour is the commonest lesion of the pituitary body. If it is composed of chromophil cells (i.e., cells staining well with eosin) it results in *hyperpituitarism*—gigantism or acromegaly. Simple hyperplasia of the eosinophil cells may have a

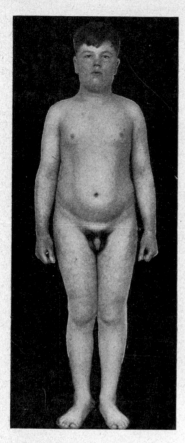

Fig. 39.—Pituitary adiposity. Boy aged 16 years. The fat is distributed in feminine sites. There is little genital hypoplasia. (Fearnside's 'pudding-face' type.)

similar result. Occasionally basophil adenomata are found causing adiposity and hirsutism with genital dystrophy (*Cushing's syndrome*), a syndrome which bears a close resemblance to suprarenal virilism. Tumours of the chromophobe cells (not staining with eosin) tend to cause hypopituitarism by pressure effect upon the other cells. Hypopituitarism is also associated, however, with hypofunction of the gland without tumour formation. In such cases the pressure effects common in acromegaly are absent.

Hyperpituitarism. — This term is applied primarily to overactivity of the alpha cells of the *anterior* lobe of the pituitary, as little is known about excess of posterior lobe secretion.

As in hypothyroidism, the age of the patient modifies the result. *Gigantism* occurs in patients in whom the gland is overactive before the epiphyses have united. The giant may have eunuchoid or acromegalic features, and the clinical characteristics may change as pituitary overfunction gives place to pituitary exhaustion.

Acromegaly occurs with hyperpituitarism in adult life. The changes in this disease are insidious, but when it is fully developed the facial aspect is most characteristic. The supra-orbital ridges, nose, cheek bones, and lower jaw are greatly enlarged, with thickening of the overlying subcutaneous tissues, giving the patient a simian appearance (*Figs.* 36, 37). The lips are thickened and often pendulous ; the teeth separated by enlargement of the lower jaw ; the hands and feet enlarged. Kyphosis is common, adding to the simian aspect. Sexual function may be increased for a short while, but is usually diminished quite soon, and the patient shows abnormal tolerance to glucose.

Pressure effects from expansion of the sella turcica may be present, e.g., pressure on the optic chiasma causing hemianopia, and radiological evidence of enlargement of the sella turcica and erosion of the clinoid processes. These signs, though not of endocrine origin, are important in diagnosis and prognosis.

Hypopituitarism.—The usual type of pituitary underactivity is known as *dystrophia adiposo-genitalis.* The name describes the presenting signs, namely obesity and genital infantilism (*Fig.* 38). Children at puberty are generally affected, though the signs persist to adult life. The child, like Dickens' character, is " a fat and red-faced boy " (or girl), and the fat is distributed in feminine sites. Secondary sex characters fail to make their appearance at puberty and the child remains infantile. All grades of the condition are seen, and some can scarcely be considered pathological. Similar pituitary dystrophies may also occur before and after puberty, and have various minor distinguishing characters (Fearnside's ' pudding-face type ' (*Fig.* 39) ; eunuchoidal type.)

A less common variety of hypopituitarism is the *Lorain type.* The child remains undersized, though of normal proportion and without any obesity.

Deficiency of anterior lobe pituitary secretions also results occasionally in *pituitary cachexia,* one type of which is *Simmonds' disease.* This is commonly due to infarction

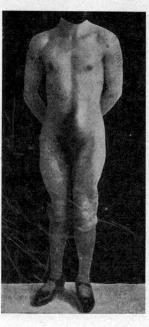

Fig. 40.—Suprarenal virilism. Muscular masculine build, small breasts, male distribution of hair to umbilicus. (*L. R. Broster and H. G. Hill's case, from ' The British Journal of Surgery '.*)

of the gland. The main characteristics are emaciation and exhaustion leading to an appearance of premature senility. Genital functions are decreased and there is gradual loss of pubic and axillary hair. The mental processes are impaired.

Diabetes Insipidus.—Interference with the posterior lobe of the pituitary or with the tuber cinereum (congenital and acquired causes) may result in this condition. The clinical characteristics are polyuria and polydipsia. The patient may pass 10–20 pints of urine of low specific gravity, daily. The urine contains no sugar or albumin and the renal efficiency is normal. These points serve to distinguish diabetes insipidus from diabetes mellitus and renal disease.

Suprarenal Diseases.—The classification of suprarenal diseases according to hyper- or hypo-function is not so satisfactory as in the case of thyroid or pituitary disease, and is complicated by the little understood function of the cortex and by the difficulty of separating cortical from medullary effects.

Two diseases are fairly well defined, *suprarenal virilism* and *Addison's disease*, both recognized principally by external appearances.

Suprarenal Virilism.—This is almost invariably the result of tumours of the adrenals, thought to arise from the cortex. Masculine characteristics develop in the female or become intensified in the male child. Hair appears in profusion in masculine sites, especially over the moustache and beard area of the face, and on the chest, abdominal wall, and thighs (*Figs.* 40, 41). The voice deepens.

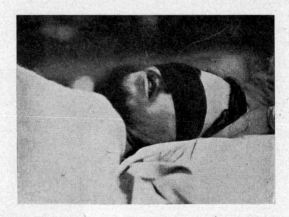

Fig. 41.—Same case as *Fig.* 40, showing facies with heavy beard and moustache.

In the female the genitalia may become modified so as to result in pseudo-hermaphroditism, and the normal development of feminine attributes such as the breasts and menstruation is absent.

In male children the genitalia may resemble both in structure and function those of the adult. In the adult male genital atrophy occurs. Obesity is present in many cases, both male and female.

Sexual precocity may also result from pituitary tumours (*see* p. 42), and more rarely from lesions of the *pineal gland*.

Addison's Disease.—Destruction of the suprarenal tissue by tuberculosis or other rarer causes results in a peculiarly characteristic clinical picture known as Addison's disease. Some of the symptoms result from the disturbance of salt metabolism which accompanies these suprarenal changes.

The salient physical sign is excessive *pigmentation*, present as a dark brown colouring on the face, hands, and other parts of the body exposed to light, and also in places where pigment normally abounds, such as the axillæ, beneath the breasts, and round the genitalia. Darkening of the oral mucous membrane is an important confirmatory sign.

The diagnosis is often difficult, but is supported by the presence of muscular and cardio-vascular *asthenia*. The patient complains of great weakness, out of proportion to the slight wasting which generally accompanies the disease, and the cardio-vascular asthenia is shown by the steady decrease in the blood-pressure, the systolic values of which may fall as low as 60 mm. Gastro-intestinal disturbances (vomiting and diarrhœa) are often present.

Gonadal Defects.—Primary *testicular* defects may be responsible for *eunuchoidism* (e.g., absence or infantile character of testes), but a similar clinical picture results from secondary testicular atrophy in pituitary and other endocrine dyscrasias. The patient lacks the secondary sex characteristics of the male. The voice is high pitched, the skin smooth and hairless, and there is often obesity and a tendency to genu valgum. Sexual functions are in abeyance.

In women deficiency in *ovarian* function is not so apparent, though it may result in masculine appearance and amenorrhœa.

Parathyroid Diseases.—The most important of these is *tetany*, a disease resulting from hypocalcæmia, which may be due to a deficiency of parathyroid secretion, but occurs in other diseases which disturb the normal calcium-phosphorus balance, e.g., rickets, alkalosis, gastro-intestinal diseases, osteomalacia, etc. A clinical syndrome called *generalized osteitis fibrosa* due to overaction of the parathyroids has also been more recently described.

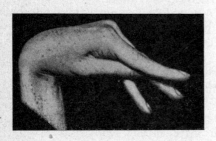

Fig. 42.—Tetany. Carpal spasm producing the ' main d'accoucheur '. Note flexion of wrist, adduction of thumb, and hyperextension of terminal phalanges.

Tetany.—The diagnosis of this disease is generally made by the observation of carpopedal spasms. In these the hands are in a state of *painful* spasm with the fingers tightly apposed, the thumb adducted across the palm, the terminal phalanges hyperextended, and the wrist flexed —the ' main d'accoucheur ' (*Fig.* 42). The spasms are less obvious in the feet, but these and the toes are plantar-flexed and the whole foot is inverted. The spasms in the hands and feet are merely an expression of increased nervous excitability, which may manifest itself by spasm in other muscles (e.g., larynx and ocular muscles), and by an excessive response to mechanical or electrical stimulation. Several signs are used to demonstrate this increased excitability. Two in clinical use may be mentioned :—

1. *Trousseau's sign* consists in squeezing the arm or leg and evoking carpopedal spasms which are latent.

2. *Chvostek's sign* is elicited by tapping over the facial nerve as it emerges from the stylomastoid foramen. This causes a contraction of the facial muscles on one side and the angle of the mouth is drawn up.

Hyperparathyroidism.—The possibility of this uncommon condition should be considered in patients presenting themselves with tender swellings over bones, and tenderness of the hands, or with spontaneous fractures. The disease is called *generalized osteitis fibrosa,* and is usually associated with a parathyroid tumour and with gross disturbances of calcium-phosphorus metabolism.

Diabetes.—As one of the commonest symptoms of this disease is *wasting* it may conveniently be described in the present chapter.* Apart from wasting, the disease is generally suggested by thirst, polyuria, pruritus, or furunculosis, which leads the physician to examine the urine for the presence of sugar.

Diabetes is an endocrine disorder dependent upon a deficient production of insulin by the islets of Langerhans of the pancreas. The deficiency leads to defective utilization and storage of carbohydrates, and the blood-sugar values rise above the level of the renal threshold for sugar, so that some escapes into the urine and causes the cardinal physical sign of the disease, namely, *glycosuria.*

The presence of glycosuria alone is not pathognomonic of diabetes, and in the absence of other conclusive signs the possibility of *renal glycosuria* must be excluded by a glucose tolerance test. Renal glycosuria is the name given to the passage of sugar in the urine when the blood-sugar values are not above normal. It depends upon a low renal threshold for sugar, i.e., the kidney secretes sugar before the usual level of 180 mg. per cent has been reached. (*See* GLUCOSE TOLERANCE TEST, p. 434.)

2. DISEASES CHARACTERIZED BY A RASH

The most important diseases of which a rash is the presenting physical sign are the exanthemata, various forms of purpura (primary and symptomatic), and urticaria. The macular rashes of typhoid and typhus fever, cerebrospinal fever, and syphilis have already received brief consideration, and the many skin lesions which have no very obvious link with general medicine cannot be described here.

The Exanthemata.—Especially in the examination of children, the possibility of infectious diseases must be considered in all febrile illnesses. Sometimes a diagnosis is possible before the rash appears (e.g., by Koplik spots in measles), but more often the first pathognomonic sign is the rash.

Measles.—The *rash* occurs fourteen days after exposure to infection, usually four days after the fever began. It consists of blotchy patches (maculo-papular) of a red or purplish character distributed over the face, especially round the forehead and ears, spreading soon to the trunk and

---

* N.B.—No special chapter has been devoted to metabolic disorders.

limbs. It begins to fade on the day it appears, but lasts in a modified form for a few days. The pyrexia increases with the eruption of the rash.

Measles has other suggestive signs besides the rash. The *catarrhal symptoms*—discharge from the eyes and nose, sneezing and coughing—are almost invariably present, and *Koplik spots* may establish an early diagnosis. These are bluish-white spots on the buccal mucous membrane, generally opposite the lower second molar teeth (*Fig.* 43), and occur on the second day of the disease.

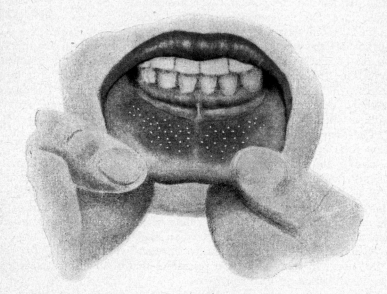

Fig. 43.—Koplik's spots. (*From French's 'Index of Diagnosis'.*)

Scarlet Fever.—The *rash* appears on the second day of the illness, and is punctate on a diffuse erythematous base, i.e., consists of pin-point dark-red spots on a general reddening of the skin. It appears especially on the chest, neck, and scapular regions, but affects the trunk and legs later. The rash is followed by *desquamation,* at first of powdery, then of coarser flakes. Desquamation may begin even whilst the fever is present, and continues for several weeks. It may be a valuable sign if the patient has not been seen during the febrile period of the illness.

The collateral evidence of scarlet fever is found in the sudden onset with *vomiting* (sometimes a rigor or convulsion), high temperature (104°–105°), and *sore throat.* The tongue is heavily furred and the reddened papillæ show through, giving it a *strawberry* appearance. The area round the mouth by contrast with the redness of the face appears unusually pale (circum-oral pallor).

German Measles.—The *rash* may be the first sign to draw attention to this disease. It is usually described as having some of the characteristics of measles and of scarlet fever, but it resembles the latter more closely than the former. It consists of rose-coloured spots distributed discretely on the face, but fusing together on the trunk.

The constitutional symptoms of German measles are mild—slight pyrexia and conjunctivitis—but the most signficant sign apart from the rash is the *enlargement of the occipital glands.*

Small-pox.—The *rash* in small-pox appears on the fourth day of the illness. It consists of several distinct elements changing from one to another in a definite sequence—macules, papules, vesicles, and pustules. The macules only last a few hours and are replaced by firm papules. On the sixth day the papules become vesicles, and on the eighth day the fluid in these becomes turbid, forming pustules. The vesicles are frequently dimpled in the centre (umbilication); this characteristic is lost in the pustules, which in their turn burst to form crusts. Fusion of the pustules sometimes takes place, converting large areas of skin into abscesses (confluent small-pox).

The distribution of the rash is of great importance in diagnosis. It occurs first on the face, wrists, and hands, then on other distal parts of the limbs ; and although it may spread later to all parts of the body, the elements remain fewer on the trunk than on the parts described.

The *constitutional* symptoms are profound and of great diagnostic import. The onset is sudden, with headache, vomiting, and lumbar pain. The temperature rises to 100°–102°, falls when the rash appears, and rises again when the rash reaches the pustular stage (maturation).

Chicken-pox.—The rash usually appears within twenty-four hours of the onset. In many respects it resembles that of small-pox, from which it is all-important to distinguish it.

Papules appear first, but change *within a few hours* to vesicles. In thirty-six to forty-eight hours these become pustules, which shrivel and form crusts by the fourth day. All elements of the rash may be present at the same time, as several crops usually occur. The individual elements remain *discrete*, and there is no umbilication of the vesicles. The rash is essentially distributed *on the trunk*, and to a much lesser extent on the limbs, though the forehead may be an early site.

The *constitutional symptoms* are similar to those of small-pox—pains in the back, vomiting, and pyrexia—but of a much milder character.

3. DISEASES OF BONES AND JOINTS

Many diseases of bones and joints are so rarely encountered in the medical wards that it is not possible to describe them here. A few are essentially medical rather than surgical, and a few are common to medical and surgical diagnosis.

Osteitis Deformans (*Paget's Disease*).—Pains in the limbs or an increase in the size of the patient's hats may first call attention to this comparatively rare disease.

The *head is enlarged*, due to great thickening in the tables of the skull, well shown by X-rays. The long bones are also thickened, and their *bowing* gives a characteristic appearance to the thighs and legs. Usually there is a moderate degree of kyphosis, giving the patient an attitude of flexion (*Fig.* 44).

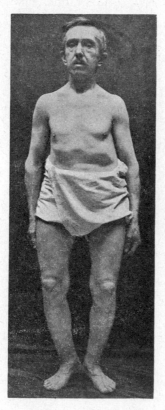

Fig. 44.—Osteitis deformans. Note the large head and bowing of the legs. (*H. Wallace-Jones and C. Thurstan Holland's case—from ' Archives of Radiology and Electrotherapy '.*)

Achondroplasia.—This condition is more a clinical curiosity than a disease, but it is essential that it should not be confused with the effects of severe rickets.

The patient is a *dwarf*, but in strength and intelligence equals a normal adult. The distinguishing features are the *short arms and legs*, with a normally developed trunk (*Fig.* 45). When the patient stands with the arms to the side, the fingers reach very little below the crests of the ilia. There is often an apparent curvature of the long bones due to peculiarities

4

of articulation. This still further diminishes the stature. The facial appearance is made characteristic by the prominence of the forehead and the depression of the bridge of the nose.

Arthritis.—

1. *Rheumatic Fever* (*Acute Rheumatism*).—Multiple joints are attacked in this disease, but the active signs of inflammation usually manifest themselves in one at a time, and remain twenty-four hours on an average, before they appear in another joint. The arthritis, however, does not pass away

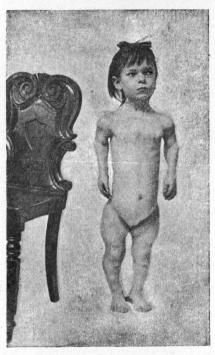

Fig. 45.—Achondroplasia. Age 15. The trunk is almost of normal length, and the limbs very short, the proximal being shorter than the distal segments. The epiphyses are enlarged, the forearms and legs curved. The nose is deficient at the bridge. In this case there is infantilism as well as dwarfism. (*From French's 'Index of Diagnosis'.*)

completely from the joint first affected, but remains in a subacute form. Thus it is common for one joint to show acute inflammatory signs whilst several others are affected to a lesser extent. *Each affected joint is hot, swollen, and exquisitely tender.* The skin over it may be reddened.

The onset is sudden, with high *fever* (100°–104° F.), *sore throat*, and malaise. Profuse *sweating* is a notable feature, and signs of cardiac involvement may take place at an early stage. The course of the disease is much modified by the treatment with salicylates which is almost invariably instituted.

Subacute forms of rheumatism are more common than fully developed rheumatic fever. All grades are found, but each is characterized by multiple arthritis, fever, sweating, and a tendency to other rheumatic infections (tonsillitis ; cardiac lesions ; chorea ; rheumatic nodules).

2. *Rheumatoid Arthritis.*—In its *acute form*, the symptoms and signs of rheumatoid arthritis are not dissimilar from those of acute rheumatism. Pyrexia, sweating, and multiple arthritis occur in both. In rheumatoid types the *smaller joints* are, however, more especially affected, those of the wrists and fingers suffering most. The temporo-maxillary and vertebral joints are also more often involved.

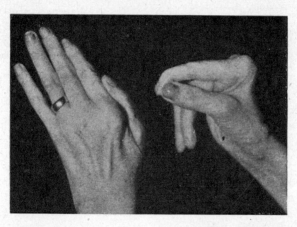

Fig. 46.—Rheumatoid arthritis. Shows crippling deformities. The *left* hand shows moderate ulnar deflection, swelling and deformity of the first metacarpo-phalangeal joint, and wasting of the interosseous muscles. The *right* hand shows extreme deformity which produces marked limitation of movement.

Rheumatoid arthritis differs in two other respects from acute rheumatism. It usually leaves *permanent changes* in the joints, progressing in severe chronic forms to serious crippling (*Figs.* 46, 47). On the other hand, it *does not damage the heart.*

The diagnosis of rheumatoid arthritis is incomplete unless an attempt has been made to discover an aetiological factor. Whereas acute rheumatism is probably a specific infection due to a streptococcus, rheumatoid arthritis may take origin in a *septic focus.* Sepsis should be sought especially in the teeth, tonsils, nasal sinuses, and alimentary and genito-urinary tracts. Certain types of rheumatoid arthritis are apparently associated with metabolic changes, e.g., the menopause.

3. *Osteo-arthritis.*—Osteo-arthritis is considered by many authorities to be a type of rheumatoid arthritis in which the bony changes are much in advance of those in the synovial membrane and periarticular tissues.

From a clinical point of view it occurs in older people, is not infrequently associated with trauma, and is *often confined to one joint,* especially a hip. Pain, limitation of movement, and bony irregularities of the joint are the salient features. Radiological examination shows the bony changes to the best advantage.

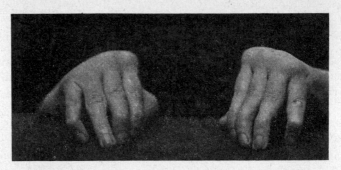

Fig. 47.—Rheumatoid arthritis. Shows crippling of hands with ulnar deviation. (*Professor Henry Cohen's case.*)

4. *Specific Forms of Arthritis.*—Many seeming cases of rheumatoid arthritis prove on fuller examination to be due to some specific organism.

Gonococcal arthritis is perhaps the most important example. It usually affects several joints at first, but as it becomes subacute the arthritis is generally limited to one or two joints. In every case of arthritis, especially in young adults, inquiry should be made for a history of venereal disease. If doubt exists as to the cause, the urethra and prostate in the male, and the vagina and cervix in the female, should be examined for signs of gonococcal infection.

Painless forms of arthritis may be produced by *syphilis.*

Tuberculous arthritis is common and important. It is usually limited to one joint. For fuller description the student should consult a surgical text-book.

Other specific forms of arthritis are rarer, but during the course of, or following, typhoid fever, dysentery, and pneumonia, the possibility of arthritis due to these diseases must be considered.

5. *Metabolic Forms of Arthritis.*—The commonest of these is *gout.* The localization of the trouble in the great toe is always suggestive of gout, though other joints may be affected (*Fig.* 48). Other signs of clinical value are the sudden onset after a short period of malaise and irritability, the sharp rise of temperature, and the short duration of the attack. The signs of inflammation in the joint are generally more severe than in other forms of arthritis. The discovery of tophi (*see* p. 28) is an important confirmatory

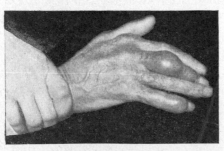

Fig. 48.—Gouty arthritis. The affected joints are swollen and the skin over them shiny. Aspiration of one showed it to contain a thin chalky fluid. A tophus was present in one ear.

sign. In doubtful chronic cases, X-ray examination is helpful, and a family history of gout is always suggestive. The patient's habits as regards alcohol and food should also be considered.

Other forms of metabolic arthritis are the rachitic changes in the bones and joints in certain cases of renal disease in childhood, *renal rickets,* and the effusions of blood into the joints in cases of *scurvy* and *hæmophilia.*

6. *Neuropathic Joint Lesions.* — In tabes and syringomyelia gross degenerative changes may take place in the joints.

The *Charcot's joint of tabes* (*Fig.* 49) is recognized by the complete disorganization of the joint (usually a knee or hip), which shows all the changes of an advanced arthritis, but *remains painless.*

Similar changes occur in *syringomyelic joints,* but the shoulder and elbow are the most commonly affected.

Arthritic changes are sometimes seen in the joints of a *hemiplegic limb.*

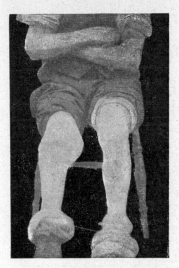

Fig. 49.—Charcot's disease of the right knee-joint in association with tabes dorsalis. Showing distension of the joint and also displacement of the tibia to the patient's right. (*From French's 'Index of Diagnosis'.*)

CHAPTER III

THE RESPIRATORY SYSTEM

SYMPTOMS OF RESPIRATORY DISEASE

THE symptoms which point specially to the respiratory system as the seat of disease are *cough* (with or without *expectoration*), *breathlessness*, and more rarely *pain*. Occasionally the patient may report such objective features as *cyanosis* and *clubbing of the fingers*, but more often these are observed by the examiner.

The symptoms mentioned have not always a respiratory origin, and the possibility of cardio-vascular, nervous, and hæmic causes must not be overlooked. The details which follow are applicable particularly to the symptoms as they are found in diseases of the organs of respiration.

Cough.—Perhaps the most pathognomonic of all respiratory symptoms, cough may be an expression of disease in the upper respiratory passages or in the bronchi or lungs. It is usually a reflex act through the coughing centre in the medulla by which an attempt is made to remove irritant material from the air-passages. If the attempt is successful expectoration of sputum results. The student should note particularly whether or not the cough is productive of sputum, how frequently it occurs, whether in paroxysms or as a constant tickling, and finally its character. A 'dry' cough occurs when the bronchial mucous membrane is congested with little or no exudate, as in the early stages of acute bronchitis and pulmonary tuberculosis. A 'loose' cough occurs when the exudate increases and is free in the bronchi, as in chronic bronchitis, bronchiectasis, and pulmonary cavities. Paroxysmal coughing is particularly common in chronic bronchitis and whooping-cough. A foreign body may be responsible for the abrupt onset of paroxysmal cough, and this possibility must be considered, especially in children, in whom no history may be forthcoming. In bronchiectasis paroxysms also occur, but at longer intervals. Cough which appears suddenly suggests acute respiratory disease—e.g., tracheitis, bronchitis, or broncho-pneumonia. A cough which causes pain, for example in pneumonia with pleurisy, is usually 'suppressed' in order to diminish the pain. Cough may result from mechanical causes such as a long uvula or enlarged heart, or by trickling down of secretions from the nose and nasopharynx. Sinusitis should always be considered as a possible cause of cough. Lastly, it should be observed whether the cough is of such severity as to cause vomiting and symptoms of collapse. Vomiting is particularly common in whooping-cough.

These remarks apply to cough originating in the bronchi, but irritability of the larynx from catarrhal processes and the irritation of tobacco are also very common causes, and before attaching too much significance to a cough, the effect of stopping smoking should be observed. Intrathoracic tumours, especially aneurysm, may cause special types of cough. If they press on the trachea the cough has a metallic hard quality described as ' brassy '.

If the tumour involves the recurrent laryngeal branch of the vagus and interferes with the normal movements of the vocal cords, the cough loses its explosive character and becomes prolonged and wheezing like that of a cow. It is then known as the ' bovine ' cough.

Diseases of the larynx responsible for cough (e.g., tuberculosis or neoplasm) are sometimes identified by associated voice changes (aphonia) and stridor.

Sputum.—Quite apart from the laboratory examination of sputum, much important information can be gained by naked-eye inspection. The patient should be instructed to spit into a sputum cup, and the amount be measured after twenty-four hours. · The student should *note the amount, smell, and appearance of the sputum.* Large amounts, ten to twenty ounces, may be found in bronchiectasis and pulmonary abscess or when an empyema ruptures into a bronchus. The expectoration of large quantities of sputum *on change of posture* is particularly characteristic of bronchiectasis and pulmonary abscess. Offensiveness is usually suggestive of bronchiectasis, more rarely of pulmonary suppuration due to a spirillum infection or to gangrene of the lung.

The constituents should then be observed. The common varieties are :—

a. Mucoid Sputum.—Jelly-like material, often grey or black owing to admixture with carbon of the atmosphere, especially in town-dwellers.

b. Pus.—In pure form only occurs in pulmonary abscess, empyema, or extrinsic abscesses rupturing into a bronchus.

c. Muco-pus.—One of the commonest types of sputum. It may be recognized by its creamy yellow gelatinous appearance. If it is coughed up in rounded coin-shaped masses, it is known as *nummular* sputum, seen sometimes in phthisis.

d. Hæmorrhagic Sputum.—This may consist entirely of blood (*see* HÆMOPTYSIS, *below*) or merely be stained with it. In pneumonia the intimate mixture of small quantities of blood with the sputum gives it a classical ' rusty ' appearance. Similarly, but rarely, the mixture of mucus and blood in the sputum of pulmonary neoplasms gives it a red-currant-jelly appearance. In other circumstances small amounts of blood merely appear as streaks.

e. Fœtid Sputum.—This has an evil smell and is usually greenish-black in appearance. It is found in bronchiectasis and gangrene of the lung, and in the latter may contain disintegrated lung tissue which is recognizable microscopically.

f. Pus Resembling Anchovy Sauce.—Sometimes discharged through the diaphragm from an amœbic liver abscess, and may be expectorated if a communication with a bronchus is established.

g. Fibrinous Casts.—These are casts of the bronchi which are expectorated in rare cases of fibrinous bronchitis.

h. Watery Sputum.—Several pints may be expectorated in the uncommon condition called bronchorrhœa serosa.

Hæmoptysis.—Spitting of blood is known as hæmoptysis. The amount may vary from streaks to several pints, and may consist of pure blood or be mixed with sputum or salivary secretions. From the patient's history it is not always easy to determine whether the blood has been coughed up or vomited, though his opinion should be given due consideration. The important differences between hæmoptysis and hæmatemesis may be summarized in tabular form.

Hæmoptysis	Hæmatemesis
Cough precedes hæmorrhage	Nausea and vomiting precede hæmorrhage
Blood frothy from admixture with air	Generally airless
Sputum bright red in colour and may be stained for days	Blood often altered in colour by admixture with gastric contents, usually dark red or brown
Alkaline in reaction	Acid in reaction
History is suggestive of respiratory disease	Previous history of indigestion

The staining of the sputum for some days after the hæmorrhage is perhaps the most convincing point of distinction between hæmoptysis and hæmatemesis.

If it is definitely established that the blood has been spat up, the mouth and throat should be examined for any local cause, such as bleeding gums or a congested pharynx, which may cause small amounts of blood to appear in the mouth.

In true hæmoptysis, where the blood comes from the bronchi or lungs, coughing is rarely absent. In all cases the first suspicion should be of *pulmonary tuberculosis*, which is the commonest cause ; but hæmoptysis is not infrequently found in other acute and chronic inflammatory diseases of the bronchi and lungs, especially pneumonia, pulmonary infarct, bronchiectasis, and pulmonary neoplasm. The symptom may also arise from extra-pulmonary conditions, such as mitral stenosis, congestive heart failure, aneurysm of the aorta, primary blood diseases, and injury to the chest. *Tuberculosis and mitral disease are the commonest causes of hæmoptysis.*

Dyspnœa (difficult breathing).—This symptom implies undue effort in respiration, often extreme enough to cause great discomfort. It is described by the patient as breathlessness, short-windedness, fighting for breath, etc. The *breathing is usually more rapid* than normal (tachypnœa), though this is not an essential feature. In some cases the patient is unable to lie down because of the aggravation of the dyspnœa—*orthopnœa.*

Dyspnœa is an accompaniment of many respiratory diseases, yet it is remarkable how frequently serious changes are present in the bronchi or lungs without it, though in many types of heart disease it is rarely absent. If a patient complains of breathlessness the observer should note whether it is present at the time of examination, and if it is increased by movement or alteration of posture. Inquiry should be made as to whether it is continuous or paroxysmal in nature.

Obstruction of the upper respiratory passages—e.g., of the larynx or trachea, by foreign bodies or extrinsic pressure—causes dyspnœa by impeding the passage of air both to and from the lungs. The respiratory rate is not usually increased and is *often diminished*, but there is a great increase in muscular action to overcome the obstruction. Similar obstruction results from spasm of the smaller bronchi in asthma. Emphysema and pleurisy also cause dyspnœa by mechanical interference with the intake of air, in the one case by permanent over-distension of the lung alveoli, in the other by the restricted movement of the chest from pain.

Most important, however, is the dyspnœa due to diminished function of the lung alveoli brought about by consolidation or collapse of the lung. Pneumonia, pleural effusion, pneumothorax, pulmonary collapse, and infarction provide examples. Whenever an organ or tissue is put out of action rapidly, the effects are more dramatic than if this occurs gradually. The lungs illustrate this rule, for *dyspnœa is proportionate to the rapidity with which the lung tissue becomes functionless*, a rapidly developing pleural effusion or pneumothorax, for example, causing much greater dyspnœa than one which slowly compresses the lung. In whichever way the dyspnœa is brought about, its ultimate cause appears to be deficiency of oxygen or excess of carbon dioxide or other organic acids in the blood, which nature attempts to rectify by more rapid or deep respirations. Often several factors are at work in the same patient.

Dyspnœa is an important symptom in heart disease (p. 95) and may also occur in cardio-renal failure, in ketosis, and rarely from intercostal or diaphragmatic paralysis.

Pain.—Lung tissue is insensitive and pain in the chest is always the result of conditions which affect the surrounding structures. In many respiratory diseases pain is an uncommon symptom. In acute tracheitis and bronchitis, for example, the rawness and burning behind the sternum scarcely amount to real pain, whilst in pulmonary consolidation due to bronchopneumonia, tuberculosis, and other causes, pain may be entirely absent.

When the pleura is involved, however, pain is a prominent feature, and has the same characteristics and distribution whether it is caused by inflammation (dry pleurisy—lobar pneumonia with pleurisy), new growth, or mechanical affections such as pneumothorax. The pain is usually described as cutting, stabbing, or tearing, and is of great severity, preventing sleep. Its site is important. Most commonly it is felt in the axillæ and beneath the breasts, regions where pleurisy is common, but it may occur in regions remote from the chest and cause difficulty in diagnosis. The parietal pleura, including that covering the outer portion of the diaphragm, is innervated through the thoracic roots (intercostal nerves), the lower six of which are responsible for the supply of skin areas on the abdominal wall and back. *Pleural pain is, therefore, frequently referred to the abdomen and lumbar regions*, and, as it is often accompanied by hyperæsthesia, has given rise to mistaken diagnosis of acute abdominal lesions. Less commonly abdominal lesions may cause referred pain in the chest (*see* ABDOMINAL PAIN, p. 162 et seq.). In lesions of the apex of the lung such as Pancoast's syndrome (usually bronchial carcinoma causing Horner's syndrome with involvement of the 8th cervical and 1st dorsal nerve roots) all the pain may be referred to the arm, and its origin overlooked unless appreciated.

The innervation of the central portion of the diaphragm by the phrenic nerve (3rd and 4th cervical) occasionally leads to referred pain in the neck, with tenderness on pinching the trapezius muscle, in diaphragmatic pleurisy.

Finally it must be mentioned that many pains occur in the chest which are not associated with respiratory disease. Amongst these may be mentioned pains due to disease of the heart (p. 97), affections of the ribs, sternum, and intercostal muscles (periostitis, fibrositis, neuralgia), herpes zoster, and diseases of the breast.

Added to these chief respiratory symptoms, are those such as hoarseness and aphonia suggesting laryngeal involvement, sneezing and nasal discharges indicative of nasal or sinus disease, and constitutional signs (especially of tuberculosis) such as loss of weight, night sweats, and dyspepsia. Any of these may be mentioned firstly by the patient and it is important that their relationship to respiratory disease should be borne in mind.

PHYSICAL SIGNS : EXAMINATION OF THE RESPIRATORY SYSTEM

Certain signs may be noted before the systematic examination of the chest is made—namely, the character of any sputum (p. 55), the presence of cyanosis or clubbing of the fingers, and the condition of the neck.

Cyanosis (blueness of the skin and mucous membranes) (*see also* CARDIO-VASCULAR SYSTEM, p. 101).—Though rarely seen to such an extreme degree as occurs in certain types of heart disease, cyanosis is a familiar characteristic of many respiratory diseases. The *lips, cheeks, ears, and nose* show changes in colour shading from a dusky red to a deep purple plum colour. Cyanosis should also be sought beneath the *finger and toe nails.*

Cyanosis results from a relative disproportion between oxyhæmoglobin and reduced hæmoglobin in the blood, the former decreasing, the latter increasing. Decrease of available oxygen may be the sequel of those causes already described under dyspnœa. The entering air may be actually limited by obstruction of the air-passages, or, having gained access, it may be prevented by exudate in the alveoli or by their collapse from coming into relationship with the blood in the capillaries, and the normal interchange of gases is thus impaired.

Cyanosis is increased by cold weather, which diminishes the rate of capillary circulation and allows more time for dissociation of oxygen. Similarly, effort aggravates cyanosis by the increased consumption of oxygen by the tissues. Rarer causes of cyanosis include polycythæmia,

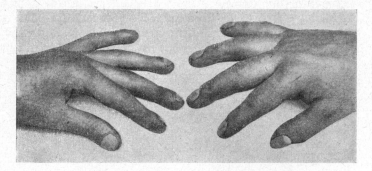

Fig. 50.—Slight clubbing of the fingers. Looked at laterally slighter degrees of clubbing are more obvious than in the antero-posterior view. The right hand is a normal one.

poisoning with trinitrotoluene, enterogenous cyanosis, etc., which may have to be borne in mind when the condition of the respiratory or cardiovascular system does not explain the symptom.

Clubbing of the Fingers (*Figs.* 50, 51).—This sign is frequently present in chronic diseases of the lungs and heart. It is seen most often in bronchiectasis and congenital heart disease, and in the latter often to

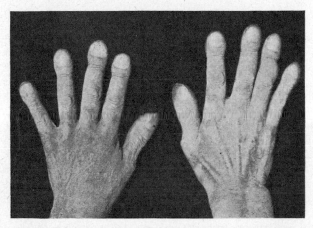

Fig. 51.—Clubbing of the fingers from a case of bronchiectasis.

an extreme degree. Occasionally the clubbing is associated with similar changes in the toes, and sometimes with swelling of the wrist-joints and ankles, when it receives the name of 'hypertrophic pulmonary osteo-arthropathy'. The sign may be recognized by a bulbousness of the soft terminal portions of the fingers and by an excessive curvature of the nails. The curvature may be longitudinal or from side to side, or both. The exact causes of clubbing of the fingers remain uncertain. It has been suggested that in its early stages it is due to œdema of the soft tissues and later on to fibrotic changes. Clubbed fingers are usually cyanotic.

The Neck.—This should be inspected for engorged jugular veins, enlarged glands, and the position of the trachea. The jugular veins may be overfilled, not only in congestive heart failure (p. 112), but in superior

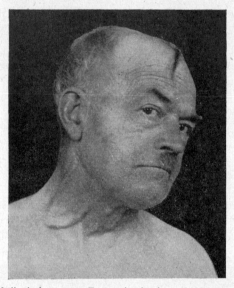

Fig. 52.—Mediastinal tumour. Engorged veins in neck. Laryngeal paresis.

mediastinal obstruction—e.g., tumour (Fig. 52). Glands may be enlarged from tuberculous, lymphadenomatous, leukæmic, or malignant infiltration, and may be a leading feature in the diagnosis.

Tracheal Tug.—The pulsations of an aortic aneurysm may pull at the bifurcation of the trachea. This may be detected clinically by extending the neck and pulling the larynx gently upwards, when a tug will be felt corresponding with each systole of the heart.

The Larynx.—Examination of this structure should be made in all cases of chronic respiratory disease. Changes in the voice and special types of cough should be noted. The laryngoscope may show tuberculous ulceration in association with phthisis, or vocal cord paralysis, especially in cases of mediastinal tumour and malignant disease of the lung.

The Chest.—It is necessary for the patient to be stripped to the waist if faulty examination of the chest is to be avoided. The *sitting posture is the one choice*, as a good view may be obtained of the chest as a whole, but in many diseases the patient is unable to get out of bed, and may even be entirely recumbent. Good lighting is essential, and the light should fall evenly on the chest to exclude shadow effects which confuse the observer.

The order of examination by *inspection, palpation, percussion*, and *auscultation* is particularly suitable for the respiratory system.

Inspection shows the configuration of the chest, the degree of movement and any inequalities on the two sides, the type and rate of respiration, and any special variety of breathing which may be present.

Palpation confirms the impressions of inspection, especially the movements of the chest and any abnormal prominence or recession in the chest wall. It also detects abnormal pulsation and areas of tenderness, and a special sign called *vocal fremitus*.

Percussion is used to demonstrate changes in the character of the lung tissue, its contained bronchi, and the surrounding pleura, and shows whether these tissues contain less or more air than normal. It serves also to define the air-containing lungs from the adjacent solid viscera, the heart and liver.

Auscultation enables the observer to suspect changes in the calibre of the bronchi by variation in the intensity of the breath-sounds, and modification of the lung substance by changes in the character of the breath-sounds. It also reveals the presence of abnormal exudates in the bronchi and lung alveoli which cause special adventitious sounds. Finally, it may give evidence of interference in the normal movements of the layers of the pleura on one another.

These methods of examination may now be considered in detail.

INSPECTION

This method of examination yields more information to the experienced eye than most others. The inspection should be systematic, the observer regarding the chest in every case from the front, back, and side, and viewing it from above downwards by looking over the shoulders.

In recumbent patients the chest should be inspected by looking from the head of the bed over the clavicles, or from the foot of the bed towards the neck. If the patient is too ill to sit up, the back may be examined by rolling the patient on each side in turn. This is necessary to compare the physical signs at the two bases, which are modified on the side on which the patient is lying. However well-developed the subject may be, some slight asymmetry is generally to be seen, but *gross differences on the two sides suggest deformities of the chest wall or disease of the underlying structures*.

The skin over the chest wall should be noted as in the inspection of any part of the body. Particular attention should be directed to the presence of engorged veins (*Fig.* 53) or subcutaneous nodules.

Position of the Apex Beat and Trachea.—These should be observed carefully, as they may be modified by respiratory disease. Palpation is necessary to confirm their position. The heart and trachea may be displaced to the opposite side by pleural effusion or pneumothorax, or drawn to the same side by pulmonary fibrosis. Displacement of the heart towards the left axilla may give a false suggestion of cardiac enlargement. Displacement to the right causes the cardiac impulse to appear well within the nipple line, and the maximal pulsation may even be to the right of the sternum.

Normal Characteristics of the Chest.—In the normal chest the intercostal spaces are broader in front than behind ; there is a depression running down the sternum which becomes most marked at its lower end ; and the shoulders and bony prominences of the thorax should be approximately at the same level on the two sides. The subcostal angle is normally about 70° to 110°, and pronounced acuity or obtuseness is pathological.

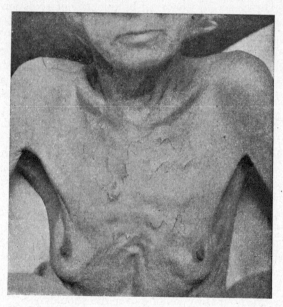

Fig. 53.—Dilated veins on the chest from a case of mediastinal tumour.

Minor variations are frequent. Thus the clavicles, scapulæ, ribs, and angle of Louis are more prominent in men, as in women they are covered by thicker subcutaneous tissues. These bony landmarks are also obscured by thick muscular coverings in athletic men.

Character of Respiratory Movements.—

Expansion of the Chest.—The degree of the expansion of the chest may be measured by placing a tape measure just below the nipples with its zero mark at the middle of the sternum, instructing the patient to breathe in and out as deeply as possible. It is important that *several readings should be taken,* as the initial respiratory efforts are often shallower than subsequent ones.

Particular note should also be made of the *equality of expansion* of the two sides (*Fig. 54*). Although poor expansion of the chest as a whole may occur in health, a *definite inequality signifies disease of the bronchi, lungs, or pleuræ.* The affected side always moves less than the sound side. Amongst the commoner causes of unilateral defective movement should be mentioned obstruction to a main bronchus by foreign bodies and new growths ; consolidation of the lung by pneumonia, tuberculosis, and new growth ; fibrosis of the lung ; and air and fluid in the pleural cavity which collapse the corresponding lung. All these conditions prevent the normal tidal air from entering the lung.

Generalized restriction of expansion is most commonly seen in emphysema, though it occurs in extensive bilateral disease such as fibrosis, consolidation, or pleural effusion.

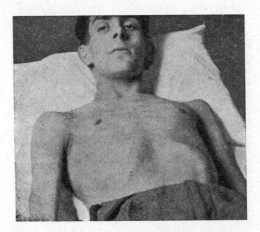

Fig. 54.—Unequal expansion of the lungs. The patient has taken a deep breath and the left side of the chest has expanded well, but the right side shows flattening at the apex. The observation is made from the foot of the bed.

Manner of Breathing.—The manner of breathing should next be noted. In men the diaphragm is more freely used than the intercostal muscles, and its downward excursion with inspiration leads to free movements of the abdominal wall—*abdominal respiration.* Similar breathing is characteristic of children.

In women, on the other hand, the movements of the chest are greater than those of the abdomen, because respiration is chiefly accomplished by use of the intercostal muscles—*thoracic respiration.* Various mixtures of these two types of breathing—diaphragmatic and costal—are found in health, but a *sudden change in the type of breathing may be significant of disease.* Thus, acute peritonitis by limiting the abdominal movements produces a costal type of breathing, whilst pain from pleurisy or other cause may lead to restriction of the chest movements. Breathing modified by pleural pain, in this way, is often jerky and irregular.

Rate of Respiration.—The rate of respiration should be observed without the patient's knowledge, as consciousness of the act of breathing tends to make it irregular. The rate varies in normal individuals between 16 and 20 per minute, but is faster in children and slower in old age. *It bears a definite ratio to the pulse-rate of about 1 : 4, which is usually constant in the same individual.* Increase in the respiratory rate (tachypnœa) is frequently present in diseases of the heart or lungs, and more rarely in other conditions of anoxæmia. It results from the body's attempt to obtain a greater supply of oxygen. A decrease takes place during sleep, coma, obstruction to the air-passages, and in certain types of poisoning, e.g., opium.

Abnormal Types of Breathing.—Particular attention should be paid to the ease of respiration and to whether more effort seems to be expended on inspiration or expiration. When great dyspnœa is present the accessory

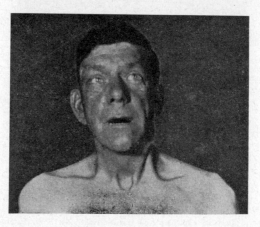

Fig. 55.—Use of the extraordinary muscles of respiration. The patient has emphysema. He has taken a deep breath and the prominent bellies of the sternomastoid and trapezius muscles are seen. Similar use of the extraordinary or accessory muscles of respiration is seen in acute respiratory disease such as pneumonia.

muscles of respiration are nearly always called into play, and care should be taken to *note any movement of the sternomastoid,* trapezius, or other neck muscles (*Fig.* 55) and of the *alæ nasi.* The depth of respiration should also be taken into account.

Normal breathing should be quiet, but in comatose and dying patients it is often noisy—*stertorous breathing*—due to the vibrations of the soft tissues of the nasopharynx, larynx, and cheeks. The death rattle combines the features of stertorous breathing with the bubbling noise produced by vibrations of mucus in the trachea and large bronchi.

A special variety of breathing known as *Cheyne-Stokes respiration* consists in a temporary cessation of breathing (apnœa) followed by respirations which gradually increase in magnitude to a maximum and then diminish until apnœa occurs once more. This phenomenon is of serious omen, and rarely found except in grave illnesses such as cerebral hæmorrhage, meningitis, uræmia, and advanced heart disease.

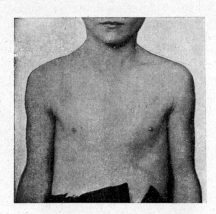

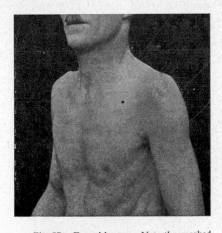

Fig. 56.—Harrison's sulcus. The lower ribs, especially on the left side, appear 'caved in '.

Fig. 57.—Funnel breast. Note the marked hollowing-out of the lower end of the sternum. The patient was a cobbler and had no respiratory disease.

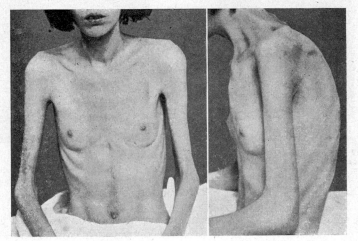

Fig. 58.

Fig. 59.

Fig. 58.—Phthinoid chest. Note the obliquity of the ribs and narrow subcostal angle. The patient is suffering from advanced phthisis ; hence the emaciation.

Fig. 59.—Phthinoid chest. Lateral view of the long flat chest. The antero-posterior diameter is rather greater than usually found in this type of chest, owing to slight kyphosis. Note especially the marked obliquity of the ribs, which almost reach the iliac crest.

In thin persons it is possible to see in the lower axillary regions a shadow about 1 cm. in breadth which moves up and down with respiration. It is caused by the reflection of light from the chest wall at

5

the points of contact of the diaphragm, and consequently moves down as the diaphragm becomes 'peeled' from the chest wall during inspiration. This phenomenon is known as *Litten's sign*, and is useful in judging of the equality of movement of the two sides of the diaphragm.

Chest Deformities.—*Abnormalities of the chest wall are not infrequently present without disease of the thoracic contents.* The softness of the bones in childhood renders the chest liable to deformities if the normal relationship between the pressure of air in the lungs and that of the atmosphere is disturbed. Thus, nasal obstruction due to adenoids or other conditions causing defective filling of the lungs often produces gross alteration in the configuration of the chest. Many types of chest deformity

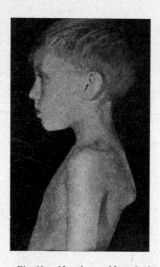

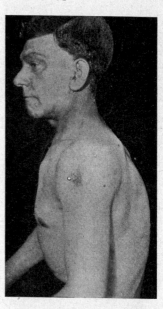

Fig. 60.—Alar chest. Note the long flat type of chest with decrease in the antero-posterior diameter and the wing-like appearance of the scapula. No actual lung disease was found in this child, but a chest of this kind may predispose to respiratory disease. The facies is somewhat adenoid in type.

Fig. 61.—Barrel-shaped chest of emphysema. Note especially the great increase in antero-posterior diameter, the gentle kyphosis, and the prominent angle of Louis.

exist, amongst which may be mentioned : (1) *Harrison's sulcus*, a groove running horizontally from the sternum outwards in the lower part of the chest (*Fig.* 56) ; (2) *Pigeon-breast*, in which there is marked bulging of the sternum ; and (3) *Funnel breast*, an exaggeration of the normal depression seen at the lower end of the sternum and sometimes found in cobblers from the continual pressure of the last (*Fig.* 57). Combinations of these three are frequently present. Rickets favours their production by making the bones abnormally soft, and sometimes leaves further traces as a 'rickety rosary', a series of knob-like projections on the chest wall at the junction of the ribs with the costal cartilages. *Such deformed chests predispose to respiratory disease,* owing to their interference with the full expansion of the lungs, and with the circulation through them. Another type of chest deformity not necessarily dependent on previous disease but rendering the patient prone to tuberculosis is the *long, flat chest (Figs.* 58, 59). In this the ribs are placed so obliquely that at their lower part they approach the crest of the ilium, the subcostal angle is unusually acute, and the scapulæ prominent. If the scapulæ stand out in a fancied resemblance to wings, the term ' alar ' is applied (*Fig.* 60). The *flat and alar chest, apart from predisposing to phthisis, may result from this disease.* In contrast to these types is the *barrel-shaped chest of emphysema,* in which the antero-posterior diameter is so increased that a section of the chest appears cylin-

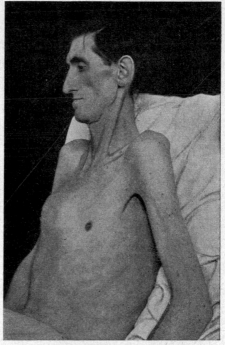

Fig. 62.—Sarcoma of the sternum.

drical (*Fig.* 61). The ribs are also more horizontally placed, and the subcostal angle obtuse. Apart from these primary defects in the chest wall, there

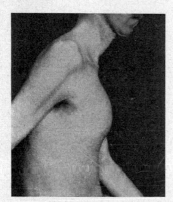

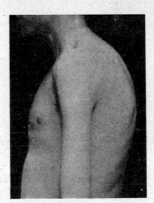

Fig. 63. Fig. 64.

Fig. 63.—Bulging of the chest wall (empyema necessitatis). Prominent bulging of one side of the chest is unusual apart from old chest deformities. It is seen most commonly in cases of aortic aneurysm. In this case an empyema has ruptured through the intercostal spaces and produced an abscess on the chest wall. (*By courtesy of Mr. C. A. Wells.*)

Fig. 64.—Chest deformity from heart disease in a child. Note increased antero-posterior diameter and the sharp precordial bulge. Such a deformity rarely results from heart disease in adult life.

may be noted bulging or recession, secondary to such causes as aneurysm, empyema, cardiac hypertrophy, local disease of the ribs or sternum, fibroid changes in the lungs and pleura, Pott's disease, etc. (*Figs.* 62–66).

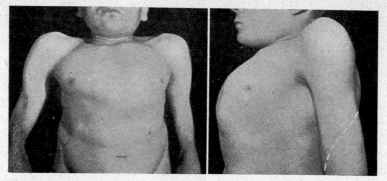

Fig. 65.   Fig. 66.

Fig. 65.—Chest deformity in Pott's disease (antero-posterior view). The shape of the chest and the position of full inspiration give the chest a superficial resemblance to that in emphysema. The neck appears very short and the head sunken into the chest, which bulges unduly.

Fig. 66.—Chest deformity in Pott's disease. The anterior bulge of the chest is particularly noticeable in this view. Note the sharp slope back from the angle of Louis to the neck. The kyphosis is marked by the broken line.

Anatomical Landmarks (*Figs.* 67, 68).—It will be convenient before leaving the examination of the chest by inspection to recall a few important facts in thoracic anatomy.

The *angle of Louis* is formed by the junction of the manubrium with

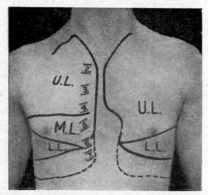
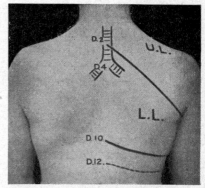

Fig. 67.   Fig. 68.

Fig. 67.—Anatomical landmarks of the lungs and pleuræ as seen from the front. The lobes of the lungs are marked out by plain black lines. The lower limit of the pleura is marked by the dotted line. The numbers between lines indicate the position of the ribs. U.L., Upper lobe ; M.L., Middle lobe ; L.L., Lower lobe.

Fig. 68.—Anatomical landmarks of the lungs and pleuræ as seen from the back. The right side only is marked. The plain lines indicate the upper and lower boundaries of the lower lobe of the lung. The dotted line indicates the lower limit of the pleura. The trachea and its bifurcation, and the positions of the spines of the second, fourth, tenth, and twelfth dorsal vertebræ are shown. U.L., Upper lobe ; L.L., Lower lobe.

the body of the sternum, and corresponds with the attachment of the second costal cartilage to the sternum. It is a convenient bony point from which to count the ribs and intercostal spaces. It serves as a guide to the position of the thoracic viscera by marking the level of the bifurcation of the trachea, the meeting of the lung borders, and the upper limit of the auricles.

Posteriorly, the *scapulæ* cover a large area of the chest which is relatively inaccessible to examination. The spine of the scapula is usually at the level of the second dorsal vertebra, its angle reaching to the seventh vertebra. The roots of the lungs lie in the interscapular region at the level of the spines of the fourth, fifth, and sixth dorsal vertebræ.

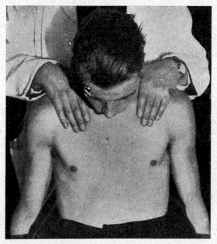

Fig. 69.—Palpation of the apices. The observer's hands should be placed in identical positions on the two sides. The patient's head should be well dropped on the chest so that the observer can see expansion of both apices at the same time. The patient is in the position of choice.

The *lobes of the lungs* may be marked out by drawing a line from the spine of the second dorsal vertebra to the junction of the sixth costal cartilage with the sternum. The line crosses the fifth rib in the axilla. Below it on each side lies the lower lobe, above it the upper lobe, and on the right side the small middle lobe. The upper margin of the last may be defined by taking a line from the junction of the fourth costal cartilage with the sternum to the centre of the previous line, which it meets in the axilla. It will be recognized at once that *the upper lobes and middle lobe are principally accessible from the front, and the lower lobes almost entirely from the back. In the axillæ parts of all lobes are open to examination.*

The apices of the upper lobes rise about one inch above the clavicles. From this point the inner margins of the lungs and their covering pleuræ slant towards the sternum, meeting each other in the mid-line at the angle of Louis. On the right side this margin of the lung continues down the sternum as far as the sixth costal cartilage, where it turns outwards and downwards to meet the mid-axillary line about the eighth rib, the scapular line at the tenth rib, and the para-vertebral line at the spine of the tenth dorsal vertebra. On the left side the landmarks are the same, with the exception that the lung border turns away from the sternum at the fourth instead of the sixth costal cartilage, owing to the position of the heart, which lies closely in contact with the chest wall over this region. At the apices, and along the inner margins of the lungs, the pleura lies so close to the lungs as to follow the same surface markings, but *at the lower borders of the lungs the pleura extends farther*, lying an inch and a half to two inches below the lung borders anteriorly and posteriorly, and as much as three and a half to four inches below in the axillæ. This potential pleural space may be filled up with lung substance during deep inspiration.

PALPATION*

For successful palpation the hands must be warm and used as gently as possible. They should be placed over the two apices, and by looking over the patient's shoulders, with his chin dropped on the chest, the movement of the upper lobes can be compared (*Fig.* 69) ; when the patient

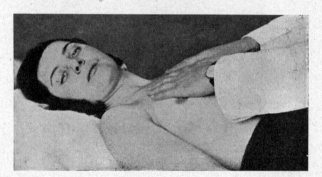

Fig. 70.—Palpation of the apices. The position of the hands used when the patient is unable to sit up.

cannot sit up, the apices are palpated as shown in *Fig.* 70. The lower lobes may similarly be examined by placing the hands round the costal margins, in the lower parts of the axillæ, or over the bases of the lungs at the back (*Figs.* 71, 72).

An examination of the vocal fremitus may then be made at the same areas.

The *position of the apex beat and of the trachea* should be confirmed by palpation. To determine the position of the trachea, the finger should be inserted above the jugular notch. The finger will slip to one side if the trachea is deviated.

The axillæ and supraclavicular fossæ should be examined for glands which may be the only evidence of malignancy. Palpation also detects

---

* L. *palpare*, to touch gently.

subcutaneous emphysema, which has a characteristic spongy feeling. Air in the subcutaneous tissues is not uncommon in artificial pneumothorax or after exploration of the chest. If it is overlooked and the area auscultated, crepitations may be wrongly diagnosed.

Vocal Fremitus.—This special sign consists in detecting vibrations transmitted to the hand from the larynx through the bronchi, lungs, and chest wall. The patient is asked to say ' ninety-nine ', or ' one, one, one ', and the *same hand* is placed on the chest in identical places on the two sides

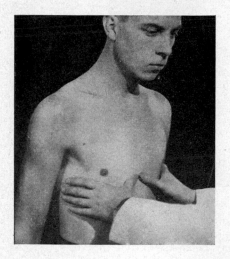

Fig. 71.—Palpation of the bases in front. The thumbs are placed in apposition in the mid-line and the fingers spread over the lower ribs in both axillæ. The patient breathes first quietly, then deeply, and the expansion is compared.

Fig. 72.—Palpation of the bases behind. The thumbs meet at the vertebral spines and the fingers extend towards the axillæ.

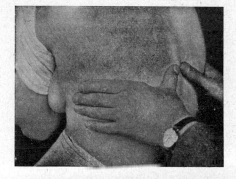

in turn. The flat of the hand may be used, or for more accurate localization the ulnar border of the hand (*Fig.* 73). The intensity of vibration felt will depend on the portion of the chest examined, and the character of the media through which the vibrations are transmitted. Certain physiological differences occur. The higher-pitched voices of women and children do not produce vibrations so easily felt as those from the lower tones of the male voice. Over those areas of the chest, such as the interscapular region and second right costal cartilage, *where the trachea and bronchi come nearer the surface, fremitus is more intense,* and due allowance must be made for this before changes in vocal fremitus are considered pathological. An unusually thick chest wall from fat or muscle will tend to diminish vocal fremitus.

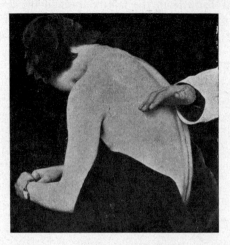

Fig. 73.—Vocal fremitus. For accurate comparison of the vocal fremitus in different parts of the chest the ulnar border of the hand should be used. Compare ribs with ribs, and intercostal spaces with intercostal spaces.

Pathologically, vocal fremitus may be *diminished* if the voice is feeble as in debilitating illnesses, or when interference to the passage of the vibrations occurs from blockage of the bronchi (foreign bodies, spasm in asthma, compression of new growths), or in conditions such as pleural effusion or pneumothorax which damp down the vibrations of the chest wall and lead to alteration in diffusion or reflection of the vibrations. *Diminished or lost vocal fremitus is one of the most constant signs of pleural effusion.*

Increase in vocal fremitus occurs when the vibrations are better conducted, as through solid lung (pneumonia, new growth), or collapsed lung in intimate contact with the trachea or bronchi.

PERCUSSION*

General Considerations.—Percussion consists in setting up artificial vibrations in a tissue by means of a sharp tap, usually with the fingers. The second finger of the left hand (pleximeter finger) is placed in close contact with the tissues, in this case the chest wall. A blow is then made on the second phalanx of this finger with the second finger of the right hand (plexor finger). The plexor finger must be kept at right angles to

---

* L. *percutere,* to strike.

the pleximeter finger as it falls, and the blow must be made by movements of the wrist only ; no movement of the shoulder is necessary (*Figs. 74–76*). *If the organ or tissue to be percussed lies superficially, percussion*

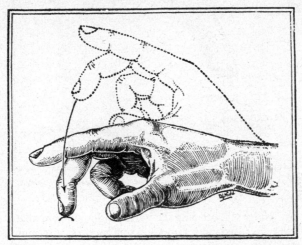

Fig. 74.—Correct method of percussion. Note : (1) Movement at the wrist ; (2) The vertical position of the terminal phalanx of the percussion finger as it strikes the pleximeter.

should be light, but if it lies deep or should it be desired to set into vibration a large mass of tissue such as the base of one lung, heavy percussion must be employed. Percussion on the clavicles (*Fig.* 77) is a useful method of

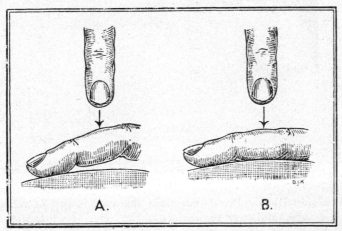

Fig. 75.—Errors in percussion. A, Incorrect—the pleximeter finger is not making close contact with the tissue to be percussed ; B, Correct position for pleximeter finger.

determining changes in the character of the lung substances at the apices. Heavy percussion may be accomplished by using two plexor fingers instead

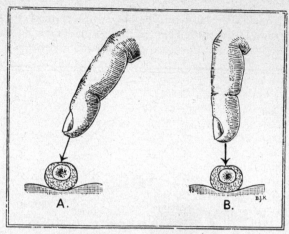

Fig. 76.—Errors in percussion. A, Incorrect—the plexor finger is not vertical as it strikes the pleximeter ; B, Correct method.

of one, or by using several fingers without any intermediate pleximeter finger (*Fig.* 78). Artificial pleximeters and plexors, although occasionally useful, produce notes of their own, and cannot be applied closely to the surface ; they are therefore much inferior to the fingers. Percussion needs constant careful practice before the student will find it a method yielding accurate and valuable information.

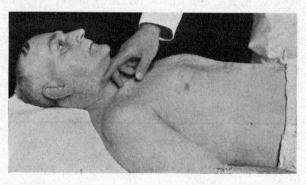

Fig. 77.—Percussion on the clavicle. Sometimes changes in the character of the lung tissue at one apex, e.g., consolidation, produce a change of note on percussion over the corresponding clavicle.

Percussion Data.—Percussion needs skill, and is only of value when the lesion is large, and near the surface of the lungs. Its limitations must be appreciated. In general terms it may be 'stated that *air-containing organs yield the note called resonance*, or some modification of this. True resonance is found only over lung tissue, in which the air is contained in millions of small pockets. Excessive resonance (hyper-resonance) is found when the air spaces in the lungs contain more air than normal, as in emphysema, whilst *tympany, an extreme form of hyper-resonance,* is met with over viscera containing gas without loculation, e.g., the stomach and intestines.

At the opposite extreme there comes the characteristic *lack of note* called *dullness.* This is found normally over solid viscera such as the liver and heart, and is due to vibrations of such frequency and high pitch that they are scarcely detectable by the human ear. An *extreme form of dullness,* often called *flatness,* is found by percussion over the thigh. Between the two extremes of tympany and flatness there exist innumerable shades of percussion note.

Modifications of the Percussion Note in Disease.—The percussion note is frequently altered by change in the structure of the underlying tissues. Thus *tympany is found when air fills the pleural sac* (pneumothorax), or is contained unloculated in a large lung cavity. A form of

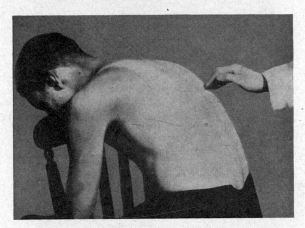

Fig. 78.—Heavy percussion. The fingers are used without an intermediate pleximeter.

tympany may also be found over the relaxed lung above a pleural effusion and is called Skodaic resonance. *Dullness may be found when the normal air-containing lung tissue becomes solidified,* as in pneumonia, new growth, fibrosis, tuberculous consolidation, etc. ; whilst *absolute dullness or flatness is present over pleural effusions* or occasionally over solid lung if the bronchi are blocked, and rarely over a pneumothorax in which the tension of air is so great as to limit the vibrations of the chest wall normally set up by percussion.

When flatness is found it is accompanied by an increased sense of resistance to the fingers due to loss of resilience in the tissues. This is particularly noticeable over pleural effusions, and to skilled fingers is valuable in distinguishing this condition from pneumonia.

Two special types of percussion may be mentioned briefly :—

Cracked-pot Sound.—This is a characteristic note described by its name. It is most commonly heard over phthisical cavities which communicate with a bronchus through a narrow opening, and is said to be caused by the expulsion of air through this opening. *It is best elicited by percussing fairly heavily with two fingers towards the end of expiration.* It is usually magnified by instructing the patient to keep his mouth open, the examiner's ear being close to the mouth. The elicitation of this sign is not free from risk, as a hæmoptysis may be induced.

Coin Test.—A peculiar metallic note is produced in cases of pneumothorax when percussion is made using coins as the plexor and pleximeter. The stethoscope should be held at a distance from the coins at identical places on the two sides of the chest in turn (*Fig.* 79).

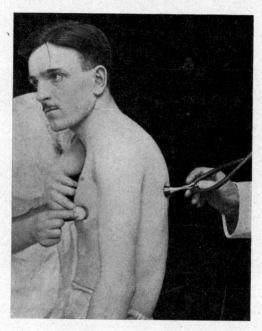

Fig. 79.—The coin test. Two coins are used as plexor and pleximeter respectively. The stethoscope is applied to the chest at a distance from the area percussed.

AUSCULTATION*

The Stethoscope.—Direct auscultation by applying the ear to the chest wall is rarely used now. Since the discovery by Laennec in Napoleon's time that the breath- and heart-sounds could be heard more clearly and comfortably through a roll of parchment, various types of stethoscope have made their appearance. The monaural stethoscope is still used by certain physicians, but with some doubtful exceptions is inferior to the binaural instrument. In choosing a stethoscope the student is advised to select one with a *bell-shaped chest-piece* which does not distort the sounds in any

---

* L. *auscultare,* to listen.

way. The rubber tubing should be thick to avoid kinking, and about 18 in. in length. Particular attention should be paid to the ear-pieces, which should fit comfortably into the external auditory meatus. If they are too large they cause discomfort, and the examiner may be conscious of arterial pulsation from his own body ; if they are too loose, extrinsic sounds will lead to confusion.

Practical Points in Auscultation.—Quietness is essential for good auscultation, and some experience is necessary in learning to disregard noises which come through the stethoscope but which are not the direct result of respiration or cardiac contraction. Hair on the chest produces crackling noises which may be mistaken for adventitious sounds, but can be removed by wetting the hair or plastering it down with soap. Unless all clothes are removed from the chest, sounds will inevitably be heard from their friction against the chest wall, and care should be taken to see that blankets put around the shoulders are not allowed to move. If the patient is nervous or cold, shivering will produce sounds similar to those heard over a contracting muscle, so that the patient should be reassured and kept quite warm before auscultation. The bell of the stethoscope should be placed firmly on the skin to prevent sounds resulting from its movement, but note should be made of any modification of breath- or heart-sounds occurring with varying pressure. Lastly, the student must learn to disregard the heart-sounds while auscultating the lungs, and the breath-sounds whilst listening to the heart. It cannot be too strongly impressed on the student that he must familiarize himself with the normal, both as regards the breath- and heart-sounds, before he can recognize the abnormal.

As in other methods by which the chest is examined, *identical points on the two sides must be compared,* and should it be necessary to auscultate with the patient lying on his side the effect of posture must be taken into consideration. On the side on which the patient is lying the breath-sounds are relatively decreased. *As much information as possible should first be gained during quiet breathing, as deep breaths not infrequently modify the physical signs.* The examiner first determines the character of the breath-sounds over many different areas of the chest, but particularly beneath the clavicles and in the supraspinous fossa to examine the upper lobes, and over the lower ribs (7th to 10th) at the back for auscultation of the lower lobes. It is most essential to be systematic in listening at many areas, so as to avoid overlooking small areas of consolidation or cavitation. *In very sick persons the axilla provides easy though limited access to all lobes.* When the character of the breath-sounds has been compared at these areas, attention may be paid to any adventitious sounds.

Auscultation must be carried out with definite objects in mind : (1) To determine if the breath-sounds are equal on the two sides ; (2) To ascertain the character of the breath-sounds ; (3) To detect any added sounds and decide their nature, and whether they are intra- or extra-pulmonary ; (4) To compare the voice-sounds over different parts of the lungs.

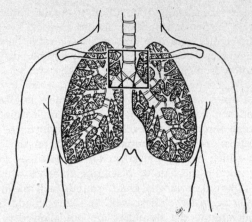

Fig. 80.—Breath-sounds in normal lung, anterior aspect. The square marks the area of broncho-vesicular breathing. Over other areas normal vesicular breath-sounds are heard.

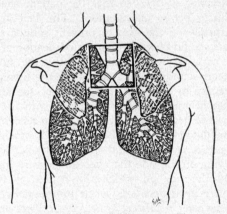

Fig. 81.—Breath-sounds in normal lung, posterior aspect. The square marks the area of broncho-vesicular breathing. Over other areas normal vesicular breath-sounds are heard.

Breath-sounds.—The breath-sounds are composed of two elements : (1) The vesicular element, a soft, rustling sound caused by the passage of air into millions of alveoli ; (2) The laryngeal element, a loud harsh sound, due to the vibrations of the vocal cords and neighbouring structures in the nasopharynx and trachea. The laryngeal element is frequently described as the bronchial element, as by passage of the sound waves into the bronchi it rapidly becomes less intense.

Under normal circumstances the *breathing over most areas of the chest is vesicular*, and sometimes so *faint* as scarcely to be heard except during deep respiration. The inspiratory sound is always longer than the expiratory ; indeed, the latter is frequently inaudible. In the interscapular region, and over the second right costal cartilage, *where the trachea and bronchi come near to the surface, the vesicular element is modified by the bronchial element*

(*Figs.* 80, 81). This *broncho-vesicular* breathing is harsh in character, has a short pause between inspiration and expiration, and a prolonged expiration ; the areas where it occurs must be remembered, lest they be mistaken for patches of consolidation.

In children the breath-sounds are normally harsher than in adults—*puerile breathing*—and a similar type of breathing may be produced by exercise. An interrupted type known as *cog-wheel breathing* may occur in normal people, but is more frequently found in early phthisis. The interruptions are often synchronous with the heart-beats.

Diminution or absence of breath-sounds may merely be due to defective transmission of these through the chest wall to the stethoscope, as in cases of obesity and great muscular development. It also occurs in feeble or

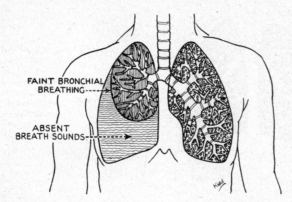

FAINT BRONCHIAL BREATHING----->

ABSENT BREATH SOUNDS----->

Fig. 82.—Breath-sounds in pleural effusion. Lung compressed, therefore relatively solid. Bronchi narrowed by compression. (*See also Fig.* 88 for other signs of pulmonary collapse.)

dying patients in whom the actual production of the sounds is diminished by the decreased movement of the tidal air. In all these cases the decrease involves every part of the chest.

More important and significant is the diminution or loss of breath-sounds which is present only in one lung or one portion of the lung (*Fig.* 82). This may result from the varied causes which obstruct a main bronchus or one of its branches.

PATHOLOGICAL BREATH-SOUNDS : BRONCHIAL BREATHING.—Apart from diminution or exaggeration of the breath-sounds, abnormalities are generally due to a predominance of the laryngeal over the vesicular element. *In effect they are all varieties of bronchial breathing,* and receive the names of bronchial, tubular, amphoric, and cavernous breathing according to variations in their quality.

Bronchial breathing has already been mentioned in dealing with the laryngeal element of the breath-sounds, of which it is but a fainter edition. Its characteristics are its *clear harshness, the equality in length of inspiration and expiration,* and the *pause* between these. A type of breathing closely resembling it may be heard over the occiput when the patient breathes through the nose. Bronchial breathing is caused by the *suppression of the vesicular murmur* and the *better conduction of the laryngeal element*, and therefore occurs when the alveoli are put out of action by such diseases as pneumonia, new growths, or tuberculous caseation. The solidification of the lungs by these diseases also renders them better conductors of sound.

Tubular breathing, regarded by some as synonymous with bronchial breathing, is usually somewhat higher pitched. It is the usual variety of breath-sound over pneumonic consolidation (*Fig.* 83).

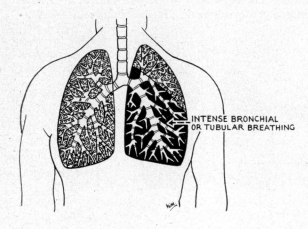

INTENSE BRONCHIAL OR TUBULAR BREATHING

Fig. 83.—Breath-sounds in solid lung, such as occurs in pneumonia or neoplasm. Lung alveoli airless, bronchi patent, breath-sounds bronchial or tubular. Lower lobe only shown as affected.

Amphoric breathing is a still more intense and high-pitched form of bronchial breathing, with a metallic quality, best imitated by blowing over the narrow neck of a bottle. It is heard over cavities, and occasionally over a closed pneumothorax. In these conditions the alveoli are collapsed or destroyed but the laryngeal sounds are well conducted through the resonating cavity (*Fig.* 84).

Fig. 84.—Breath-sounds in pneumothorax. Amphoric breath-sounds. Lung collapsed. Bronchi partially obliterated. Communication at arrows between lung and pleural sac. (For other effects of pneumothorax, such as mediastinal displacement, *see Fig.* 88.)

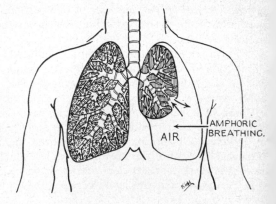

AIR

AMPHORIC BREATHING.

Cavernous breathing is a low-toned form of bronchial breathing typically heard over cavities or an open pneumothorax (*Fig.* 85). It may be imitated by breathing into a tumbler. It is produced in a similar fashion to amphoric breath-sounds.

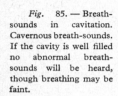

Fig. 85. — Breath-sounds in cavitation. Cavernous breath-sounds. If the cavity is well filled no abnormal breath-sounds will be heard, though breathing may be faint.

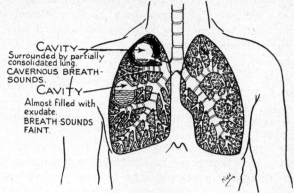

CAVITY—
Surrounded by partially consolidated lung.
CAVERNOUS BREATH-SOUNDS.
CAVITY—
Almost filled with exudate.
BREATH SOUNDS FAINT.

Vocal Resonance.—Just as the laryngeal and other sympathetic vibrations are palpable on the chest wall as vocal fremitus, so they are audible through the stethoscope as vocal resonance, though high-pitched sounds are appreciated by the stethoscope, whereas only low-pitched ones are able to cause palpable vibrations. In those areas where the trachea or bronchi come nearest the surface—the interscapular region and the right apex—the resonance is loudest, just as in the case of vocal fremitus. Similarly vocal resonance is fainter in women than in men, because the thorax is not so favourably adapted as a resonator of the laryngeal sounds as in men, and the voice-sounds are higher pitched.

Increased vocal resonance, or *bronchophony*, is heard over solid lung tissue, e.g., pneumonia and tuberculous consolidation, because the medium conducts sound better than the normal air-containing lung tissue. Bronchophony may occur over tuberculous and other forms of cavity which have resonating qualities. In cases of pulmonary tuberculosis it is said to occur over the spinous processes at a lower level than in health. This is known as *d'Espine's sign*. If the bronchophony is so intense that the actual syllables can be identified, the term *pectoriloquy* is used. This physical sign may be found under similar circumstances to bronchophony, and may be detected even with the whispered voice—*whispering pectoriloquy*—a sign of great value in the diagnosis of consolidation or cavitation as it can be elicited without the fatigue which loud speaking entails. A peculiar form of vocal resonance known as *ægophony* is sometimes heard over solid lung, but more frequently at *the upper limit of a pleural effusion*. It has a high-pitched nasal quality, and is likened to the bleating of a goat or lamb ; it is due to the interception of the low-pitched elements of the voice-sounds.

6

Adventitious Sounds.—Sounds which are not an essential part of the respiratory murmur are known as adventitious sounds, *and frequently accompany abnormal types of breath-sound.*

With few exceptions they are produced by the passage of the air current through a narrowed or partially blocked respiratory tract.

Confusion has been caused by the different terminology employed in various schools. The classification adopted here is that used in many English teaching centres.

CONTINUOUS	INTERRUPTED
Stridor	Râles
Rhonchus	Crepitations
Pleural friction	

The alternative names used by some authorities are given below in brackets.

CONTINUOUS SOUNDS.—

Stridor.—A noisy type of breathing generally found when the larger air-passages—trachea and main bronchi—are obstructed, e.g., by a foreign body, diphtheritic membrane, or tumour. It may be heard without a stethoscope and even at a distance.

A fainter type of stridor may be heard as the wheezing of asthmatic subjects, in whom the smaller bronchi are obstructed.

Rhonchus (dry râle ; sibilus).—A musical sound caused by passage of the air current through bronchi obstructed by exudate or congested mucous membrane. Rhonchi may have a deep-toned note, *sonorous rhonchi*, when produced in the large bronchi, or a high-pitched squeak, *sibilant rhonchi*, when arising in the smallest bronchi. All degrees of sounds may occur between these two extremes, but for convenience rhonchi are often classified as sonorous, medium, and sibilant.

They are present most often in bronchitis where the bronchial mucous membrane is congested and the lumen partially obstructed by viscid muco-pus.

Pleural Friction (pleural crepitus).—A grating or creaking sound is produced when the roughened, inflamed surfaces of the pleura ride over one another during respiration. This sound is called pleural friction or pleural rub. It is heard where areas of pleurisy are most frequent, namely in the *axilla* and *beneath the nipples.* The examiner should never neglect to auscultate over a wide area including the *area of the pain*, otherwise a pleural rub may remain undiscovered. The sound is generally continuous, but may be interrupted, especially as it is disappearing, when the remnants may even resemble râles or crepitations.

The intensity of a pleural rub is often increased by firm pressure of the stethoscope, and the sound has a curious *superficial quality.*

INTERRUPTED SOUNDS.—

Râles.—These sounds vary considerably in quality, but originate in the *bubbling of the respired air through a fluid medium* such as mucus, muco-pus, or other exudate present in the bronchi or alveoli. Their character is *modified by the condition of the surrounding lung, and their depth from the surface.* Râles may be subdivided as follows : (1) Bubbling râles, which are coarse, low-toned, and ' moist ', especially when produced in the larger bronchi, but may have a somewhat crackling quality if they emanate from the smaller bronchi. They are commonly found in bronchitis affecting the larger tubes, and over cavities. (2) Crackling râles (subcrepitant râles, coarse crepitations) have a drier quality and are heard over congested or œdematous lung tissue, e.g., in congestive heart failure, and in bronchitis affecting the smaller tubes. It is probable that they can be produced both in the bronchi and alveoli.

Crepitations (crepitant râles).—These arise in a similar manner to râles, by the passage of air through exudate in the alveoli or bronchioles, though in this instance the exudate has led to partial collapse of these structures and the crepitations are produced as the air enters and separates the adherent walls. Their quality is modified by changes in the lung tissue such as congestion or consolidation, which impart a sharper ' metallic ' element not possessed by râles as defined above, though the coarser varieties closely resemble crackling râles. They have a high pitch, and may be imitated by rolling hairs between the fingers. *Their presence generally denotes actual involvement of the lung substance* by consolidative processes such as those of pneumonia, tuberculosis, or pulmonary collapse. *They are nearly always heard during inspiration.* As a *temporary* phenomenon they may appear when some of the alveoli have collapsed (marginal crepitations or râles), e.g., in bed-ridden patients, old persons, and shallow breathers.

It is very important, therefore, that distinction should be made between crepitations which persist and those which disappear after a few deep breaths. The effect of deep breathing and coughing on adventitious sounds should always be observed, for if the sounds are abolished by these acts, the structural changes in the lung or bronchi are probably less than when they remain. To illustrate this it is only necessary to note the disappearance of noisy sonorous rhonchi in cases of bronchitis after vigorous coughing, whilst the sibilant rhonchi present when the smaller tubes are affected do not vanish so readily.

Conversely, in definite structural disease of the lung, adventitious sounds, e.g., crepitations in early phthisis, may be brought out by coughing.

SPECIAL INVESTIGATIONS

When a provisional diagnosis has been made based on the symptoms and physical signs described, special methods of examination may give fuller information, and may occasionally establish a diagnosis which is not possible on ordinary clinical grounds.

The more important accessory methods of examination are : radiological examination ; examination of the sputum ; laryngoscopy ; bronchoscopy ; examination of the nasal sinuses ; paracentesis. (*See* Chapters XII—XIV.)

THE DIAGNOSIS OF RESPIRATORY DISEASES

The symptoms and signs which have been described, when pieced together in a certain way, form a composite picture of some pathological change in the respiratory tissues, and the student's object in eliciting the signs should be to form such a picture in his mind. This is not always easy, for the different ways in which the signs may be combined are numerous, owing to the extreme variability in the grade and type of pathological change. For convenience in describing their signs the common diseases of the respiratory organs may be grouped under the following headings—those affecting (1) the bronchi, (2) the lungs, (3) the pleura.

1. THE BRONCHI

Diseases of the bronchi yield more abnormal signs by auscultation than by other methods of examination unless the lung is secondarily involved.

Bronchial Obstruction.—The bronchi may be narrowed or occluded in any part of their course by exudate, foreign bodies, or growth within the lumen, or by pressure from without by tumours or conditions causing collapse of the lungs. The best examples are seen in blockage of the lumen by neoplasm (carcinoma) and blockage by pressure from without by pleural effusion and pulmonary collapse.

In all forms of bronchial obstruction the breath-sounds will be diminished over the area of lung to which the affected bronchus is distributed, and in cases of complete obstruction to a main bronchus no breath-sounds will be heard. The diminished air entry leads to complete or partial collapse of the lung, with corresponding lack of movement on the affected side (*see also* COLLAPSE, p. 88).

If the obstruction is partial, the breathing may also be altered in character—e.g., stridor in partial obstruction of the trachea or a main bronchus, and *wheezing respiration in asthma* in which the small bronchi and bronchioles are in a state of spasm.

Bronchitis.—In bronchitis the mucous membrane is at first congested, and later there is an exudate of mucus or muco-pus. Both factors narrow the lumen of the bronchi, causing at the beginning of the attack the dry sounds described as rhonchi, to be followed shortly by râles due to the bubbling of the air through the exudate of muco-pus. The combination of râles and rhonchi ('bubble and squeak') without evidence of involvement of the lung is characteristic of bronchitis. Further, the signs are bilateral. The patient's principal symptom is cough. Fever is also present in acute cases.

Bronchiectasis.—In bronchiectasis the bronchi are dilated either diffusely or by local bulging of parts of the bronchial wall. The bronchi involved are generally in the lower lobes, where the signs should be specially sought.

The extra capacity of the bronchi leads to accumulation of secretions, which become infected, especially when pressure on the bronchi from without favours retention. The secretions are coughed up periodically as a characteristic offensive sputum. In classical cases, on standing it separates into three layers : (1) on top, brownish froth, then (2) fluid consisting of mucus and muco-pus, and (3) at the bottom a greyish-black semi-solid deposit containing pus and crystals. This type of sputum is present in only a small percentage of cases, but the *large amount and offensive smell* of the sputum are fairly constant features.

The weakening of the walls of a dilated bronchus by infection which also spreads into the surrounding lung frequently leads to the formation of a *cavity*, and for signs of this search should be made carefully, especially at the bases of the lungs (*see* CAVITATION, p. 87).

The examiner should also look for *clubbing of the fingers* in every suspected case of bronchiectasis.

Diagnosis of this condition is frequently difficult on clinical grounds, but has been made easier since the use of lipiodol, which can be injected through the trachea, and outlines the bronchial tree, showing up on X-ray examination any abnormal dilatation (*see* Chapter XIII, RADIOLOGY).

Asthma.—The characteristics of *bronchial asthma* are attacks of respiratory distress due to bronchial spasm, in which laboured wheezing respiration occurs. This is most noticeable in auscultation. The attacks are nearly always nocturnal at first, but later may be continuous, with exacerbations.

It has been said that " all is not asthma that wheezes ", to emphasize that bronchial obstruction may be due to many causes other than allergic spasm. Paroxysmal dyspnœa of an asthmatic type is common in left ventricular failure (p. 96). Localized wheezing respiration (determined by auscultation) may occur in bronchial obstruction due to neoplasm or foreign body.

True bronchial asthma usually *starts* in childhood or youth. Other causes of asthmatic breathing are commoner in older persons. Bronchial asthma is generally associated after some years with emphysema and bronchitis.

2. THE LUNGS

The more important pathological changes which may take place in the lungs are congestion, œdema, consolidation, cavitation, collapse, and fibrosis. These changes are found in various combinations in different lung diseases.

Congestion.—

Acute Congestion.—The lung may be acutely congested at the onset of pneumonia or from irritant gases, but the structural changes are so slight that physical signs are usually equivocal. The diminution in calibre of the bronchi and the encroachment on alveolar space may cause fainter breath-sounds and impairment of percussion note. Exudate may lead to the production of râles or crepitations. Constitutional signs, especially fever, may be present.

Chronic Congestion.—Chronic congestion (hypostasis, hypostatic pneumonia) as a part of congestive heart failure is more easily recognized than acute. Cough and dyspnœa are the usual symptoms. Hæmoptysis may occur. The lung, although not consolidated, contains less air than normal. This leads to *impairment of percussion note.* The breath-sounds are diminished. The œdema which accompanies the congestion acts as an exudate in the bronchi and alveoli and causes *râles,* usually crackling in character, and sometimes crepitations.

Œdema.—Like congestion, œdema may occur in an acute or a chonic form.

Acute Œdema.—Consists of sudden flooding of the bronchi and alveoli with serous fluid. The exact causes of the condition are uncertain, but it may occur in certain types of myocardial disease, and high blood-pressure.

The lungs are rendered relatively airless, and *intense dyspnœa* occurs, with expectoration of *copious frothy sputum.* Limited movement and impairment of percussion note may result, but the principal physical sign is the abundance of *fine moist râles.*

Chronic Œdema.—Occurs in cardiac failure as a part of chronic congestion, and the signs are similar, though more profuse expectoration may occur.

Consolidation.—If the alveoli are filled with solid material, or destroyed and replaced by this, the signs are characteristic, and depend partly on the lack of function in the affected portion of the lung, and partly on its property of conducting sound better than the normal air-containing tissue.

Inspection shows decreased movement. The entering air cannot expand the already filled or obliterated alveoli.

Palpation confirms this deficient movement and reveals an increase in vocal fremitus. The laryngeal vibrations are transmitted better through solid lung.

Percussion gives a dull note, as over solid viscera, but not quite so flat, as air is still present in the bronchi and in unaffected portions of the lung.

Auscultation generally demonstrates bronchial or tubular breathing—the vesicular murmur is suppressed, and the laryngeal element well conducted through the solidified lung, which has similar acoustic properties to the bronchi and chest wall, so that the sounds are not interrupted in their passage as in normal lung. Adventitious sounds may or may not be present according to the amount and character of the exudate in the bronchi and alveoli. Râles, if present, usually have a sharp crackling quality. Crepitations may also occur. The conduction of sound is better through the solid medium, and vocal resonance is correspondingly increased.

To sum up, the signs of consolidation are *diminished movement, increased vocal fremitus, increased vocal resonance, dullness* on percussion, and some form of *bronchial breathing (Fig.* 86). If the bronchus leading to the consolidated area is not obstructed, *these signs are present whatever the cause of the consolidation,* but if the bronchus is blocked, e.g., by exudate within or the pressure of a tumour without, the signs may resemble those of a pleural effusion, with the exception that there is no displacement of the mediastinum, and the heart remains in its normal position. Blockage of the bronchus also

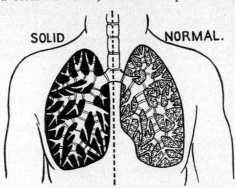

Fig. 86.—Pulmonary consolidation. Lung solid, bronchi patent. No mediastinal displacement. Signs : limited movement ; increased vocal fremitus and vocal resonance ; percussion note dull ; bronchial or tubular breathing.

results in absorption of any remaining air in the alveoli, and the signs of pulmonary collapse may be added to the picture.

The commonest causes of consolidation in the lung are : (1) Pneumonia, an inflammation involving the lung parenchyma in which the alveoli are filled by an exudate of blood elements ; (2) Tuberculosis, causing destructive changes (caseation) rendering portions of the lung solid ; (3) New growth, in which portions of the lung are replaced by the solid neoplasm ; (4) Pulmonary infarction—a hæmorrhagic infiltration of a portion of a lung due to blockage of a pulmonary vessel.

Cf. also PULMONARY COLLAPSE, p. 88.

Cavitation.—The signs of a cavity in the lung vary with its size and proximity to the surface, whether or not it communicates with a bronchus, the character of the surrounding lung, and the fullness or emptiness of the cavity.

Frequently, owing to small size or considerable depth from the surface, or the abnormal signs produced in the neighbouring lung, the characteristic signs of cavitation are obscured, but solid lung surrounding a small cavity will amplify the signs. When present the *most pathognomonic are those found on auscultation,* dependent on the resonating qualities of the cavity. The *breath-sounds* are *amphoric* or *cavernous,* but not infrequently fainter than normal. Adventitious sounds, usually *rales with a metallic quality,* are common owing to the fluid contents. They are more often found in an active than a quiescent lesion. *Bronchophony and whispering pectoriloquy* are important but not characteristic, as they occur over consolidated lung.

A special sign called *post-tussive suction* is said to be pathognomonic

After the patient has given a cough, the air can be heard to re-enter the cavity with a hissing noise.

The non-auscultatory signs of cavitation are frequently bound up with those of the disease causing the cavity.

Inspection often shows flattening if the cavity is at an apex, and diminished movement owing to the surrounding fibrosis.

Percussion elicits a dull note in most cases owing to the retracted lung tissue, and the fact that the cavity generally contains fluid. Rarely tympany may be found over a large empty cavity near the surface.

The cracked-pot note may be demonstrated in some cases.

Cavities in the lung may be caused by bronchiectasis, as already explained, and are usually located in the lower lobes. Because of their greater depth from the surface and the bulk of lung overlying them, the signs are often difficult to elicit.

Phthisis is the commonest cause of a cavity. This is generally found in the upper lobe, and is therefore easier to diagnose than a bronchiectatic cavity. It must be mentioned that the cavities of phthisis and bronchiectasis are not always found in their classical position ; those of tuberculosis may be at the base and those of bronchietasis at the apex.

Rarely cavitation results from abscess formation, gangrene, the breakdown of new growths, etc.

Collapse.—Pulmonary collapse or atelectasis may occur as a congenital abnormality, but will be discussed here only in its acquired form.

It results from many causes, which act either by preventing the air from entering the lungs normally (e.g., bronchial obstruction, feeble respiratory movements), or by squeezing the air out of the alveoli by external pressure as in pneumothorax or pleural effusion. Under these circumstances, whatever air may be left in the lungs will be absorbed.

A special form—massive collapse—occurs suddenly—after operations, in trauma to the chest, and other conditions—and involves the whole of one lung, or a whole lobe.

The *symptoms* vary in intensity according to the rapidity with which the collapse occurs. *Breathlessness* is the principal symptom owing to diminished oxygenation, and in cases of sudden collapse of the lung, e.g., in pneumothorax and massive collapse, is extreme. In the usual gradual collapse from pleural effusion or partial bronchial obstruction, dyspnœa may be hardly noticeable except on effort.

The *signs* of collapse vary with the cause of the condition, and are frequently obscured by this, as in the case of pleural effusion or pneumothorax.

They are characteristically found in massive collapse. The chest wall accommodates itself to the lung and is *retracted*. The *heart is displaced to the affected side, a most valuable sign*, but not pathognomonic, as it occurs also in pulmonary fibrosis. The retraction and the denser character of the collapsed lung cause *dullness* on percussion. The limited air-entry results in *faint breath-sounds*. These are often *bronchial*, and other signs of consolidation may be present as the collapsed lung is virtually consolidated. There is usually an increase in the respiratory or pulse-rate and a rise in temperature.

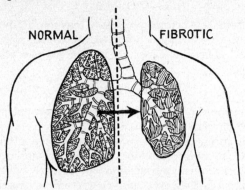

NORMAL | FIBROTIC

Fig. 87.—Pulmonary fibrosis. The shoulder is lower and the chest wall retracted on the affected side. The lung is shrunken and the bronchi compressed. The signs are therefore : limited movement ; diminished vocal fremitus and vocal resonance (variable) ; percussion note impaired ; breath-sounds faint (sometimes bronchial) ; mediastinal contents (trachea, heart, etc.) displaced in direction of arrow.

The possibility of collapse should be considered in cases when doubtful physical signs of pleural effusion or consolidation are present, especially when the signs appear a day or two after operation or injury.

Fibrosis.—The eventual results of fibrosis of the lung are in some ways comparable with those of pulmonary collapse, for the lung becomes shrunken in volume, contains little air, and draws in the chest wall on the affected side and the mediastinum from the opposite side. The results are, however, produced in a much more gradual manner, and although the chief symptom is again *breathlessness*, it is rarely so urgent as in acute forms of pulmonary collapse. Cough and expectoration are also usual.

The *signs* of fibrosis (*Fig.* 87) depend on the shrinkage of the lung and its consequent drag on surrounding tissues, and on the diminished amount of air entering and contained in the lung. The *chest is retracted and smaller in volume* and the *heart and trachea are pulled towards the affected side.* The ribs are often closer together, and *expansion is limited* or absent.

The *percussion note is dull* because of the relatively airless state of the lung.

The *breath-sounds are faint* and may be bronchial as in the case of pulmonary collapse.

Adventitious sounds are not a distinctive feature, and when present are generally due to associated diseases of the lungs and bronchi, e.g., bronchitis, tuberculosis, or bronchiectasis.

Pulmonary fibrosis may be the result of almost any inflammatory or any irritant disease of the lung. The more important causes are :

tuberculosis (fibroid phthisis), industrial diseases associated with inhalation of irritant dust (silicosis, siderosis, etc.), lobar pneumonia, and broncho-pneumonia.

Two important and common diseases may be used to illustrate the way in which these pathological processes are found together in one and the same disease. These examples are pneumonia and phthisis.

Pneumonia

Lobar Pneumonia.—The symptoms in lobar pneumonia are often in advance of the physical signs.

The *onset* is abrupt with a rigor in adults or convulsions in childhood and a rapid rise of temperature to $104°-105°$. Pain in the chest, 'the side,' as the patient often calls it, also occurs early when the pleura is involved (*see* p. 57). Dyspnœa and cough are invariably present, and the sputum is frequently blood-stained—'rusty sputum'. The *constitutional signs* of a high fever are present, namely, rapid pulse, dry skin, furred tongue, constipation, and as the fever persists a varying degree of delirium. Cyanosis results from the diminished oxygen-carrying power of the lungs.

The *local signs* are at first those of acute congestion. Perhaps the most important are faintness in the breath-sounds and slight impairment of percussion note, but no certain diagnosis can be made at this stage. Within twenty-four to forty-eight hours, *signs of consolidation* usually appear and have already been described (p. 86). These signs persist not only during the febrile stage of the illness but for a few days or weeks after the constitutional signs have disappeared (unresolved pneumonia).

In this phase it is most important to watch carefully for any changes in the signs from those of consolidation to those of fluid.

In pneumonia of the upper lobes the only signs may be found high in the axilla, which always deserves special examination.

The fever and constitutional signs continue in most cases for a week, and the pyrexia then subsides by crisis.

Broncho-pneumonia.—This form of pneumonia is commoner in children and old persons, and is often secondary to some other condition, e.g., one of the exanthemata or anæsthesia.

Its onset and its termination are more gradual than those of lobar pneumonia. The fever subsides by lysis. Dyspnœa and cough occur, but pain is unusual, as the pleura frequently escapes. Cyanosis is often pronounced. Fever is of a slighter grade than in lobar pneumonia, but the toxæmia is often considerable and the pulse-rate unduly high. In many cases the condition is suggested by aggravation of the existing symptoms of respiratory infection—e.g., in whooping-cough or bronchitis.

The *physical signs* result from two pathological lesions, bronchitis and consolidation. These are diffusely scattered through the lungs, and the signs are accordingly widespread. Adventitious sounds are much more frequent than in lobar pneumonia owing to the bronchitis.

Crackling râles and coarse crepitations are common, probably produced partly in the bronchi and partly in the consolidated patches of lung.

If the area of solid lung is large the signs resemble closely those of lobar pneumonia.

Pulmonary Tuberculosis

(*Phthisis* ; *Consumption*)

This disease is undoubtedly the best illustration of the manner in which the pathological processes described—congestion, œdema, consolidation, cavitation, collapse, and fibrosis—may exist side by side in the same lung. Consolidation and cavitation are destructive processes ; fibrosis and to some extent pulmonary collapse are reparative, and the general condition of the patient and the constitutional signs will depend upon the balance between these opposing changes.

The *symptoms* of phthisis, like the physical signs, are protean. In the acute forms of the disease, pneumonic phthisis and tuberculous broncho-pneumonia, they are similar to those of pneumococcal infections of the lungs.

In the commonest type—chronic pulmonary tuberculosis—the onset is usually insidious. Cough is the most important local symptom, at first dry, later with expectoration of muco-pus, and, most significant when it occurs, of blood.

The other symptoms are of a constitutional type dependent on the toxæmia caused by the tubercle bacillus. They are, therefore, common to all forms of tuberculosis in the lungs and elsewhere.

Fever is usually present, with a characteristic evening rise and morning fall. The latter is often accompanied by profuse sweating in the early hours of the morning. Loss of weight, languor, anorexia, and anæmia are other notable symptoms, but by no means exhaust the manifold symptomatology of this disease. Symptoms may exist without physical signs, and the early diagnosis can often only be made by X rays.

The *signs* are found especially at the apices of the lungs, and the examination of the infraclavicular and the suprascapular regions should be most careful, but must systematically include all parts of the lungs.

In early cases the signs, when present, are usually those of bronchitis, pulmonary consolidation, or small areas of collapse. Later as the disease advances consolidation becomes more extensive, and signs of cavitation may be added.

When repair processes take the upper hand a common combination of physical signs is that of cavitation and fibrosis.

Valuable information is afforded by radiographs of the chest. (*See* Chapter XIII, RADIOLOGY.)

3. THE PLEURA

Dry Pleurisy.—This term is applied to inflammation of the pleura without the formation of fluid. It occurs as an almost invariable feature of lobar pneumonia, as a tuberculous infection, and frequently without obvious cause and without any clue to its aetiology.

The movements of the inflamed pleura give rise to *pain*, which is aggravated by breathing, coughing, sneezing, or other efforts leading to greater excursion of the inflamed layers. (*See also* PAIN, p. 57).

The only local physical *sign* is a *pleural rub*, which has already been described. Occasionally this friction may be perceptible to the hand.

Constitutional symptoms—especially fever and tachycardia—are usually present.

Pleural Effusion.—Fluid may collect between the layers of the pleura in amounts varying from a few ounces to several pints, as a result of transudation in heart failure and renal disease, or as a result of pleurisy, especially when caused by the tubercle bacillus. The fluid is generally a clear straw-coloured liquid ; purulent effusions are described under the separate term of *empyema*, a common complication of pneumonia. Effusion also occurs with neoplasm, and is blood-stained in some cases.

The *signs* of pleural effusion are similar whatever its origin, though the symptoms vary. They are due in part to the collapse of the lung, the degree of which is proportionate to the amount of the fluid, and in part to the special characteristics of fluid as a medium of conduction of laryngeal vibration. They may be conveniently considered in the usual order.

Inspection.—Although the lung is collapsed, the affected side of the chest has a *normal or greater volume*, as it is filled with fluid. *The heart is displaced to the opposite side.* In cases of left-sided effusion the cardiac impulse is usually found nearer the sternum, and in extreme cases may even be present to the right of the sternum. In right-sided effusion the apex-beat is displaced towards the left axilla, and the altered position of the heart is more easily recognised. *Movement of the affected side is limited or absent*, as little or no air is entering the lung.

Palpation.—The defective movement of the chest and the position of the apex-beat are confirmed. *Vocal fremitus is reduced or absent*, owing to the increased reflection and diffusion of the vibrations in their passage through the media of air-containing bronchi, relatively solid lung, and fluid. The fluid also damps down the vibrations of the chest wall.

Percussion.—The characteristic note is *flat*, accompanied by an *increased sense of resistance*, but all grades of note are found, and in small effusions the note is only dull and confined to the back, for the fluid pushes the lung upwards and forwards. The fluid level falls as it extends to the front of the chest, though it is often high in the axilla, giving the percussion line an S shape (Ellis's S-shaped line).

A triangular area of dullness may occur on the opposite side of the vertebral column to the effusion (Grocco's triangle), said to be due to displacement of the mediastinal contents.

Auscultation.—The *breath-sounds are diminished* in proportion to the degree of collapse in the lung, but as the lung generally contains some air the respiratory murmur frequently comes through as a *faint form of bronchial breathing*. This will be louder if the lung behind the fluid is consolidated. In large effusions the breath-sounds are often completely absent. The remnants of a pleural rub may be heard occasionally just above the level of the fluid.

From the description of the signs of consolidation and of fluid in the pleural cavity, the student will gather that while the diagnosis between the two conditions is generally simple, it may be confusing or even impossible. *To settle any doubt, exploratory aspiration is necessary,* and even in unequivocal cases of effusion it should be used to establish the nature of the effusion and exlude the possibility of pus.

Pneumothorax.—Air in the pleural sac is known as pneumothorax. The air generally enters through a communication between a bronchus or pulmonary cavity and the pleural sac, such as may occur from the destructive processes of tuberculosis, bronchiectasis, and other diseases. The condition usually occurs suddenly, with the production of *intense dyspnœa, pain,* and *collapse.* If it occurs by gradual leakage the symptoms are much less marked.

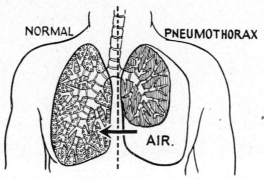

Fig. 88.—Pneumothorax. The lung is shown collapsed. Mediastinum displaced to opposite side (indicated by arrow). Lung and bronchi are compressed. Signs are : defective movement ; breath-sounds faint (amphoric with pneumothorax) ; diminished vocal fremitus and vocal resonance ; percussion note varies with cause e.g., dull with fluid, usually resonant with air. Similar signs, with modifications, are found in collapse due to other causes—e.g., fluid, massive collapse.

The effects of pneumothorax (*Fig.* 88) are similar to those of a rapidly produced pleural effusion. The lung is collapsed on the affected side, with *displacement of the mediastinal tissues, including the heart, to the opposite side.*

There is *lack of expansion* on the affected side, though the chest appears fully expanded irrespective of respiratory movements. *Vocal fremitus is diminished* because of the collapsed lung and loss of vibrations at the interface between lung and air. *Breath-sounds and vocal resonance are faint* for similar reasons, but may have an *amphoric character* owing to the resonating properties of the pneumothorax. Adventitious sounds, for a similar reason, take on a metallic quality, and the ' *metallic tinkle* ' may be produced by râles evoked by coughing, sneezing, etc. It would sometimes appear that the metallic tinkle is synchronous with cardiac contractions. Metallic tinkling is often heard at the end of inspiration and is peculiarly suggestive of pneumothorax. It is likened to the sound caused by tapping with a pin on a glass vessel. It is present in a hydropneumothorax, and is thought to be due to a bursting of air-bubbles at the surface of the fluid from a concealed fistula below. It may also be caused by splashing into the fluid of drops from the surface of the cavity above.

Of the special signs of pneumothorax, the *coin test* has been described (p. 76). Another of great antiquity is *Hippocratic succussion*, a splashing sound produced by shaking the patient, who should be in the sitting posture. *It occurs only when fluid and air are present in the same cavity.*

CHAPTER IV

THE CARDIO-VASCULAR SYSTEM

SYMPTOMS OF HEART DISEASE

THE patient with heart disease may complain of many different symptoms, any or all of which may be unconnected with the cardio-vascular system. Often there are *no* symptoms and a cardiac lesion is found by routine examination.

Certain symptoms are, however, very constantly found in cardio-vascular disease, and though they may have other causes, careful attention should be paid to them in order to eliminate or confirm their cardiac origin. The patient should be encouraged to give a full and spontaneous description of his symptoms, and detailed questioning on the part of the examiner left until he has no more to say.

Dyspnœa (*see also* RESPIRATORY SYSTEM, p. 56).—This is the most common and perhaps the most important symptom occurring in heart disease. It does not point to any special structural defect in the cardio-vascular system, but to cardiac failure—early or late, according to its degree, character, and associated symptoms and signs.

Alone it must not be taken as evidence of heart failure, unless other causes (e.g., respiratory diseases and anæmias) have been excluded, and unless the examiner is satisfied that the patient is genuinely more breathless than he should be under the circumstances described. This applies especially to dyspnœa on exertion. A genuine dyspnœa is characterized by more rapid and deeper breathing than normal, in severe cases interfering with normal speech. Everyone is familiar with such dyspnœa, occurring in health, after severe or unaccustomed effort. It must be distinguished from the sighing and desire for deeper breath so often manifested by neurotic patients.

Dyspnœa on Effort.—This is the commonest type of dyspnœa and it may long precede other evidence of heart failure. It occurs independently of the cause of this failure, and many causes which ultimately provoke cardiac failure may long exist without dyspnœa. This is well seen in aortic regurgitation, hypertension, and other lesions in which dyspnœa may occur late. In other conditions, e.g., mitral stenosis, the symptom is commonly found much earlier.

The grade of dyspnœa is a most valuable guide to the heart's capacity. Other things being equal, the greater the dyspnœa, or the less exertion needed to provoke it, the greater the encroachment upon the heart's reserve of power. Due allowance must be made for the wide variation in cardiac reserve in different individuals, and it is more valuable to know how the patient's breathing responds to physical tasks to which he has been accustomed than to compare his response to some special test against that of a healthy man. If he is aware year by year, or month by month, that his breathing is more embarrassed by the same hill, a gradual depletion of the cardiac reserve may be presumed, unless other factors causal of dyspnœa be present. When he is breathless even walking on the level, a more serious reduction of the heart's reserve has occurred, and sooner or later dyspnœa may be expected to occur at rest in association with evidence of venous congestion. A close analysis of some of these cases may reveal that the dyspnœa was brought on by very minor exertion such as alteration of position in bed.

Orthopnœa ("upright breathing"; dyspnœa on lying down).—This is often seen in patients who have dyspnœa on slight exertion accompanied by other signs of congestive heart failure. Such a patient seeks comfort in the adoption of a semi-sitting posture during sleep, and slipping out of this posture not uncommonly causes a type of nocturnal dyspnœa which must be distinguished from cardiac asthma. It is often associated with left ventricular failure.

Paroxysmal Dyspnœa (dyspnœa at rest).—Attacks of dyspnœa occurring during sleep and awakening the patient are often found in hypertensive heart disease and less commonly in coronary artery disease, arteriosclerosis, and specific aortitis. In these conditions, left ventricular failure, which causes the attacks, is common. Men are usually affected.

The patient wakes with a sense of oppression or suffocation and sits up often by the open window to seek relief. The breathing is laboured and wheezing and in severe cases distress is very great, the patient sweating profusely and showing signs of collapse. The attack may continue for a few hours, though it is often reckoned in minutes. Pulmonary œdema may ensue and a cough with frothy and blood-tinged sputum follows.

These attacks are commonly called 'cardiac asthma,' though a similar phenomenon is seen in uræmia.

Cheyne-Stokes Breathing (*see also* p. 64).—In heart disease this type of respiration, also known as periodic breathing, is commonest in similar affections to those in which cardiac asthma occurs. The waxing and waning of the respiration, periods of hypernœa and apnœa, are particularly common during sleep, which they may interrupt.

Any or all of these types of dyspnœa may be found in the same patient.

Palpitation.—By this term is meant that the patient is conscious of his heart-beats, which he may describe as bumping, throbbing, or fluttering in the chest or peripheral vessels. Several factors may be responsible for the symptoms—namely, increased force, increased rate, and irregularity of the heart—but unless the nervous system is sensitive they may not result in palpitation. For this reason the symptom is more common in excitable states of the nervous system, such as hyperthyroidism and anxiety states, than in organic heart disease. It is not uncommon for a placid patient with a heaving apical beat or with an abnormal rhythm or tachycardia to be quite unaware of the heart's action.

If palpitation occurs in *attacks*, careful attention must be paid to the patient's story. In simple sinus tachycardia, it will usually be found that emotion or exercise causes the heart to beat faster, and as the precipitating cause diminishes so the heart-rate and the palpitation lessens. By contrast, in abnormal rhythms such as auricular flutter or paroxysmal tachycardia, the onset and offset of the attacks are instantaneous. The patient often states that he was conscious of the heart missing a beat or " turning over " and then the palpitation was in full swing. Similarly the attack passed away by a sudden consciousness of some disturbance in the heart-beat. Short attacks of this character are suggestive of paroxysmal tachycardia ; longer attacks, lasting many hours or days, suggest auricular flutter. Auricular fibrillation may also come in attacks, and the patient may be able to date the onset of the attack by the sudden appearance of palpitation having an irregular character. Extrasystoles are usually appreciated as occasional irregularities. The patient may be aware of a missed beat or an extra large bump corresponding with the next normal beat after the extrasystole. In most cases of palpitation the heart beats faster than normal, but occasionally, in heart block, the increased stroke volume may cause awareness of the heart's slow action.

Precordial Pain.—Pain as a symptom of heart disease is very important, but sometimes difficult to evaluate. It occurs so frequently without gross evidence of cardio-vascular disease that a diagnosis may have to rest on this symptom alone. For this reason an accurate and careful description of the site, character, and duration of the pain is essential.

Anginal Pain.—When it is fully developed this is a pain of such severity that it is the dominant clinical feature and has led to the symptom of angina pectoris being regarded almost as a disease. The pain is *situated beneath the sternum*, usually in its upper part, though sometimes as low down as the xisphisternum, especially in coronary thrombosis (*see below*). It is described as crushing or *gripping in nature*, or as a sense of weight or tightness in the chest. Not uncommonly the patient refers to it as " indigestion ". It is a continuous pain ; never sharp or interrupted. From its substernal position it radiates, if sufficiently severe, towards the cardiac apex, and often down the inner aspect of the left arm as far as the elbow or finger-tips. In more severe cases it spreads into the right arm, neck, jaw, or back. Sometimes the pain occurs first in one of these unusual sites, and diagnosis is difficult until the substernal pain develops later. The occurrence of pain or constriction at the root of the neck led to the term angina.

The wide spread of anginal pain still requires much investigation, but depends upon the elaborate innervation of the heart by the sympathetic and vagus nerves. The afferent fibres from the sympathetic enter the cord through the first five dorsal nerve-roots in the rami communicantes.

7

Their connexion with the corresponding somatic nerves would appear to account for the usual distribution of anginal pain over the upper part of the chest and arms. Rarer types of pain such as those in the jaw and neck may be due to the connexion between the cardiac branches of the vagus and the fifth cranial and second and third cervical nerves.

The pain is usually so severe that the patient stops whatever he is doing, and stands motionless till it passes away in two or three minutes. The symptom is characteristically *brought on by effort, and when a pain in the chest comes on only after physical exertion a cardiac origin should be suspected.* Even if the pain is confined to the arm, back, jaw, or neck, but is provoked constantly and only by exertion, angina should be suspected. The pain does not always occur in this classically severe form, though such an attack may be necessary before a satisfactory diagnosis can be made. Once a severe attack has occurred, minor types of pain, the significance of which the observer may have been unable to assess, assume great importance. Other features of angina pectoris the student will read of in his text-book of medicine. As a symptom it has been given considerable prominence here because of its importance in diagnosis.

Its actual cause is still disputed. More and more evidence goes to support the view that most types are essentially due to a deficient coronary circulation, resulting in absolute or relative myocardial ischæmia. In angina pectoris there may be actual narrowing of the coronary arteries from arteriosclerotic changes, diminishing the blood-supply to the heart muscle. Spasm of the coronary arteries, alone or acting upon such narrowed coronary vessels, may also be responsible for the pain. In *coronary thrombosis*, in which intense anginal pain lasting for many hours occurs, the coronary artery affected is occluded permanently. Even in anæmias and diabetes, although the quantity of the blood received by the heart muscle is not diminished, its quality is impoverished, and anginal pain may more rarely result. All of these conditions lead to greater or less degrees of myocardial ischæmia. When the patient is at rest the blood supplied may still be sufficient for the heart's needs, but on effort, or with increased peripheral resistance demanding more work from the heart, the supply is insufficient and pain results. In this way can be explained the characteristic occurrence of angina on effort, emotion, exposure to cold, etc.

Other Forms of Precordial Pain.—It will be useful here to mention the frequency with which pain in the chest results from non-cardiac causes which must be carefully distinguished from the type of pain just described. Pain of an aching character is common in effort syndrome, especially after fatigue. Aching or sharp pains occur in fibrositis, intercostal myalgia and neuralgia—pain commonly called ' pleurodynia '. These pains are usually worse on movement of the affected parts and are associated with localized tenderness. The pain of pleurisy is generally severe, cutting or burning in character, and constantly related to breathing. All these pains tend to be localized to the mammary, axillary, or back regions, rather than substernal. Further, they are often of long duration—hours or days.

Aneurysm may produce severe pain in the precordium, in the back, or in the upper abdomen according to the site of the dilatation. The pain is due to pressure effects on bony structures and nerves.

Gastro-intestinal Symptoms.—In cases of congestive heart failure where the viscera—liver and gastro-intestinal tract—are engorged with blood, dyspeptic symptoms are common. *Loss of appetite, nausea,* fullness after meals, and distension of the abdomen are the usual features. *Vomiting* occurs occasionally, and the bowels are usually constipated. Pain over the liver is common, owing to congestion of the organ and stretching of its capsule.

Respiratory Symptoms.—Again as a part of congestive heart failure the lungs are usually engorged with blood, resulting in *cough,* increase in the dyspnœa, and less commonly in *hæmoptysis.* In long standing cases altered blood may be found in the sputum. If there is œdema of the lungs the sputum may be plentiful and frothy.

Urinary Symptoms.—Congestion of the kidneys leads to *decrease in the secretion of urine,* sometimes to complete suppression. The urine passed is highly coloured owing to its great concentration, shows a marked deposit of urates on standing, and frequently contains albumin; blood is a rare constituent. *Oliguria,* as this decrease in urinary output is called, is one of the most important symptoms of cardiac failure, and is a useful guide to the grade of failure and its response to treatment.

Cerebral Symptoms.—The most important of these is syncope, which is considered below separately. Dizziness, headache, and mental changes are not uncommon features of hypertension or of arterial degeneration and cardiac failure, but they also occur more commonly in effort syndrome in which no organic cardio-vascular lesion can be found.

Syncope.—Fainting is commonly caused by vasodilatation which depletes the cerebral circulation of an adequate amount of blood. This is accompanied by vagal effects which cause slowing of the heart. The attacks are therefore commonly called vasovagal. They occur particularly in persons of nervous temperament from emotional causes such as fright, shock, unpleasant sights or smells, or even mental apprehension under tense conditions. In normally balanced persons they may occur as a result of severe pain as in biliary or renal colic and in coronary thrombosis. They are not particularly a feature of heart disease; but they may occur during the course of organic cardio-vascular disease, and it is important to exclude such disease in order to be able to reassure the patient of the harmless nature of the symptom. In particular, those forms of heart disease in which syncopal attacks appear to be frequent should be excluded, especially abnormal rhythms, aortic regurgitation, coronary artery disease, and hypertension.

The attacks occur whilst the patient is standing, practically never in recumbency. The patient feels giddy, often with a sense of nausea, though there is no sense of rotation as in aural vertigo. Profuse sweating sets in and the patient feels cold and weak. At this stage he commonly sits or lies down and the attack may pass away. If he persists in standing, he falls and loses consciousness, usually only for a few seconds but sometimes for many minutes. The face is ashen, the pulse slow, usually between 40 and 50, and feeble. Occasionally slight convulsive movements appear, especially in the head and neck, but incontinence is rare.

Syncopal attacks of cardiac origin, i.e., due to defective ventricular output, may bear a close resemblance to these vasovagal attacks. They occur under two particular circumstances : (1) Excessive ventricular slowing ; (2) Very rapid action of the ventricles.

The first is seen in heart-block, in which syncope may occur in degrees varying from a transient feeling of faintness to deep unconsciousness resulting in death. Such attacks known as Stokes-Adams seizures result from an excessive slowing of the ventricles usually to a rate of between 10 and 20. They do not occur in complete heart-block so long as the rate remains above 30. The milder attacks result only in loss of consciousness for a short period, but in the more severe cases this is associated with venous engorgement, cyanosis, cessation of respiration, and, later, epileptic convulsions. Death often occurs during an attack. Sometimes the ventricles stop beating completely and no pulse is perceptible.

In auricular flutter and paroxysmal tachycardia, especially where the ventricular rate is very high (usually over 250), the defective ventricular output may also result in syncope.

Syncope of cardiac origin, i.e., due primarily to failure of ventricular output rather than to vasodilatation, is often distinguished by the lack of sweating and the fact that the attack may occur in the recumbent posture. The discovery of heart-block or an abnormal rhythm may decide the diagnosis.

Other Symptoms.—Finally, it should be noted that in serious heart disease a great variety of symptoms may arise owing to malnutrition of the body as a whole or of certain special organs. *In children, wasting and lack of normal development is a common result,* and even in adults some loss of weight is usual, though obesity may also occur.

PHYSICAL SIGNS: EXAMINATION OF THE CARDIO-VASCULAR SYSTEM

The examination of the cardio-vascular system comprises a study of the heart and blood-vessels, but corroborative evidence of heart disease is so frequently present in other organs that certain signs should be looked for in every case. These may conveniently be discussed first.

Œdema (dropsy).—The patient may complain of swelling of the ankles or feet, but if this symptom does not enter into the history it should be sought purposely. Œdema is not fully understood, but it is known that certain factors are concerned in its production. Gravity plays an important part, especially in cardiac œdema, and *the swelling is found in the most dependent parts of the body*—in the feet and ankles when the patient is ambulatory, over the sacrum (sacral cushion—*Fig*. 89), lumbar region, genitalia, and backs of the thighs in patients who are sitting upright in bed. Looseness of the subcutaneous tissues also favours the accumulation of dropsical fluid, hence the occurrence of œdema in the genitalia

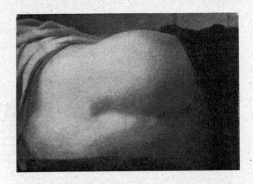

Fig. 89.—Sacral cushion of œdema. Pitting on pressure over the sacrum is common in patients who have been bedridden in the usual sitting posture adopted in heart failure. The œdema may disappear from the legs, and it is therefore important to look for it in this position.

and beneath the eyes in renal disease or extreme cardiac failure. Interference with the return of the blood to the heart also favours dropsy. This is seen in cases of localized venous thrombosis, but there is little doubt that the more generalized obstruction to venous return which occurs in many types of heart disease acts in the same way. Malnutrition of the tissues, whether produced by stagnation of blood in cardiac conditions, by impoverishment in the quality of the blood in anæmias, or by the accumulation of toxic products in renal or heart disease, is another factor at work.

Œdema is recognized by the characteristic '*pitting*' *on pressure,* and should be *distinguished from the more solid swelling of hypothyroidism* or lymphatic blockage. As a gauge of the disappearance of œdema the *weight* of the patient is generally reliable, for, with the dispersal of the fluid and its excretion through the kidneys, bowel, and skin, there is a rapid reduction in weight ; whilst, conversely, *increase in weight suggests further accumulation of dropsical fluid.* Œdema is not confined to the subcutaneous tissues, but may affect serous sacs, causing *pleural and pericardial effusion,* and *ascites.*

Cyanosis.—Blueness of the extremities, which has already been described under the RESPIRATORY SYSTEM as cyanosis (p. 58), may occur to a marked degree in certain heart diseases. In its extreme forms it is *usually seen in congenital defects,* such as pulmonary stenosis with patency of the septa of the heart, in which intermingling of the arterial and venous blood occurs. In other forms of heart disease cyanosis is not so pronounced, but it is *often a conspicuous feature in mitral disease (Fig. 90), and in heart changes secondary to respiratory disorders.* The venous congestion in these conditions leads to a defective contact between the circulating blood and the alveolar air, and the poor interchange of gases results in an increase of the reduced hæmoglobin in the tissues. Interference with the return of blood to the heart also acts by giving longer time for dissociation

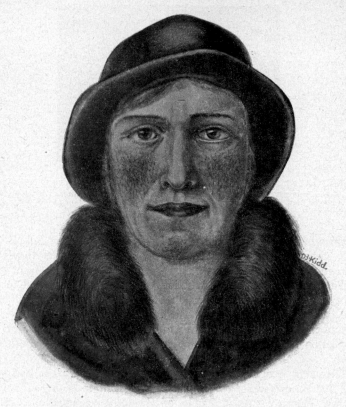

Fig. 90.—Mitral facies. The cheeks are rosy, with a bluish tinge, which on closer inspection is frequently seen to be due to dilatation of the malar capillaries. Note the cyanosis of the lips. Sometimes the remainder of the skin of the face has a creamy pallor. This was not present in the patient illustrated here.

of oxygen to occur in the tissues, and the blood eventually returned to the heart is depleted of more oxygen than usual. The *effect of cold and effort in increasing cyanosis* is to be observed in most cases.

Respiratory Distress.—Particular note should be made of the degree of breathlessness, before the patient volunteers any statement about this symptom. When heart disease is responsible for it the dyspnœa is usually proportionate to the cyanosis. The lungs should also be examined in every case, as, apart from the congestion which occurs in cardiac failure, such abnormalities as emphysema or fibrosis may be responsible for the production or aggravation of the heart condition.

Abdominal Signs.—The abdomen should be examined in all cases of heart disease, as there may be enlargement of the liver or ascites, suggestive of congestive failure, and enlargement of the spleen in cases of infective endocarditis.

Pulsation in the Epigastrium.—Epigastric pulsation may be due to : (a) The contraction of the right ventricle; it is seen as a systolic retraction in the epigastrium, and may occur in normal persons; when the heart is hypertrophied it may be felt as a systolic thrust on palpation. (b) Aortic pulsation in nervous but otherwise normal persons, especially when the abdominal wall is thin; aneurysm of the abdominal aorta may be simulated; aortic pulsation follows the heart-beat by about 1/10 second. (c) Abdominal aortic aneurysm, in which an expansile swelling bigger than the normal aorta is present. (d) Pulsation of the liver, which is more easily seen than felt; the area of pulsation extends more to the right than in the case of aortic or ventricular pulsation, and signs of congestive failure are present. It is to be noted that the enlarged liver may transmit pulsation from the heart or aorta.

Signs Pointing to the Aetiology.—As the causes of cardio-vascular disease are comparatively few, the examiner should be alert for evidence of arthritis, rheumatic nodules (*Fig.* 91), chorea, or tonsillitis which may suggest a *rheumatic* origin, for past signs of *syphilis* such as scars on the penis or old ulceration of the legs, and for clubbing of the fingers, anæmia, and petechiæ suggestive of *infective endocarditis*. Enlargement of the *thyroid* together with other evidence of thyrotoxicosis may explain cases of heart disease in which no other aetiological factors are found.

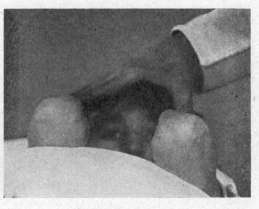
Fig. 91.—Rheumatic nodules.

We may now proceed to investigate the cardio-vascular system proper. This involves examination of : (1) The peripheral vascular system (the pulse) ; (2) The heart.

1. EXAMINATION OF THE PULSE

It is usual to examine the pulse before proceeding to the examination of the heart itself. This should include inspection, palpation and auscultation of important vessels, especially the radial, brachial, and axillary arteries, the carotids and temporal vessels, and the femorals and their distal branches. Most information is derived from the radial artery commonly called *the* pulse, and the most important method of examination is palpation, which will be considered first.

Palpation

The *pulse should be felt in both wrists*, as variations are sometimes found on the two sides both in health and disease. Marked inequality suggests either an abnormally placed artery on one side, or pressure causing defective filling of the artery. Such pressure may be exerted by aneurysm and other forms of mediastinal tumour on the subclavian arteries, or the aneurysmal sac may prevent the proper filling of the artery on one side. Thereafter the following points should be noted in sequence :—

I. Rate.—The pulse-rate normally averages about 72 per minute, but in children is more rapid (90 to 110), and in old age may become slow (55 to 65). Quite trivial disturbances are sufficient to cause an acceleration in the pulse-rate—for example, the emotion roused by a medical examination, or the effort of climbing stairs or hurrying to the consulting room. Due allowance must be made for these factors before attaching too much importance to a rapid pulse-rate, and it is useful to *take the rate at the beginning of the consultation and again before the patient leaves. The heart-rate should always be compared with the pulse-rate*, as in some cases there is a 'pulse deficit', i.e., the pulse-rate is less than the ventricular rate.

2. Rhythm.—The normal pulse-waves succeed one another at regular intervals, but respiratory variations are common in health, *the pulse quickening with inspiration and slowing with expiration*. If this variation in rate is noticeable even with quiet breathing the term *sinus arrhythmia* is applied to it. If other forms of irregularity are present the observer

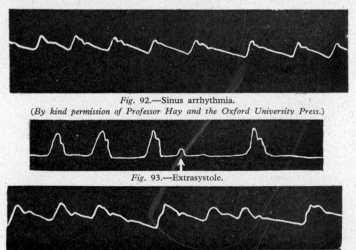

Fig. 92.—Sinus arrhythmia.
(*By kind permission of Professor Hay and the Oxford University Press.*)

Fig. 93.—Extrasystole.

Fig. 94.—Auricular fibrillation.
(*By kind permission of Professor Hay and the Oxford University Press.*)

should *note whether the pulse is completely irregular all the time or only occasionally*. Finally, the effect of effort on the rhythm should be noted. Decisions as to rhythms should always be deferred until examination of the heart has been made, as the pulse alone may be deceptive (*see* p. 136).

The commonest irregularities detectable in the pulse are extrasystoles (premature beats) and auricular fibrillation, though partial heart-block and auricular flutter may be suspected. Extrasystoles usually produce an *occasional* irregularity in which the pulse drops a beat·or in which a small pulse-wave occurs earlier than is expected. If the extrasystoles are numerous, the pulse may *appear* completely irregular. In auricular fibrillation the pulse *is* completely irregular, and this is usually easily recognized, though it may not be observed if the heart-rate is slow, so that exercise should be employed to quicken the heart. Extrasystoles, on the other hand, often disappear with exercise. (*Figs*. 92–94.)

3. Blood-pressure.—If the index finger of each hand is placed on the radial pulse and an attempt is made to obliterate this with the upper finger, the disappearance of the pulse can be noted by the lower finger, and some idea of the pressure necessary for this will be gained. This gives a rough idea of the force necessary to obliterate the intra-arterial pressure (systolic and diastolic) and is useful in cases where instrumental estimation of the blood-pressure seems unnecessary. At the same time it prevents the physician from overlooking unsuspected high blood-pressure.

INSTRUMENTAL ESTIMATION OF BLOOD-PRESSURE.—This is accomplished by use of a *sphygmomanometer*. Many instruments are on the market, some of mercurial pattern and some of the aneroid type.

The arm band should be about four inches in width, as narrower ones are known to give false readings.

The band is wrapped *firmly and evenly* round the arm about *three inches above the elbow*, which should be quite free to move, so that the bell of the stethoscope can be placed in the antecubital fossa. The arm band contains a rubber bag which is blown up until the brachial artery is occluded. At this point the radial pulse disappears.

The Systolic Pressure (i.e., the maximum pressure during the propagation of the pulse-wave).—This may be estimated by :—

1. *The palpatory method* : The armlet is pumped to a greater degree than is necessary to obliterate the radial pulse. The air is then slowly released until the pulse is once more palpable. The reading on the manometer at this point represents the systolic pressure.

2. *The auscultatory method* : The bell of the stethoscope is placed over the brachial artery at the bend of the elbow, and the armlet pumped up until all sounds disappear. It is then gently released until a soft puffing noise is first heard. This point represents the systolic pressure (*Fig*. 95).

It is preferable to use the auscultatory method for the systolic as well as the diastolic pressure, but the systolic should be checked by the palpatory method, by which it may be found 5 to 10 mm. lower.

The Diastolic Pressure (i.e., the constant pressure in the artery between each systole).—This is only roughly measurable.

The *auscultatory method* is now usually employed. The procedure is the same as for obtaining the systolic pressure ; the observer listens for sounds over the brachial artery at the elbow. Following the puffing noise heard at and below the systolic reading, there occurs a knocking or thudding sound which increases in intensity, and then passes suddenly into another softer sound. *The sharp transition from the loud knocking to the soft blowing sound is taken as the diastolic pressure* in England, though in America the cessation of all sound is held by many to be the correct diastolic reading. Sometimes it is impossible to record the diastolic pressure owing to lack of any distinction between the knocking and soft sounds.

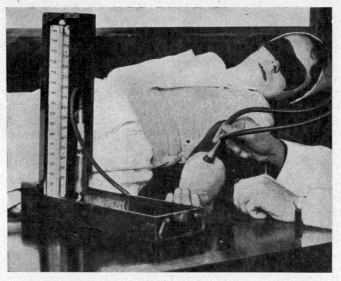

Fig. 95.—Auscultatory method of estimating systolic blood-pressure.

A useful confirmation of the diastolic pressure is obtainable by noting that it corresponds with the *maximum oscillation of the mercurial column*.

4. Form.—Under this heading may be considered the *volume and variations in the type of the pulse-wave*, which can really be best appreciated by graphic methods. Considerable experience is necessary before much information can be obtained by the use of the fingers alone, but by careful comparison of a series of normal and abnormal pulses the student will learn to distinguish a thin thready pulse from a full bounding one, and with experience the slighter grades of these extremes. Similarly, he will be able to appreciate certain special varieties of pulse. The more important of these are the *anacrotic pulse* and the *plateau pulse* in which the summit of the pulse-wave has a longer duration than normal (the anacrotic differs from the plateau pulse only in having an extra wave on the upstroke of the main wave); the *collapsing pulse* in which the peak of the pulse-wave is rapidly produced, of very brief duration, and rapid descent; and the *dicrotic* or *hyperdicrotic pulse* in which the dicrotic notch and wave are so pronounced as sometimes to give the impression of two separate pulse-waves, the second being smaller than the first. The anacrotic and plateau pulses

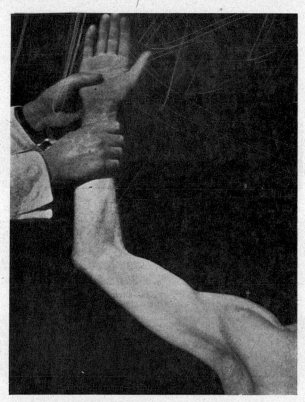

Fig. 96.—The collapsing pulse. To elicit the collapsing pulse the patient's arm should be raised well above the head and the wrist grasped so that the palm of the examiner's hand lies over its anterior aspect. This intensifies the collapsing sensation felt in the arteries after each systole of the heart.

are found in conditions of increased peripheral resistance and in aortic stenosis where the systole of the heart is more sustained than usual. The collapsing pulse, *best elicited by placing the hand round the patient's wrist with his arm held vertically (Fig.* 96), is found in conditions where, the diastolic pressure is so low as to produce an emptiness of the arteries and a flaccidity of their walls, and therefore occurs in aortic regurgitation, anæmias, fevers, thyrotoxicosis, and other conditions causing vasodilatation. The patient may complain of throbbing headache or pulsation in the finger-tips. If, as in the case of aortic incompetence, there is also a high systolic pressure resulting in a big pulse-pressure, the collapsing or ' water hammer ' pulse is intensified. The 'water hammer' pulse derives its name from a toy, and is also called Corrigan's pulse after the physician who described

PULSE TRACINGS (*see also Figs.* 92-94).

(*Figs.* 97 *and* 99 *by kind permission of Professor Hay and the Oxford University Press.*)

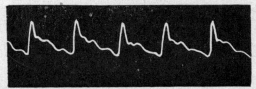

Fig. 97.—Normal spnygmogram

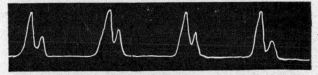

Fig. 98.—Dicrotic pulse.

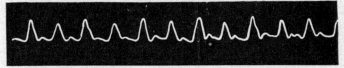

Fig. 99.—Pulsus alternans.

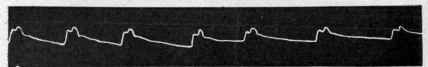

Fig. 100.—Aortic stenosis—anacrotic pulse.

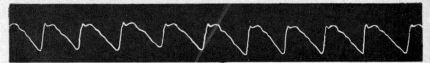

Fig. 101.—Aortic stenosis—plateau pulse.

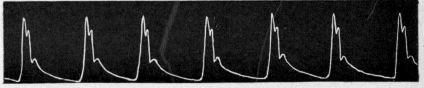

Fig. 102.—Aortic regurgitation—collapsing pulse.

some of the vascular phenomena of aortic incompetence (1832). The collapsing pulse is perhaps the most common designation, and implies a rapid fall of the pulse-wave. Actually the phenomena by which this pulse is recognized are due chiefly to the steep *rise* of the pulse-wave, especially in aortic regurgitation, in which the ventricle must throw out its normal quota of blood, augmented by that which has poured back into it during diastole. None the less the pulse gives the impression of ' collapsing ', especially when the wrist is grasped with the whole hand.

The dicrotic pulse is frequently found in acute infections, especially in typhoid fever. In these the systolic force of the heart is diminished, so that the initial pulse-wave is smaller than normal, whilst on closure of the aortic valves the dicrotic wave produced is relatively greater than normal. In studying the form of the pulse *invaluable knowledge may be acquired by comparing pulse tracings (Figs. 92–94, 97–102) with the results of palpation.*

Alteration in the volume of the pulse may occur from beat to beat. In the normal person the volume becomes greater with inspiration, but occasionally it happens that the reverse obtains—a phenomenon known as the *pulsus paradoxus.* This may be seen physiologically if the breathing is thoracic in type or if the chest is held rigidly with the shoulders braced backwards. When these conditions have been excluded the pulsus paradoxus is sometimes found in *pericardial effusion or adherent pericardium* —conditions which interfere with the normal return of blood to the heart and produce a diminished filling of the pulses at the height of inspiration.

In *pulsus alternans* there is an alternate variation in the size of the pulse-wave, said to be due to a defective myocardium in which not all the fibres are capable of contracting at each heart-beat. It is often found, there-fore, in *serious myocardial disease, and is a sign of grave omen.* It is important, however, to realize that pulsus alternans *may occur without serious myo-cardial disease if the ventricular rate is rapid*, as, for example, in paroxysmal tachycardia. It is also sometimes found after the exhibition of digitalis.

5. **Condition of the Arterial Wall.**—The examination of the pulse is completed by observations on the wall of the artery. An attempt should be made to roll the vessel under the index and second fingers. In many young persons the arterial wall is so thin that with pressure of this kind it seems to merge into the surrounding tissues and to have no separate entity. In middle age it becomes distinctly palpable, and in the later decades can usually be felt as a cord-like structure. No hard-and-fast rule can be laid down as to what should be considered physiological and what pathological arterial thickening. Again it is only by experience that the examiner can form suitable standards for comparison.

Whilst palpating the arterial wall *note should also be made of any irregularity in its surface and of any tortuosity in its course.* Irregularities are chiefly associated with those types of arteriosclerosis where calcareous material is deposited in the vessel wall, the ' pipe-stem ' arteries of old age, and in certain cases hard ring-like structures can be felt along the course of the vessel, giving it a semblance to the trachea. Thickening of the tibial vessels with diminished or absent pulsation is of considerable diagnostic value in peripheral arterial disease such as thrombo-angiitis obliterans, intermittent claudication, and gangrene. The condition of these vessels must be carefully compared with the temperature and colour of the limb.

Special tests have been devised to estimate the competence of the periperal arteries. Some are laboratory procedures and will not be described here.

Reactive Hyperæmia Test.—This is a clinical test of some value though in its employment the chances of inducing thrombosis in diseased arteries must be considered. The leg is raised above the horizontal with the patient recumbent. The veins are emptied by light massage towards the trunk, and a sphygmomanometer band is applied above the knee and pumped up to obliterate the popliteal vessels (160–250 mm. Hg. or more according to the patient's blood-pressure). The limb below the constriction is blanched, and the pressure is maintained for 5 minutes. On release there is an immediate intense flushing of the skin down to the toes in a normal person. With sclerotic and narrowed vessels the hyperæmia is much less (faint pink and slowly produced) and may take a considerable time to reach the foot.

Inspection and Auscultation of the Peripheral Vessels

Inspection.—Although the principal examination of the pulse is by palpation, useful information may be derived from inspection and auscultation. All the important peripheral vessels should be inspected. In those conditions in which the collapsing pulse is found, notably aortic regurgitation, the arteries pulsate vigorously and in a jerky manner. This is well seen in the carotids, causing the head to nod or the ears to move with each systole of the heart.

Arteriosclerosis may often be recognized by the *tortuosity* of the

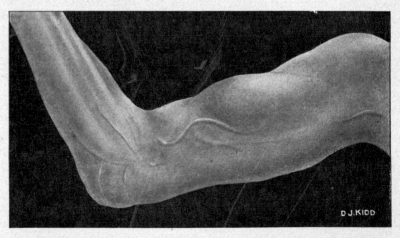

Fig. 103.—Locomotor brachial (arteriosclerosis). Note the prominence and tortuosity of the brachial artery in the axilla, and just proximal to the elbow. The angle between the arm and forearm must be greater than a right angle in looking for this sign, otherwise a false locomotor brachial may be produced.

superficial vessels (e.g., temporal, brachial, and axillary arteries) due to their lengthening whilst remaining more or less fixed at their proximal and distal points. In particular when the arm is flexed at the elbow to about 110°, the tortuosity of the brachial artery becomes most noticeable (*Fig.* 103), and the snake-like movements of the tortuous vessel with each systole have earned for this phenomenon the name of ' locomotor brachial '. *It is important that the elbow shall not be flexed beyond a right angle*, otherwise spurious tortuosity may be apparent.

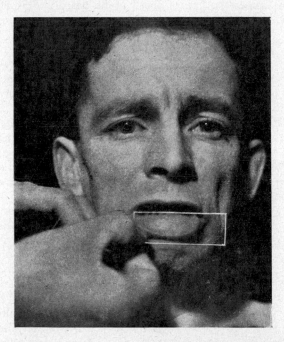

Fig. 104.—Capillary pulsation (aortic regurgitation). The lower lip is everted and the glass slide pressed on the mucous membrane sufficiently firmly to produce an area of blanching. With each systole of the heart the blanched area becomes pink. This can be seen particularly at the junction of the blanched area with the normal mucous membrane. Note also the anxious facies so common in aortic regurgitation.

The *retinal vessels* should be specially examined. In hypertension they are commonly narrowed and tortuous, kinking the veins where they cross. In advanced cases these changes are associated with papilloedema and exudate into the surrounding retina.

Capillary pulsation is found where there is marked vasodilatation, particularly if there is also a big pulse-pressure. It is therefore most frequently seen in *aortic regurgitation*, but may be found in normal persons if the skin is warm and in hyperthyroidism in which the skin is usually warm. It may be observed by pressing with a glass slide on the finger-nail, or lip, sufficiently heavily to cause partial blanching (*Fig.* 104). The blanched area becomes pink with each systole of the heart.

Auscultation.—This method of examination of the arteries is of less importance than inspection or palpation, but certain interesting facts may be observed. Murmurs are not uncommonly propagated into the great vessels. The harsh systolic murmur of aortic stenosis is usually transmitted into the carotids. A systolic and diastolic murmur is heard on pressure of the stethoscope over the great vessels (especially the femorals) in aortic regurgitation (Duroziez's murmur). Similarly, in this disease, the sudden output of a large quantity of blood from the left ventricle into the relatively empty arteries causes the 'pistol shot' to be heard. This has the same significance as the 'water hammer' pulse.

Examination of the Veins

This should include inspection and palpation of the superficial veins for evidence of engorgement, varicosity, and the presence of thrombi or evidence of inflammation.

Venous Engorgement.—Venous engorgement is most easily observed in the neck (*Fig.* 105), though other veins than the jugulars may exhibit evidence of it. In judging whether veins are over-distended, it is necessary to fix a zero level. This is taken to be the manubrium sterni, for in whatever position the patient may be, sitting, standing, lying, or in intermediate postures, it represents the zero position in the venous system, the level, in other words, of the blood in the right auricle. Veins above this level are collapsed: veins below filled to varying degrees. Whether a vein is pathologically over-filled, therefore, will depend upon the *height above the manubrium sterni* at which the distension can be recognized. Normally, when the patient is supine with the head on pillows, the level of the blood in the jugular veins reaches about one-third of the way up the neck. This level will

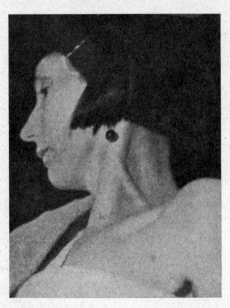

Fig. 105.—Engorged jugular vein. The tense engorged vein forms a triangle with the sternomastoid to the left and the clavicle as its base. Engorgement of this kind is seen in congestive heart failure, and for its observation the patient should be in the sitting posture, as some degree of jugular filling may be present in a healthy person lying flat.

be found to coincide with the level of the manubrium. In early cases of congestive failure in the same position, the jugular column rises to half way to the jaw, and, in more severe cases, right to the jaw. Now if the patient sits gradually more upright, the column of blood will fall, in normal subjects, to such an extent that it can no longer be seen (it has sunk to the level of the manubrium and is no longer filling the jugular veins). In cases of congestive failure, however, the column may still be visible above the clavicle for several centimetres or even throughout the course of the veins.

The filling of the veins should be bilateral and roughly equal. A local obstruction may cause minor degrees of unilateral distension, often removed by turning the head.

Pulsation of the Veins.—This should be noted carefully. It often helps to localize the upper limit of jugular engorgement. In itself it is not pathological, but it may indicate that the level of venous distension is above the manubrium. It must be distinguished from arterial pulsation, which is more obvious in the erect posture, whilst venous pulsation, from what has already been said, will diminish or disappear as the venous column falls with the assumption of an erect posture. It is difficult to *feel* venous pulsation, and then only with lightly placed fingers, but arterial pulsation pushes the fingers away forcibly. None the less, the distinction between the two is sometimes difficult.

Pulsation in the jugular veins affects both external and internal vessels. The former is more easily recognized in the normal person, but the latter is more often found in congestive failure.

When the engorgement is due to non-cardiac causes such as mediastinal tumours, there is often *no* pulsation, as the pressure of the tumour interferes with the movement of blood between the jugular veins and right auricle. This and other evidence of congestion help to distinguish cardiac jugular distension from other causes.

2. EXAMINATION OF THE HEART

The examination of the heart should follow the usual routine of inspection, palpation, percussion, and auscultation.

Inspection enables the examiner to see the position and extent of the apex-beat, its forcibility, and its rhythm. The presence of abnormal pulsation is noted over the precordium, over the great vessels in the neck, and in the epigastrium. Some of these points have been considered under the EXAMINATION OF THE PULSE.

Palpation confirms the position of the apex-beat, and gives more information about the force of the cardiac thrust. Thrills, a special form of vibration, are communicated to the hand. Expansile pulsation may be detected in cases of aneurysm.

Percussion is valuable in defining the outline of the heart, and is complementary to inspection and palpation, as it limits those borders of the heart which produce no appreciable pulsation of the chest wall. It is of less value in defining the limits of the aorta.

Auscultation is of great value in the detection of valvular abnormalities,

8

which commonly produce both changes in the heart-sounds, and added sounds called murmurs. It is also of some importance in diseases of the heart muscle which alter the character of the heart-sounds, and in pericarditis where a friction sound is present. The rhythm of the heart is determined by examination of the pulse and auscultation of the heart. These points will now be considered more fully.

Inspection

This method of examination is of greatest value in studying the position, character, and rhythm of the cardiac impulse (p. 115). Abnormal pulsations, especially of aneurysms, may also be visible. The patient should be in a good light, and the cardiac and other pulsations examined with him both in the erect and recumbent posture.

Palpation

Palpation also should be carried out with the patient first in the recumbent and then in the erect posture. The *flat of the hand* should be placed systematically over the apex beat and over the base of the heart (*Figs.* 106, 107). The extent of the cardiac impulse already defined by

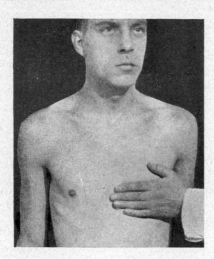

Fig. 106.—Palpation of apex beat. The flat hand should first be placed over the probable position of the cardiac apex. Later one or two fingers may be used for more accurate localization (*see Fig.* 108).

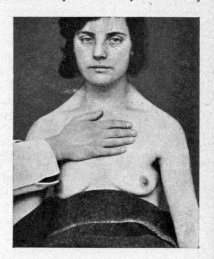

Fig. 107.—Palpation of the base of the heart. The flat of the hand should be placed across the manubrium sterni, so as to cover the aortic and pulmonary areas.

inspection should be confirmed and the *force* of the cardiac thrust can also be appreciated. The hand should then be placed on all areas of the precordium in order to detect any abnormal pulsations or vibrations.

As the cardiac impulse is normally circumscribed the palm of the hand is too large for accurate palpation, and the information gained by it should be supplemented by the use of *two fingers allowed to rest lightly over the cardiac thrust (Fig. 108).* In this way the area of the cardiac impulse and its forcibility can be defined more carefully.

Palpation is the most reliable method, apart from X rays, of estimating the size of the heart. It is essential, however, that the position of the apex beat should be measured from the sternum *to the farthest point towards the axilla at which the palpating fingers are actually lifted.* With a normal heart this distance varies from 3 to 4 in. according to the patient's stature or build.

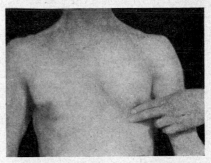

Fig. 108.—Localization of the cardiac apex. After the flat of the hand has been employed to determine the area of cardiac pulsation, the apex beat may be more accurately localized by placing two fingers over the intercostal spaces until they rest on the point of maximum pulsation.

It should be noted that in the normal adult little or no pulsation is communicated to the hand from the heart base or great vessels. Undue pulsation in this region is suggestive of aneurysmal enlargement of the great vessels, especially of the ascending part or arch of the aorta, more rarely of the pulmonary artery. Pulsation in the 2nd left intercostal space may, however, be seen normally in children.

The student should make it a practice to place the hand on both sides of the chest in turn, especially when the cardiac impulse is not easily palpated in its normal position on the left side. In this way he will avoid overlooking *dextrocardia.*

The Cardiac Impulse.—The cardiac thrust is maximal normally at the apex beat and can be examined by inspection and palpation. Two separate aspects must receive attention : (*a*) The position ; (*b*) The character.

Position.—The normal impulse is visible and distinctly palpable 3–4 in. from the midline and generally in the 5th intercostal space. It is circumscribed and can usually be covered by a penny. It is almost invariably within the nipple line except occasionally in children and adolescents. In women this landmark for obvious reasons is of no value, but in men it is useful, as the nipple is generally further from the midline in sthenic individuals whose hearts are also proportionately larger. The systolic thrust is caused by the contact of the contracting left ventricle with the chest wall. Internal to the thrust may be seen an area of systolic retraction caused by movements of the right ventricle, and it is necessary that this systolic retraction should not be confused with that of pathological origin. With changes of posture (lying on one side) the apex beat may move $\frac{1}{2}$–$\frac{3}{4}$ in. If the impulse is abnormal in position particular care should be taken to look for causes of cardiac displacement such as scoliosis, and pleural and pulmonary diseases (e.g., pleural effusion and pulmonary fibrosis). When these causes have been eliminated an abnormal position generally signifies cardiac enlargement.   If the impulse moves downwards into the 6th or 7th spaces (and usually outwards at the same time), left ventricular enlargement is probably responsible.   Right ventricular enlargement is more difficult to detect, though it may result in movement of the apex beat towards the axilla, and increased dullness to the right of the sternum.   If the apex beat is $4\frac{1}{2}$ in. or more to the left in the 5th interspace, it can be considered abnormal in position.

Character.—In normal persons the apex beat raises the palpating fingers without an undue thrust.   The strength of this thrust can only be judged by experience.   It is diminished in health by a thick chest wall (muscle or fat) or by emphysema, and is more noticeable in thin persons.

When very strong *it may move the ribs or sternum*, which almost invariably indicates *cardiac hypertrophy.*

If the impulse is feeble, less significance can be attached to it, unless it has been watched from day to day, and known to have changed.   In this case a feeble diffuse impulse, combined with change in position towards the axilla, may suggest *dilatation.*   Diffuseness alone often results from simple overaction of the heart as in nervous persons, after exercise, or in hyperthyroidism.

The position and character of the cardiac impulse thus give valuable information as to the presence of cardiac enlargement and whether this is due to hypertrophy or dilatation.   It will be convenient here to consider briefly the clinical significance of these phenomena.

Hypertrophy.—The presence of hypertrophy indicates that the heart is working under an extra load.   The clinical examination is therefore directed primarily to the discovery of this load, which may include hypertension, arteriosclerosis, valvular disease, pulmonary diseases, and others. The degree of the hypertrophy is also a rough indication of the extent of the load, i.e., the seriousness of the condition causing hypertrophy.   Moreover, it appears from clinical experience that hypertrophied heart muscle is not so sound as normal.   Both ventricles hypertrophy together, though one chamber may be more affected than the other.   Left ventricular hypertrophy, as already stated, can generally be recognized clinically. Right ventricular hypertrophy and enlargement of the auricles cannot easily be detected except radiologically.   They occur commonly in mitral stenosis, in which the position of the apex beat may be normal, though its character is often distinctively tapping.

Dilatation.—This accompanies hypertrophy in most cases and the one cannot be separated from the other in chronic heart disease.   In acute processes such as abnormal rhythms with tachycardia (flutter and paroxysmal tachycardia) and in toxic diseases such as diphtheria and pneumonia, enlargement of the heart may develop from day to day.   Dilatation is caused by distension of the heart by returning blood, when the cardiac output is impaired by rapid action or a feeble myocardium, and if these causes disappear (e.g., on cessation of an attack of flutter) the cardiac impulse soon returns to its normal position.

Thrills.—When vibrations are communicated to the palpating hand from the heart or its great vessels, they are spoken of as thrills. *A thrill is the analogue of a murmur*, and is usually produced in the same way, though as a rule the conditions necessary for its production must be more exaggerated than in the case of a murmur. Of these conditions the main one is the passage of blood from a smaller cavity into a greater one, but the thrill will be intensified if the chest wall is thin, if the blood flow is rapid, and if the site of production is comparatively near the surface. Like murmurs, thrills may be systolic or diastolic in time, or more rarely may occur continuously throughout the cardiac cycle. For the novice it is often difficult to time a thrill accurately, and it is justifiable to consider the timing in conjunction with that of the murmur which nearly always accompanies it. *The presence of a thrill is more certain evidence of organic disease of the heart than the presence of a murmur.*

At the base of the heart thrills are more commonly systolic. In *aortic stenosis* and in aneurysm of the great vessels at the root of the neck a powerful systolic thrill may be palpable over the 2nd right interspace, usually spreading upwards towards the neck. To the left of the sternum in the 2nd interspace *congenital pulmonary stenosis* gives rise to a similar type of thrill. Lower down the sternum, usually in the 3rd or 4th interspace, systolic thrills are occasionally felt due to congenital lesions of the heart, particularly infundibular stenosis (a type of congenital pulmonary stenosis in which the obstruction is at the origin of the pulmonary artery from the right ventricle) and patency of the heart septa. Very rarely systolic thrills are found at the apex alone, due to mitral regurgitation, but it is not uncommon for a thrill arising at the other areas mentioned to spread into the region of the apex.

By contrast, diastolic thrills at the apex are relatively common and usually due to *mitral stenosis*. They may occupy any part or the whole of diastole, but are more common in the early part, and again just before the commencement of the first sound (presystolic thrill). The latter type often ends in a forcible systole which imparts to the hand a systolic shock.

The combination of a systolic and diastolic thrill is rare. It sometimes occurs over the base of the heart, spreading from the aortic to the pulmonary area, in cases of *patent ductus arteriosus*. If such a thrill exists care should be taken not to overlook the possibility of vascular swellings, such as an enlarged overactive thyroid gland, a vascular mediastinal tumour, or still more rarely an arteriovenous aneurysm.

Percussion

Although percussion cannot compete with the radiological examination of the heart for accurate determination of its size, it remains a method of value which can be helpful to all who employ it carefully. Many of the technical details of percussion described under the respiratory system are applicable to the heart. Certain special points, however, need consideration. Light percussion is rarely of value, and equally so very heavy percussion, which gives inaccurate results owing to the vibration set up in the chest wall and in viscera other than the heart. A mean should be chosen between these two extremes, and constant practice is necessary before the student is able to determine the exact force required in the percussion stroke. *The position of the apex-beat can be defined equally well, if not better, by palpation than by percussion,* but the left border of the heart

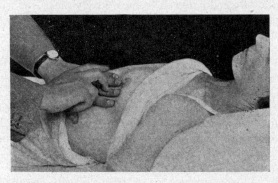

Fig. 109.—Percussion of the heart. The *orthodox* method is shown in which the pleximeter finger is kept approximately parallel with the expected border of the heart.

above the apex and the right border of the heart cannot easily be determined by palpation, while in certain cases percussion may give a rough idea of their position.

In percussing the outer limits of the cardiac impulse the pleximeter finger should be kept parallel with the sternum, and *percussion should be*

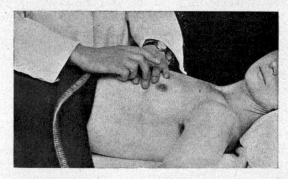

Fig. 110.—Percussion of the heart. By this *unorthodox* method of percussion it is possible to obtain better results in women. The pleximeter finger is placed in the 5th intercostal space and the percussion finger strikes the first phalangeal joint each time. The finger is moved one-quarter of an inch at a time from the axilla towards the midline. The orthodox method of percussion with the pleximeter finger parallel with the heart border is impossible in many women owing to the size of the breasts.

commenced well into the axillary region lest the heart extends so far out. The pleximeter finger should then be moved inwards along the 5th intercostal space a quarter of an inch at a time until a change of note is obtained. It may then be moved into the 4th and 3rd intercostal spaces in turn and the process repeated, but in this case the finger should be inclined at an angle corresponding with the slope of the heart from the sternum towards the apex so that it is roughly parallel with the heart margin (*Figs.* 109, 110, 111). The upper limit of the cardiac dullness cannot be defined with any great accuracy, but usually some change of note is obtained in the 3rd intercostal space if percussion is made from above downwards in the 1st, 2nd, and 3rd interspaces. The lower limit of the cardiac dullness is usually in the 5th intercostal space, but may be masked by the stomach resonance. Similarly, it is often *difficult to detect any change of note in percussing the right margin* of the heart. Before this is attempted *the liver dullness should be defined* by percussing downwards in each intercostal space until a change of note is found, usually in the 5th interspace. The pleximeter finger should then be placed above this level but parallel with the sternum and moved inwards a quarter of an inch at a time until a change of note is found. If no change of note is found because of the resonance produced by the sternum itself, a record should be made of this fact. From the various points of dullness found in this way a rough idea is obtained as to whether the heart margins extend farther than normal in a particular direction, but the true shape of the organ cannot be accurately appreciated.

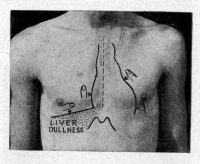

Fig. 111.—Diagram to show the different positions of the pleximeter finger in percussing the margins of the heart and the upper margin of the liver.

The significance of extension of the heart margins has been partly discussed under inspection, but further information is given by percussion. Increased dullness in the 3rd or 4th left interspaces occurs in right ventricular enlargement. Normally this area of dullness should not extend more than 2 in. from the mid-sternal line. Dullness to the right of the sternum may be part of a general cardiac enlargement or due particularly to enlargement of the right auricle. If it is marked in the upper intercostal spaces (2nd and 3rd) the possibility of aneurysmal dilatation of the aorta should be considered, especially if the dullness extends beneath the manubrium sterni. The possibility of dextrocardia should not be overlooked if extensive dullness occurs to the right of the sternum. In cases of pericardial effusion there may be increased dullness both to the right and the left of the sternum, but diagnosis of this condition from cardiac enlargement cannot be made by percussion alone. Lastly, when the area of cardiac dullness is altered, it must not be assumed that this is due to cardiac enlargement until the *possibility of cardiac displacement* has been excluded. The cardiac dullness is lost in well-established emphysema.

Auscultation

Auscultation ranks with inspection as a most important method of examining the cardio-vascular system. By means of it the rate and rhythm of the heart may be confirmed and compared with those of the pulse, but its main value is in the information it yields concerning the functions of the heart valves and to a lesser extent of the myocardium and pericardium. The patient should learn to *concentrate first on the auscultation of the heart-sounds* before turning his attention to any additional sounds, called murmurs, which may be present.

THE HEART-SOUNDS

Even in perfect health considerable differences exist in the intensity and character of the heart-sounds in different individuals. To form some idea of the limits of these variations the beginner should examine as many normal hearts as possible. In obese persons, in emphysema, or in those with well-developed musculature, the sounds are diminished in intensity. Conversely, thin coverings of muscle or fat on the chest wall allow the sounds to be conducted more clearly and loudly to the stethoscope. For this reason it is usually easy to define the heart-sounds at all areas of the precordium in children.

Before describing the character of the heart-sounds and their mode of origin, it is necessary to recall that the four valves of the heart—aortic,

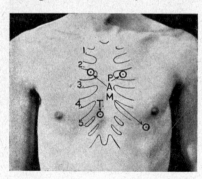

Fig. 112.—Areas of auscultation. The letters indicate the approximate position of the heart valves: P, Pulmonary valve; A, Aortic value; M, Mitral valve; T, Tricuspid valve. The circles indicate the areas at which sounds from these valves are best heard. The ribs are numbered.

pulmonary, tricuspid, and mitral—are situated close together behind the middle of the sternum, and direct auscultation over this area leads to confusion as to which valve is responsible for the sound. To obviate this difficulty the heart is examined at regions some distance from the valve itself, but to which the sound is conducted. The sounds from the mitral valve are conducted towards the cardiac apex, those from the pulmonary valve to the 2nd left intercostal space, those from the aortic valve to the 2nd right intercostal space, and those from the tricuspid valve to the lower end of the sternum at its junction with the 6th right costal cartilage. These regions are, therefore, called respectively the mitral, pulmonary, aortic, and tricuspid areas (*Fig.* 112). *It must be clearly understood that the sounds produced in the heart have a common origin,* and in speaking of the mitral first sound or the aortic second sound, for example, we are merely describing the first and second sounds of the heart as they are heard at the mitral and aortic areas.

How the Heart-sounds are Produced.—The *first sound* is due chiefly to the closure of the mitral and tricuspid valves at the commencement of systole. This valvular element has a somewhat sharp snapping quality, but is toned down by a superadded sound caused by the actual contraction of the ventricular muscle. Even the muscular element of the first sound has two parts—(a) a sharp sound of short duration, and (b) a more prolonged roaring sound, such as may be heard by listening over a contracting muscle.

The *second sound* is probably entirely valvular in origin, caused by the closure of the aortic and pulmonary valves at the commencement of diastole.

A third sound is sometimes heard and may cause confusion in deciding whether or not a mitral diastolic murmur is present.

When these sounds are examined at the four cardiac areas described it is usually found that the *first sound is louder at the apex* and that the *second sound is louder at the base* of the heart. The basal second sound can be further compared at the aortic and pulmonary areas, and the relative intensity will be noticed to vary according to age: *in young persons the pulmonary second sound is louder than the aortic, and vice versa in old age* ; between the two extremes of childhood and old age all grades of sound may be detected, and frequently the second sound is of the same intensity in both areas.

The heart-sounds are usually imitated by the syllables ' *lub-dup* ', the more prolonged ' lub ' of the first sound indicating its combined valvular and muscular nature, the shorter ' dup ' of the second sound pointing to its valvular origin.

Just as the pulse-rate and the blood-pressure should be examined at the end of a consultation as well as at the beginning, in order to exclude the effects of emotion or exercise, so the heart-sounds should be compared at the beginning and end of the examination. If this is done systematically the student will learn that a *considerable modification of the sounds may take place as the result of excitement or physical effort*—both of which tend to make the heart-sounds sharper and louder than normal though the relative intensity of the sounds remains the same, i.e., the first sound is louder at the apex and the second sound at the base.

Normal Rhythm of the Heart-sounds (*Fig.* 113).—In a normal heart the first and second sounds are quite close together but the interval following the second sound is relatively long. The sequence is thus lub-dup-pause, lub-dup-pause. In disease a pendular or ' tic-tac ' rhythm may occur.

Exaggeration of the Sounds.—Exaggerated sounds occur in diseases which increase the excitability of the heart, e.g., neurasthenia, hyperthyroidism, and fevers, and, as in the case of emotion and exercise, increase is most obvious in the first sound at the apex and in the second sound at the base. The first sound is also increased when there is considerable cardiac enlargement, and in mitral stenosis, particularly at the apex. The second sound is increased at the aortic area in atheroma of the aorta, aneurysm, and arterial hypertension. At the pulmonary area the second sound is increased when there is greater tension than normal in the pulmonary circuit, as in pulmonary diseases and mitral stenosis.

Diminution of the Sounds.—Diminution in the heart-sounds is more often due to extra-cardiac than to cardiac causes. Of these, emphysema is one of the most important, as the air-containing lung spreads over the area where the heart normally comes in contact with the chest wall. Similarly, fluid or air in the pleural or pericardial cavities may form a

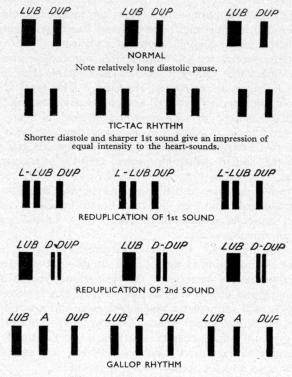

Fig. 113.—Diagram of heart-sounds.

layer preventing the heart-sounds from reaching the surface normally. Until these causes and the physiological ones mentioned earlier have been considered, feebleness of the heart-sounds does not rank as an important sign; but *if the patient has been examined previously and was known to have well-defined heart-sounds which have become feeble, the sign is of more significance*, and may suggest circulatory failure, either due to weakening of the myocardium, or, more commonly, to peripheral vascular failure as in hæmorrhage, infections, etc.

Reduplication of Sounds.—A double sound may be audible in which *the two elements are very close together*. This closeness is an essential character of reduplication, and distinguishes it from various forms of gallop rhythm in which three sounds are present but at considerable intervals one from the other. Reduplication may be imitated by the syllables ' l-lub ' and ' d-dup '. When affecting the first sound it is usually heard best at the apex, and is probably due to an asynchronous closure of the mitral and tricuspid valves. Reduplication of the second sound, commonly found at the base of the heart, is probably due to asynchronous closure of the pulmonary and aortic valves.

Reduplication is not always pathological; it may, for example, be found in the second sound at the base during deep expiration ; but it occurs with greater frequency in pathological conditions, such as delay in auriculo-ventricular conduction, bundle-branch block, and conditions causing increased tension in the pulmonary circuit, such as mitral stenosis and lung diseases. These act either by causing asynchronous contraction of the two ventricles or by altering the relative pressure in the systemic and pulmonary circulations so as to produce asynchronous closure of the valves.

Gallop Rhythm.—When three separate heart-sounds are heard, separated from one another by a considerable interval, gallop rhythm is said to be present; but the resemblance to a gallop can only be appreciated if the heart-rate is increased. There are several distinct types of gallop rhythm, varying with the position of a third sound in relation to the other two. This sound is commonly associated with auricular contraction, and occurs in presystole (presystolic gallop rhythm), but if auriculo-ventricular conduction is delayed (long P.R.) a mid-diastolic gallop appears.

ADDITIONAL SOUNDS

These include the class of sounds known as *murmurs*, originating at the valves or in the great vessels, and *friction sounds* produced in the pericardial layers and in the pleura which lies in close contact with the heart. Peculiar sounds are also heard occasionally due to impact of the heart against surrounding tissues—for example, against fluid in the pleural cavity, or through the diaphragm against the air- and fluid-containing viscera; these sounds have little importance, and, although their origin is often uncertain, they are rarely confused with the murmurs and pericardial sounds to be described.

Pericardial Friction Sounds.—A friction sound or rub is heard in cases of acute pericarditis, and is comparable with a pleural rub. It is produced by the movement of the two layers of pericardium over one another in the presence of an exudate. The sound may be heard over any part of the precordium, and sometimes over so small an area as to be overlooked, whilst at other times it is so extensive as to be present over every part of the heart. *The rub has a peculiar superficial quality, and is sometimes rough and grating in character, and at other times soft and murmuring*, so that it may be confused with the to-and-fro murmur so frequently heard in aortic regurgitation. Not uncommonly pericarditis is associated with pleurisy, and the pericardial friction rub may become continuous with the pleural rub and extend outside the limits of the precordium. In cases of organized pericarditis leading to adherent pericardium creaking sounds are occasionally heard.

Murmurs.—When the position and character of the heart-sounds have been determined the student is in a position to pay attention to any murmurs which may be present.

GENERAL POINTS FOR CONSIDERATION.—The following points should be ascertained whenever a murmur is present:—

1. *The Time Relationship* (*Fig.* 114).—This implies not only whether the murmur occurs in systole or diastole but also whether it occupies a part or the whole of these. Great care is often necessary to time a murmur successfully. If the cardiac impulse is sufficiently great to lift the bell

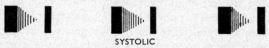

SYSTOLIC

Rough in aortic stenosis; blowing in mitral insufficiency.

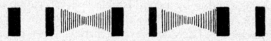

MITRAL DIASTOLIC

Starts shortly after second sound, tends to diminish in intensity in the middle of diastole and increase again before the first sound. If the last part of the murmur is the most obvious and has a barking character it is commonly called a presystolic murmur.

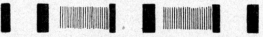

AORTIC DIASTOLIC

This murmur begins at the second sound, which it may replace. It is of fairly equal intensity throughout the greater part of diastole, but sometimes only occupies the first part of the diastole.

Fig. 114.—Diagram of murmurs.

of the stethoscope during systole, this forms an easy way of timing the first sound of the heart and thus of timing the murmur. If the impulse is feeble, reliance must be placed on the pulsation of the carotid artery and allowance made for the fact that this occurs one-tenth of a second later than the actual contraction of the ventricles (*Figs.* 115, 116). Systolic murmurs usually follow the first sound immediately, but diastolic murmurs may appear immediately after the second sound or only after an appreciable interval, and in the case of presystolic murmurs just precede the first sound. It is sometimes almost impossible to time a murmur with certainty, and its position in the cardiac cycle must then be guessed by its character, to which great attention should be paid.

2. *The Character of the Murmur.*—Murmurs may vary from a soft blowing sound to a harsh rasping one. The *loudness of the murmur is no*

criterion of the organic changes in the heart necessary to produce it, and quite soft murmurs may be significant of serious disease, though if the murmur has a harsh rough quality as distinct from loudness, it will more commonly be found to be associated with organic disease of the heart.

3. *Distribution.*—A careful record should be made, preferably in the form of a diagram, of the area over which the murmur is heard and of the *point of maximum intensity*. A record of this kind constitutes a valuable method of assessing the significance of a murmur and its place of production. Associated with this observation there should be noted—

4. *Direction of Spread.*—When the maximum intensity of the murmur has been noted, the stethoscope should be moved radially from this point in different directions to observe whether the murmur is circumscribed

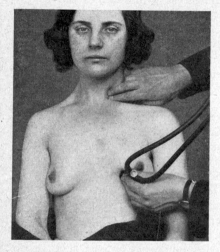

Fig. 115.—Timing murmurs. If the apex beat is not palpable, the heart-sounds and any murmurs may be timed by placing one or two fingers on the carotid artery. Allowance must be made for the fact that the carotid pulsation follows that of the apex beat by approximately $\frac{1}{10}$ sec.

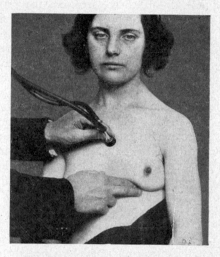

Fig. 116.—Timing murmurs. When the apex beat is palpable the finger may be placed over it. Each systolic rise corresponds with the first sound and the murmur may be timed by this. In this photograph the bell of the stethoscope is placed in position for detecting an aortic diastolic murmur.

or conducted to other parts of the chest wall. *The direction of conduction, or on the contrary the absence of conduction, is characteristic of certain types of murmur.*

5. *Relation to Respiration, Posture, and Exercise.*—Many murmurs, especially functional ones, are modified by *respiration*, often disappearing at the height of inspiration. This is particularly true of pulmonary systolic murmurs, but may occur in the case of mitral systolic murmurs.

The effect of *posture* should be observed, as some murmurs—e.g., an aortic diastolic—are best heard in the erect posture, whilst others— e.g., a mitral diastolic—are heard most clearly when the patient is recumbent.

Again, *exercise* modifies murmurs, and when there is no contra-indication (e.g., active endocarditis or heart failure) the patient should be exercised to increase the heart-rate. Presystolic mitral murmurs are often intensified by such exercise.

CAUSES OF MURMURS.—The ultimate cause of many murmurs is uncertain, but certain broad principles underlie their production. *The principal of these is that a sound is produced when blood passes from a vessel or chamber of smaller calibre to one of greater.* It must be presumed that in a normal heart the chambers bear such a relationship one to the other that the passage of blood through the communicating orifice does not cause a murmur, but if the cavity into which the blood is flowing is enlarged and the orifice remains normal, or conversely if the cavity remains normal and the orifice is narrowed, the result will be a murmur caused by the relative disproportion between the orifice and the cavity into which the blood is pouring. Undoubtedly many accessory factors are also concerned : the vibration of valve cusps, especially if these are thickened by disease, the roughening of the cavity itself as in atheroma of the aorta, the vibrations produced in the chordæ tendineæ and musculi papillares by the eddying blood-stream, may all tend to produce or increase a murmur.

In the past it has been customary to divide murmurs into functional and organic, and to explain many functional murmurs on a basis of altered viscosity of the blood (hæmic murmurs), or even to describe them as accidental. These terms are undesirable as they are without pathological proof. It is preferable to retain the term *functional* for those murmurs which are essentially *physiological*, particularly systolic bruits at the pulmonary area, or for those due to some *temporary disproportion* between the orifice and the chamber which it guards, as in the stretching of the left ventricle occurring in anæmias and infections. In the latter type of case there is no doubt that some degree of mitral regurgitation may take place, but the murmur may be correctly styled functional because there is no actual disease of the valve cusps and because as a rule the murmur is temporary and may well disappear when the conditions producing it are remedied. On the other hand, *in the case of organic murmurs the valve cusps are damaged,* so as to lead either to their fusion (causing *stenosis* of the valve, with *obstruction* to the blood flow) or to their retraction (causing *incompetence* of the valve, with *regurgitation* of the blood), and in the majority of instances these anatomical defects are permanent.

Great care and judgment are necessary to determine the significance of many murmurs. This is particularly so in the case of systolic murmurs, which are often harmless, but may raise suspicion of organic diseases when there is a history of rheumatic infection or when there are associated signs of heart disease.

The decision as to the seriousness of these murmurs is important, for on the one hand the patient may be made into an unnecessary invalid, or on the other an early valvular lesion may be overlooked, and the patient will go untreated.

Diastolic murmurs are simple. Sometimes as in the case of mitral stenosis the murmur alone suffices to make the diagnosis. Similarly the diastolic murmur of aortic incompetence is rare except in that disease, though corroborative vascular phenomena help to complete the picture.

The signs which support a diagnosis of valvular disease are considered elsewhere. It is frequently stated that wide conduction of a murmur, particularly of a mitral systolic murmur, is an indication of its organic nature, and it is therefore necessary to emphasize that *conduction merely depends upon intensity*, and it has already been stated that intensity is no criterion of the degree of deformity of the heart valves. If the patient is exercised it will be realized that *intensity may be increased by an increase in the heart-rate*.

Special details relating to murmurs may now be considered under the headings of the areas of the heart where they are found.

MURMURS AT THE CARDIAC APEX.—

Systolic Murmurs.—Systolic murmurs at the cardiac apex are common, and often difficult to evaluate as indications of organic disease. The murmurs are usually soft in character, and if sufficiently loud are conducted in a characteristic manner towards the axilla and often through to the back at the angle of the left scapula (*Figs.* 117, 118). Very loud murmurs may

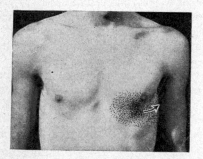

Fig. 117.—Mitral regurgitation. The systolic murmur has a wide area of conduction towards the axilla and back (*see also* Fig. 118).

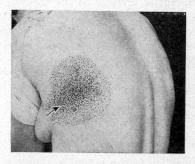

Fig. 118.—Mitral regurgitation. The systolic murmur is often well conducted to the back near the angle of the left scapula.

also spread upwards to the pulmonary and aortic regions and to the right of the sternum. *The majority of these murmurs indicate a slight or great degree of mitral regurgitation, but the murmur itself gives little indication of the degree of leakage.* Probably in a high percentage of cases the degree of leakage is so slight as to be negligible, which justifies the murmur being disregarded, unless there are other signs of heart involvement

The regurgitation may be due to stretching of the mitral orifice as a part of general dilatation of the left ventricle. This occurs in fevers, anæmias, and in conditions such as hypertension, chronic renal disease, and hyperthyroidism, where dilatation and hypertrophy of the left ventricle occur concomitantly. Some of these conditions to a greater or less degree are susceptible of improvement, with a corresponding disappearance of the systolic murmur. The murmur therefore should be described as functional. In most cases the murmur is not conducted to the axilla, but in some it is sufficiently intense for conduction to occur. The diagnosis of the true value of the murmur is made by looking for the causal disease, and, above all, by watching the patient to see if the murmur disappears. If the murmur does not disappear, as may happen for example in dilatation of the left ventricle due to hypertension, the mitral regurgitation remains as a permanent feature of the illness, and the murmur may then be regarded as no less important than if there were damage to the valve cusps.

Systolic murmurs dependent on shrinkage of the cusps of the mitral valve from rheumatic or other infections are essentially the same in character as the so-called functional murmurs. In assigning to them their correct importance much reliance should be placed upon the *history of rheumatic infections*, upon the *size of the heart*, and upon the *presence of any other valvular lesion*; but it must be admitted that it is sometimes impossible to decide whether or not a systolic apical murmur indicates the presence of organic disease of the mitral valve cusps, though the course of the disease and the subsequent development of other evidence of rheumatic damage to the myocardium or valves may establish a correct diagnosis. When it is suspected that a systolic murmur indicates organic mitral regurgitation, a persistent search must be made for *the diastolic murmur of mitral stensosis* which so commonly accompanies the disease.

It only remains to be added that murmurs originating at other areas of the heart may be conducted to the apex and imitate those due to mitral insufficiency.

Diastolic Murmurs.—When a diastolic murmur is heard only at the mitral area it is nearly always due to mitral stensosis of the organic type, in which the valve cusps are fused together and the orifice from the left auricle into the ventricle is narrowed. Only rarely is a diastolic murmur heard when the mitral valve is normal, and in such cases there is general dilatation of the left ventricle, another example of the production of a murmur by a relative disproportion in the size of communicating cavities, in this case the left auricle and left ventricle. This relative type of mitral stensosis may occur in aortic regurgitation (in which the murmur is frequently called, after its describer, the Austin Flint murmur) and in adherent pericardium, two conditions in which a diastolic murmur of this type may be found.

The mitral diastolic murmur is nearly always of low tone and rumbling in character. It is often appreciated with difficulty by the unpractised ear, and to avoid overlooking it the student should examine the patient in the recumbent posture, when it may easily be audible in cases in which it was not apparent erect. The murmur is often intensified when the patient lies on the left side so that the cardiac apex is brought into closer contact with the chest wall. Exercise may also bring out a murmur which is otherwise difficult to hear, and the stethoscope should be applied immediately the patient lies down after the effort, so that the first few heart-beats will not be missed, for it is in these, when the blood velocity is high, that the murmur is generally heard. Diastolic murmurs, in contrast with systolic, are circumscribed, and *often localized* to an area round the apex beat which could be covered by a five-shilling piece (*Fig.* 119). The murmur may commence early in diastole and last its whole length. More commonly it diminishes in mid-diastole, sometimes to increase again towards the end. If the murmur is chiefly late diastolic and becomes continuous with an accentuated first sound, it has an

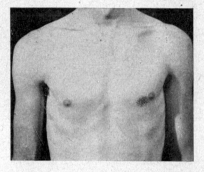

apparently crescendo character and is often called a *presystolic murmur*, though in reality it is only a part of a longer diastolic murmur. Before making a diagnosis of mitral stenosis on the presence of a presystolic murmur the observer should listen most carefully for the low-toned rumble which is generally present in other parts of diastole.

MURMURS AT THE AORTIC AREA.— *Systolic Murmurs.*—Systolic murmurs are very common at the aortic area, and are usually associated with

Fig. 119.—Mitral stenosis. Diastolic and presystolic murmurs. The murmur is localized usually just internal to the left nipple.

a slight dilatation of the aorta without any abnormality of the aortic valve or orifice. This occurs particularly in elderly persons with atheromatous changes in the aorta, and in association with aortic regurgitation when the wall of the aorta loses its tone and is stretched. The murmur in these cases is generally *soft and blowing*, and not uncommonly associated with similar murmurs over other areas of the heart. *It has no serious pathological significance.* A similar murmur may be heard in the extreme dilatation of aneurysm of the aorta.

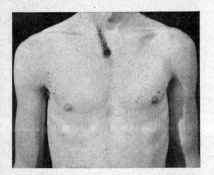

Fig. 120. Aortic stenosis. Area of thrill and murmur. The murmur is maximum over the aortic area, but is conducted upwards into the right carotid artery.

Of an entirely different kind is the systolic murmur of *aortic stenosis*, which is *harsh* in character, *conducted upwards* into the great vessels of the neck, and usually *accompanied by a thrill* (*Fig.* 120). The student should be cautious in making a diagnosis of aortic stenosis unless these characteristics are present, as systolic murmurs at the aortic area are much more commonly of the functional

9

type. If the stenosis produces much narrowing of the valvular opening, an anacrotic or plateau type of pulse will be present (*see* p. 106), without which some authorities consider a diagnosis of aortic stenosis cannot be made.

Diastolic Murmurs.—These are rarely found at the aortic area except in *aortic regurgitation.* The murmur is soft and blowing in character and is heard over a large area of the chest wall. It is propagated characteristic-

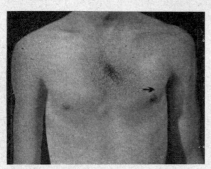

ally down the sternum and towards the apex beat. In the aortic area itself it is often faint and difficult to hear, and it reaches its *maximum intensity about the middle of the sternum* at its left border (*Fig.* 121). It may be well heard over the apex or even in the axilla, but can generally be distinguished from a diastolic murmur of mitral origin by its soft character. In listening for this murmur the student should *examine the patient in an erect posture,* and should auscultate systematically from the second right costal cartilage down the sternum and towards the apex beat.

Fig. 121.—Aortic regurgitation. The diastolic murmur is of maximum intensity about the middle of the sternum at its left border. The area of conduction is often wide, and, as indicated by the arrow, may extend towards the axilla.

A similar murmur has been reported by some authorities in cases of severe anæmia and in high blood-pressure, but such causes are extremely rare.

MURMURS AT THE PULMONARY AREA.—

Systolic Murmurs.—Systolic murmurs over the pulmonary area may be similar in character to those over the aortic zone, namely, soft and blowing. *They occur with great frequency in perfectly healthy individuals,* and are probably due to some physiological alteration in the tension in the pulmonary circuit due to respiration. The murmur is most marked when the patient is lying down. Pathological conditions which increase the tension in the pulmonary circuit— e.g., mitral disease and emphysema— aggravate the murmur. The murmur of *congenital pulmonary stenosis* (*Fig.* 122) is comparable with the murmur of aortic stenosis, as it is *loud, rasping,* and usually *accompanied by a thrill.*

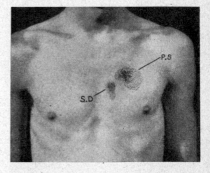

Fig. 122.—Murmurs of congenital heart disease. P.S., Pulmonary stenosis; S.D., Septal defects (generally patency of interventricular septum). These murmurs are systolic in time.

Diastolic Murmurs.—At the pulmonary area diastolic murmurs are very uncommon, and in many cases confused with those of a similar character at the aortic area. Such a murmur occasionally occurs in mitral stenosis (Graham Steel murmur), and very rarely in congenital heart disease.

MURMURS AT THE TRICUSPID AREA.—Murmurs at the tricuspid area are so commonly associated and confused with those arising from mitral disease that their discovery as a rule does not yield much useful information. Systolic murmurs may be present at the lower end of the sternum in tricuspid regurgitation, and diastolic murmurs of a low rumbling type may occur in tricuspid stenosis, but diagnosis is always difficult.

OTHER MURMURS.—Sometimes murmurs are found which do not correspond with any of the valvular areas. *In these cases the possibility of congenital heart disease always arises.* Systolic murmurs midway between the pulmonary and mitral areas, i.e., over the 3rd and 4th left inter-spaces, may be present in cases of pulmonary stenosis when the obstruction is near the origin of the artery from the right ventricle, and in cases of patency of the interventricular septum (*Fig.* 122). These *murmurs are nearly always rough, and generally accompanied by a thrill.* A murmur occupying both systole and diastole, and closely resembling the systolic and diastolic murmurs of aortic regurgitation, may sometimes be found over the base of the heart equally

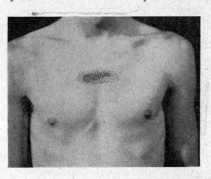

Fig. 123.—Patent ductus arteriosus. Continuous murmur in systole and diastole audible from aortic to pulmonary area.

intense in the aortic and pulmonary zones. This murmur is characteristic of a *patent ductus arteriosus* (*Fig.* 123). Murmurs may have a *vascular* origin. They are usually systolic in time and blowing in character, and may be heard over an engorged thyroid gland, over vascular tumours in the thorax, and over aneurysm of the aorta or other large vessels. Diastolic murmurs are less commonly found, but may be present in aortic regurgitation, particularly over the femoral arteries (Duroziez's murmur). The *bruit de diable* is the name given to a continuous venous hum sometimes heard over the neck in profound anæmias, especially of the hypochromic type.

SPECIAL INVESTIGATIONS

The special investigations include instrumental examination by means of the electrocardiograph, sphygmograph, polygraph, and the sphygmomanometer, and also X-ray examination. (*See* Chapters XII-XIV.)

THE DIAGNOSIS OF CARDIO-VASCULAR DISEASES

It is convenient to deal with the diagnosis of cardio-vascular disease under two headings : (1) Structural defects ; (2) Derangements of function. These are commonly found together, but one may occur without the other.

1. STRUCTURAL DEFECTS

Diseases of the cardio-vascular system producing anatomical changes may affect (a) the pericardium, (b) the heart muscle, (c) the valves, (d) the blood-vessels. The majority of them result from inflammatory or degenerative processes, and the signs by which they may be recognized overlap to a considerable extent.

The Pericardium.—

*Pericarditis.—*Inflammation of the pericardium is recognized in its acute stage by the *friction rub* already described. This usually appears during the course of an acute infection, especially rheumatic fever, but also in pneumonia, tuberculosis, and other conditions. It may be a terminal event as in chronic renal disease. The rub is usually discovered as a result of routine examination in these conditions, rather than by any special complaint of the patient, though in some cases there may be pain, especially if the diaphragm or pleura is involved in the inflammatory process.

*Pericardial Effusion.—*Some increase in pericardial fluid occurs in most cases of acute pericarditis, but may only be discovered on routine examination, and may not cause symptoms. If the tension is high, resulting in increased venous and lowered arterial pressure (tamponade), severe dyspnœa occurs.

The most important signs are: (1) An increase in *cardiac dullness* without a corresponding displacement of the apex beat. The dullness may assume an inverted pear-shaped outline in the erect posture, or globoid in recumbency, and extends into the 2nd or even 1st left interspace as much as 2 in. to the left. The basal dullness, where the effusion surrounds the great vessels, may shift with change in posture. (2) *Feebleness of the cardiac impulse* and faintness of the heart-sounds because of the separation of the impulse from the chest wall by the fluid. (3) With a large effusion, *collapse of the lung* in its left lower lobe, producing an area of dullness, bronchial breathing, and bronchophony or ægophony. Narrowing of the subcostal angle during inspiration (Hoover's sign) may also occur. (4) Pulsus paradoxus (p. 109).

Radiology confirms the heart and fluid outlines and should always be employed if possible.

*Adherent Pericardium.—*Following acute pericarditis, adhesions may partially or completely obliterate the pericardial sac and may attach the heart to surrounding mediastinal structures.

In spite of this, few signs may appear and the diagnosis is always uncertain. Amongst suggestive signs should be included immobility of the cardiac impulse (on change of posture) and great systolic retraction of the intercostal spaces.

*Constrictive Pericarditis.—*This is generally non-rheumatic and insidious in onset. It is often associated with mediastinitis, to which some of the symptoms and signs are due.

The most important signs are *intense venous congestion* with liver enlargement and ascites, in a patient in whom no valvular disease or cardiac enlargement is found. The degree of dyspnœa is relatively slight. As with adherent pericardium, systolic retraction, immobility of the cardiac impulse, and pulsus paradoxus may occur, but are of less importance than the congestive signs.

The Myocardium.—There is no conclusive symptom or sign of myocardial disease. When such exists, it is commonly associated with other cardio-vascular defects as in rheumatic carditis and coronary ischæmia. Symptoms of myocardial weakness more commonly result from an increased burden borne by the heart, as in high degrees of tachycardia, valvular disease, and hypertension, rather than from any essential change in the structure of the heart muscle, though this may exist concomitantly.

Suggestions of myocardial weakness (whether due to myocardial disease or increased load) are to be found in the presence of *pulsus alternans* and *gallop rhythm*, which sooner or later are associated with clear evidence of heart failure—especially left ventricular failure. Indications of structural changes in the myocardium are sometimes revealed by the electrocardiogram, as in bundle branch block and inversion of T I and II, and such signs may be of value in pointing to the cardiac origin of symptoms such as dyspnœa or pain.

Beyond this it is not possible to go in the diagnosis of myocardial disease save under two special circumstances : (1) Cardiac infarction due to coronary thrombosis ; (2) Acute myocarditis, commonly the result of diphtheria, but occasionally arising from other infections.

Cardiac Infarction.—The cardinal symptom of this condition—anginal pain—has already been considered (p. 97). It only remains to add that whilst the pain is usually severe, it may be slight. It is of variable duration, minutes to several days, but generally about twenty-four hours and nearly always longer than in other forms of angina. It is often accompanied by collapse, shown by pallor, sweating, a feeble pulse, and falling blood-pressure, and sometimes by vomiting.

The infarct in contact with the pericardium may result in an area of pericarditis with its sign—a friction rub—and the inflammatory processes in the myocardium may be evidenced by slight pyrexia and leucocytosis. These signs usually appear 2–3 days after the coronary thrombosis.

In some instances cardiac failure, especially of the left ventricular type, results, and more rarely the weakened area of heart muscle bulges to form an aneurysm which can be recognized radiologically.

Acute Myocarditis.—During the course of diphtheria or, less commonly, other infections (e.g., pneumonia, typhoid, septicæmias, etc.) myocarditis may be suspected by the onset of precordial oppression, rapid feeble pulse with a fall of blood-pressure, or bradycardia and cardiac dilatation. Confirmatory signs may be found in the electrocardiogram, especially in those cases with bradycardia which prove to be due to heart-block. Transient auricular fibrillation may occur. Diagnosis, which is difficult, may be made more certain by the development of signs of cardiac failure.

The Valves.—Endocarditis, or inflammation of the endocardium, results in deformities of the valves, causing incompetence of the valve or narrowing (stenosis) of the orifice guarded by the valve. Incompetence causes regurgitation of blood through an orifice which should be closed. Stenosis impedes the entry of blood into the chamber guarded by the affected valve. Any of the valves may become incompetent or stenosed, but especially the mitral and aortic valves.

The diagnosis of valvular diseases depends above all on auscultation, which reveals the characteristic murmurs and alteration of sounds already described. *Thrills* frequently accompany the murmurs.

Confirmatory evidence is furnished by *enlargement of the heart* due to the extra work put upon it by the valvular defect, and it may be possible to suspect which valve is involved from the type of cardiac enlargement. Disease of the aortic valve imposes more strain on the left ventricle, disease of the mitral valve on the left auricle and right ventricle, and some information on the *type of enlargement* may be gained by careful inspection, palpation, and percussion.

Supplementary evidence of valvular disease is found in the character of the *pulse*—for example, the collapsing pulse and capillary pulsation of aortic regurgitation, the anacrotic pulse of aortic stenosis, and the small thin pulse of mitral stenosis.

The most important valvular lesions are : (*a*) Mitral stenosis ; (*b*) Mitral regurgitation ; (*c*) Aortic regurgitation ; (*d*) Aortic stenosis.

a. Mitral Stenosis.—Diagnosed by the presence of a mitral diastolic murmur with accentuation of the mitral first sound. Confirmatory signs are the enlargement of the heart transversely, and, when present, the mitral facies (*see Fig.* 90, p. 102). The radiograph may show enlargement of the left auricular and prominence of the pulmonary arc. Electrocardiograms often exhibit right ventricular preponderance and split P waves. These graphic signs may be helpful in doubtful cases, but the diastolic murmur remains the only certain diagnostic sign.

b. Mitral Regurgitation.—Often accompanies mitral stenosis; diagnosed by the presence of a mitral systolic bruit conducted to the axilla, and enlargement of the heart. The difficulties of diagnosis between mitral regurgitation due to disease of the valve cusps, and to relative incompetence from stretching of the mitral ring, have been discussed under systolic murmurs.

c. Aortic Regurgitation.—Characterized by an aortic diastolic bruit of classical distribution. The corroborative signs in aortic regurgitation are of great value, especially the collapsing pulse, capillary pulsation, and undue pulsation of the large arteries. The heart is enlarged, principally downwards and to the left. The enlargement is confirmed by X rays, in which the left ventricle is characteristically rounded. Electrocardiography usually shows left ventricular preponderance.

d. Aortic Stenosis.—Quite a rare lesion as compared with the other valvular diseases described. The diagnosis should not be made without the presence of the rough systolic bruit conducted into the neck, and the presence either of a thrill or an anacrotic pulse or both. Aortic regurgitation of some degree generally accompanies stenosis.

Congenital Lesions.—The diagnosis of congenital lesions, like valvular disease, depends partly upon auscultation. Brief reference has already been made to some of the characteristic murmurs. It must be emphasized that no murmurs need be present even in serious congenital defects. What is more important than the anatomical diagnosis is the functional incapacity produced by the lesion, and this can be more correctly gauged by the exhibition of dyspnœa, cyanosis, clubbing of the fingers, and general under-development, than by the presence of murmurs.

Bacterial Endocarditis.—This must receive special consideration if a valvular lesion is found. It is suggested by the association of valvular murmurs with signs of septicæmia, notably splenic enlargement, pyrexia, anæmia, finger-clubbing, embolic manifestations, and the discovery of organisms in the blood-stream (blood-culture). These signs are present in varying combinations.

The Arteries.—Three conditions need mention : (*a*) Arteriosclerosis ; (*b*) Aneurysm ; (*c*) High blood-pressure.

a. Arteriosclerosis.—Arteriosclerosis produces thickening and tortuos-ity of the peripheral vessels, which may be recognized as described on p. 109 in the radial, brachial, retinal, and other vessels. When it is dis-covered in one group of vessels it should be sought in others, as the more generalized its distribution the more significant it becomes.

Atheroma, the special variety of arteriosclerosis which affects the large vessels, particularly the aorta, shows few characteristic signs, but accentuation of the aortic second sound may be of importance in the absence of high blood-pressure.

b. Aneurysm.—Aneurysm is a dilatation of an artery, usually a large one. The aorta is most commonly involved, and may be uniformly dilated or present a

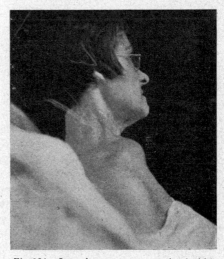

Fig. 124.—Innominate aneurysm associated with diffuse aortic dilatation and aortic regurgitation.

bulging tumour of its wall which causes pressure on the surrounding structures. By these pressure signs (e.g., engorged veins in the neck or on the chest wall, sympathetic paralysis, etc.) it is more often recognized than by any of the usual symptoms or signs of heart disease. (*Fig.* 124.)

c. High Blood-pressure.—Careful observation of the blood-pressure should be made in all cases of cardio-vascular disease, and it is important not to rely on a single reading, as a considerable increment—of the systolic blood-pressure in particular—may follow emotion or effort. The dia-stolic blood-pressure is more stable, and therefore of greater significance when it is abnormal. High blood-pressure may be a symptom of several diseases, the most important being chronic renal disease and (systolic rise only) aortic regurgitation. On the other hand, it may occur as an isolated abnormality (*hyperpiesis*), changes in the heart or other organs being secondary thereto. The blood-pressure may be considered *high when the systolic pressure is persistently over* 150 *mm. Hg, or the diastolic over* 100 *mm. Hg.* Although a rough estimate of the blood-pressure may be gained by palpation (*see* p. 105), the sphygmomanometer (*see* p. 105) should be used in every case when a rise of pressure is suspected.

2. DISORDERS OF HEART FUNCTION

Unlike the lungs, the heart may be subject to disturbance of function with little or no anatomical change. This is seen in the *arrhythmias*, or abnormal rhythms, which, although commonly associated with pathological changes in the heart muscle, may occur quite independently. *Cardiac failure* is also a disturbance of function, but is almost invariably dependent upon structural defects.

Abnormal Rhythms

Many abnormal rhythms can be identified with reasonable certainty by skilful examination of the pulse, but some are very confusing and require not only examination of the pulse and heart, but graphic methods, for their elucidation. The more important disturbances of the heart rhythm and rate are :—

1. **Extrasystoles** (premature or ectopic beats).—These are extra contractions of the heart arising away from the normal pace-maker (sino-auricular node) and interrupting the normal rhythm. As they occur prematurely before the ventricles have received their full quota of blood, the beats are small. They are generally followed by a long pause until the next normal beat. These points are appreciated by feeling the pulse, but sometimes the beat is not sufficiently strong to produce a pulse-wave, yet the heart-sounds corresponding with it may be heard.

The most characteristic feature of extrasystoles is that they are not present all the time, though if very numerous they may appear to be, and may then imitate other irregularities, especially auricular fibrillation. They have no serious significance, and tend to *disappear when the heart-rate is increased* by suitable exercise.

2. **Auricular Fibrillation.**—In this condition the auricles cease to beat properly, and produce minute contractions or 'fibrillations' at an average rate of 400 per minute which evoke an irregular response in the A.V. node. In its turn this causes irregular action of the ventricles. The results are shown in a *complete irregularity of the pulse and apex beat*, manifested by a variation in the size of the beats and in the interval between them. Auricular fibrillation generally occurs with other serious heart disease, e.g., valvular or myocardial affections, but may occur alone. It is most commonly associated with mitral stenosis and thyrotoxicosis.

The rate is generally rapid, and some of the beats may not be strong enough to open the aortic valves and allow transmission to the pulse. In such cases the ventricular rate will be greater than the pulse-rate, and in fibrillation *reliance should be placed on the heart-rate rather than the pulse-rate*.

3. Auricular Flutter.—Comparable in many ways with auricular fibrillation, flutter may exist along with other forms of heart disease, or be an isolated manifestation.

The auricles beat at a great rate (240-400), and owing to the limited conductile power of the A.V. bundle the ventricles can only respond to a smaller number of these contractions (2 : 1, 3 : 1, 4 : 1), usually half. *Flutter may be suspected clinically when a high regular ventricular rate* (120 *to* 200) *persists for a long time* (weeks or months). The usual ventricular rate is 160 or less, and this can be temporarily slowed by pressure over the carotid sinus (carotid artery at the angle of the jaw).

Occasionally the rapid contractions of the auricles communicate a pulsation to the jugular veins at a greater rate (usually twice) than that at which the ventricles are beating. Sudden doubling or halving of the ventricular rate is strongly suggestive.

4. Paroxysmal Tachycardia.—The heart beats regularly at a high rate (150 to 200, commonly over 160), and the condition may be mistaken for auricular flutter, but apart from the *higher ventricular rate* the condition is of much *shorter duration than flutter*. Its duration is usually minutes, and attacks may be stopped by simple measures such as a change of posture, or pressure over the carotid sinus or eyeball.

One of the most important signs is the *characteristic sudden onset and offset*, a sign which also applies in the case of flutter.

When the patient is not seen during an attack, great attention should be paid to the story of the mode of onset and offset, and the circumstances under which the attacks appear. Abnormal rhythms (paroxysmal tachycardia and flutter) are unexpected and unexplained, whereas simple tachycardia is often expected and provoked by emotion or exercise.

5. Simple Tachycardia.—It has already been observed that tachycardia may be produced in normal individuals by emotion, exercise, fevers, toxæmias—especially thyrotoxicosis—and other causes, and the pulse-rate may be as high as is found in paroxysmal tachycardia or auricular flutter, but rarely remains more than 140 when the patient is at rest.

In distinguishing simple tachycardia from abnormal rhythms, such as flutter or paroxysmal tachycardia, the student should *note that exercise, emotion, and other causes influencing a simple tachycardia do not alter the heart-rate in abnormal rhythms*.

6. Bradycardia.—A slow heart-rate—simple bradycardia—like tachycardia, may occur in perfect health, and is common in old people. Rates of 60 are common, and they may even be as low as 50.

Various non-cardiac conditions may be responsible for temporary bradycardia, notably the after-effects of febrile illnesses such as influenza and pneumonia, jaundice, increased intracranial pressure such as occurs in cerebral tumour, and syncope.

The most important cardiac condition in which bradycardia occurs is *heart-block*, a condition of diminished conductivity in the bundle of His which partially or completely cuts off the ventricles from auricular influence (partial or complete heart-block). The result is a *higher auricular than ventricular rate*, the latter usually varying between 30 and 50 according to the degree of block. In complete block the ventricles beat quite regularly at about 30, and this rhythm is not usually influenced by exercise, emotion, etc.; but in partial heart-block irregular action may be present, and the rate may be suddenly increased (generally doubled) by exercise.

Bradycardia (50 to 60) is also found in aortic stenosis and in high blood-pressure where the peripheral resistance is increased.

From this description of cardiac arrhythmias the student will appreciate that in every case where the heart-rate or rhythm appears abnormal, it is essential to observe carefully :—

1. *The rate at the pulse and apex beat.*
2. *The variation of these with exercise and excitement.*
3. *The mode of onset and offset of the attacks, preferably by observation; if not, from the history.*
4. *The presence of any jugular pulsations and their rate.*

Heart Failure

The examination of a heart case is not complete when a diagnosis of valvular, myocardial, or other disease has been made. The most important question still remains to be answered, namely—What is the heart's capacity for work? This question has been partially discussed in describing the symptoms of heart disease, *especially breathlessness, which, when it occurs without the customary degree of effort, is the earliest indication of cardiac failure*. Later, objective signs appear which are usually of serious import. They result from failure of the ventricles to discharge their contents adequately into the systemic and pulmonary circulations. As a result the heart is unable to receive back from the systemic and pulmonary veins the optimum amount of blood.

In general the heart fails as a whole, i.e., both left and right ventricles, but in many cases the burden is laid on one ventricle more than the other, at least for a time. It is thus customary to speak of left and right heart failure.

Left Ventricular Failure.—This is liable to occur in the increased load which the ventricle must bear in hypertension, severe arteriosclerosis, and myocardial infarction. The left ventricle fails to discharge its contents successfully and the blood from the left auricle (and pulmonary veins) cannot be accommodated. The right ventricle continues to pump blood into the lungs. Pulmonary congestion results.

The failure is often relatively sudden. Paroxysmal dyspnœa (p. 96) and clinical signs of pulmonary congestion and œdema, cough, laboured breathing, and râles at the base appear. There is little or no venous congestion. Death may occur rapidly in severe cases.

Right Ventricular Failure.—This form of failure is usually produced more gradually and occurs especially in mitral stenosis (because of pulmonary congestion), and in respiratory diseases (e.g., emphysema and pulmonary fibrosis) which cause extra work for the right ventricle.

It is this form of failure which is chiefly responsible for the common *congestive heart failure*, which is a later feature of so many types of heart disease.

Congestion is apparent in several ways. It is seen in the engorged external veins (p. 112), in the enlarged, tender, and pulsating liver (p. 187), in impairment of renal function shown by oliguria and concentrated urine, and in cardiac œdema. Breathlessness is common and severe but is chiefly precipitated by exertion or assumption of the recumbent posture. Signs of pulmonary congestion may be present, but are not so constant or rapidly produced as in left ventricular failure.

These two types of failure, as previously mentioned, are commonly found together, but in varying degrees, and any attempt to separate them strictly would be artificial.

Both types of failure may disappear with treatment, leaving the causal state behind, but the failure may be repeated from time to time.

PERIPHERAL VASCULAR DISORDERS

Under this heading are included several diseases the aetiology of which is incompletely understood. For a time some of them were described as vasomotor neuroses, or trophoneuroses, but recent work has shown them to be largely independent of the nervous system and essentially vascular in origin.

The more familiar examples are Raynaud's disease, erythromelalgia, thrombo-angiitis obliterans, and angioneurotic œdema, though many other varieties are described.

Raynaud's Disease.—This condition generally appears in young adult life and is commoner in women. The symptoms and signs depend upon arterial spasm in the extremities, especially in the fingers and toes, but occasionally in the nose, ears, etc. The spasm is *precipitated by cold*.

Four stages are described :—

1. *Local Syncope.*—The part has a waxy pallor. This may last minutes to hours. Slight pain may be present.

2. *Asphyxia.*—The part is blue to bluish-black in colour, very painful, and sometimes accompanied by the fourth stage—gangrene. This stage may last hours or days.

3. *Hyperæmia.*—In recovering from Stages 1 or 2 the part becomes red, hot, and painful. The vessels pulsate.

4. *Gangrene.*—Small patches of gangrene may occur after prolonged asphyxia. The gangrene is usually dry, but little blisters filled with fluid may precede its appearance. The resulting loss of tissue is usually

slight and affects the terminal portions of the extremities, especially the fingers (*Fig.* 125).

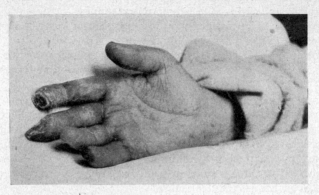

Fig. 125.—Gangrene due to Raynaud's disease.

In many cases of Raynaud's disease only the first stage is reached, and only in the severe forms is gangrene seen.

Erythromelalgia.—In this rarer disease the symptoms and signs are somewhat similar to those of the second stage of Raynaud's disease. The *feet* are most commonly affected, especially the ball of the great toe. The attack generally comes on when the part is exposed to *heat*. Severe pain is followed by local swelling, redness, and pulsation of the vessels. The pain is increased by dependency of the parts. The attack lasts minutes to hours.

Thrombo-angiitis Obliterans.—This is a disease of the blood-vessels, especially affecting men past middle life, and commoner in Jews and heavy smokers. The legs are generally involved and the patient experiences pain on walking, particularly in the calf muscles—*intermittent claudication*—or if arterial obstruction is pronounced, spontaneous pain may occur, followed in some cases by gangrene of part of the limb.

The skin shows important changes, particularly reduction of temperature, pallor in recumbency, or congestion and cyanosis when the limb is dependent. Trophic changes, e.g., shininess of the skin or loss of hair, may also occur. The pulsation in the arteries (dorsalis pedis and posterior tibial) may be diminished or absent. There is also a tendency to venous thrombosis.

Angioneurotic Œdema.—This malady is important because it may be mistaken for other conditions of which œdema is a symptom, e.g., acute nephritis and insect bites. The essential sign is the sudden appearance of pale or pink swellings in different parts of the body, sometimes on the arm or leg, on the lips or eyelids, or on the genitalia. The swellings differ from urticaria in the absence of itching, and from ordinary œdema in the absence of pitting. Serious complications occasionally arise from a visceral distribution of the œdema, especially when it affects the glottis, causing asphyxia.

CHAPTER V

THE URINARY SYSTEM

SYMPTOMS OF URINARY DISEASE

THE symptoms suggestive of urinary disease include : (1) Variation from the normal emptying time of the bladder—most commonly this means increased *frequency* of micturition, less often decreased frequency ; (2) Alteration in amount of urine ; (3) Alteration in appearance of urine ; (4) Difficulty with micturition (dysuria) ; (5) Pain—renal, vesical, or urethral ; (6) General symptoms such as œdema, headache, and vomiting due to the effects of abnormal renal function.

1. Variation from the Normal Emptying Time.—The number of times that urine is passed varies considerably in normal individuals, but micturition usually takes place every three or four hours in the day and perhaps once at night. Departure from the individual normal may be significant.

Frequency results from irritation of the bladder due to local conditions in this organ—e.g., stone, cystitis, or irritation by extrinsic pressure ; or from irritation caused by abnormal constituents of the urine—e.g., highly acid urine, blood, and pus. Frequency is, therefore, a common symptom of such diseases as pyelitis and nephritis, in which abnormal constituents are passing from the kidney into the bladder. Polyuria may also lead to frequency, especially in chronic renal disease (arteriosclerotic types) and diabetes.

The reverse state, decrease in the frequency with which urine is passed, is met with in conditions causing partial or complete retention of urine in the bladder—e.g., severe lesions of the spinal cord such as myelitis and spinal compression, and sometimes when the actual secretion of urine is diminished (oliguria or anuria).

2. Alteration in the Amount of Urine.—The urine may be increased (*polyuria*), or diminished (*oliguria*), or absent (*anuria*).

Polyuria.—Large quantities of urine may be passed as a temporary phenomenon as a result of the ingestion of large quantities of liquid, especially when these contain diuretic principles, e.g., tea, coffee, or alcohol. Polyuria may also result from nervousness, e.g., during medical examination. Polyuria of this type has no pathological significance, but when persistent it is a symptom of great importance. In chronic renal disease it is nearly always present owing to failure of the kidney concentration power. It is also found in *diabetes mellitus* in direct proportion to the thirst, and in diabetes insipidus owing to a failure of the normal regulation of water excretion.

Oliguria and Anuria.—These symptoms are grades of the same condition, namely, a decrease in the secretion of urine. The decrease may occur in *acute nephritis*, and in chronic forms of nephritis as a terminal symptom. It may also appear suddenly after severe operations, especially on the kidney or bladder, and in other conditions of shock. Oliguria has already been mentioned as a symptom of *cardiac failure*. The amount of urine may decrease to a few ounces daily or be completely suppressed. Oliguria and anuria must be carefully distinguished from retention, in which urine is present in the bladder but cannot be voided.

3. **Alteration in the Appearance of the Urine.**—This is considered more fully under the examination of the urine (p. 148 and Chapter XIV). It is only necessary here to point out that the patient may first suspect urinary disease by noticing alteration in the colour and general appearance of the urine, e.g., red in hæmaturia, or cloudy in pyuria.

4. **Dysuria (Difficulty in Micturition).**—Difficulty in micturition may be experienced without pain, though the two symptoms are often found together. The patient may complain of diminution in the force or size of the urinary stream, often culminating in complete *retention*. Dysuria may occur in local conditions of the bladder and surrounding organs which weaken the bladder wall or cause obstruction at its outlet into the urethra. Muscular weakness, for example, may occur in old age or in defective innervation of the bladder resulting from serious nervous diseases such as myelitis. Obstruction is often caused by enlargement of the prostate and stricture of the urethra.

5. **Pain.**—The purely medical diseases of the kidney are frequently unaccompanied by pain. Thus *in most forms of nephritis pain is either absent* or scarcely amounts to more than a dull ache in the lumbar regions.

Pain is particularly associated with any obstruction of the ureter, either at its origin in the pelvis of the kidney, during its course in the abdomen, or at its entrance into the bladder. Obstruction may be caused by stones, or by solid material such as blood or pus in urinary infections. An obstruction of uncertain nature is present in hydronephrosis ; hence pain is also common in this condition. Only rarely is the obstruction caused by stricture or kinking of the ureter (e.g., by an aberrant renal artery). In all such instances the characteristic pain of *renal colic* may be present. This consists of intense sharp pain generally referred in the first place to the lumbar region, radiating forwards into the abdomen and downwards into the groin, the testicle, or the thigh. Vomiting and great prostation generally accompany these attacks, which may last for several hours, especially when calculus is the cause of the obstruction. Movement generally aggravates the pain. Between attacks of renal colic a dull ache may be present in the loin, said to be due to swelling of the kidney with distension of its capsule.

Pain from diseases of the bladder is comparable with renal colic, generally occurring when the bladder holds solid material such as stones, pus, or blood, and endeavours to pass these through the urethra. The pain in this case is referred to the lower abdomen, to the perineum, and in the male to the glans penis.

6. General Symptoms.—

a. Renal Œdema.—In acute nephritis and in the more insidious forms (subacute nephritis and nephrosis) œdema is often the first symptom to be noticed by the patient or his relatives. In acute nephritis the œdema may be slight and short-lived, chiefly occurring in the face, ankles, and hands. In subacute nephritis and nephrosis, the œdema may be generalized, extreme, and long-standing. The cause of renal œdema is not yet fully understood. In the early stages it is undoubtedly due to disturbance of water and salt excretion, perhaps because of a lowering of glomerular pressure in the kidney. In the more chronic cases this is aggravated by a reduction of the amount of protein in the blood-plasma. The plasma protein is depleted by prolonged albuminuria, and this leads to a reduction in the colloid osmotic pressure of the plasma and so to increased transudation of fluid into the tissues. Renal œdema thus tends to be generalized, and not confined to the dependent parts as in heart disease, though in long-standing cases the effect of gravity is apparent and the œdema is more marked in the lower parts. Renal œdema is also more noticeable in the mornings, whereas in cardiac cases it is worse at the end of the day.

b. Symptoms due to High Blood-pressure.—Many of the symptoms occurring in renal disease are really symptoms of high blood-pressure. In acute nephritis there is often a sharp rise of blood-pressure in the early stages, so that headache is common, and symptoms of cardiac failure (dyspnœa, pulmonary œdema, or anginal pain) may occur. The *convulsions* which occasionally take place during the acute stage are also probably related to the high blood-pressure. They are not of uræmic origin. Chronic renal disease is nearly always associated with a persistently high blood-pressure, which accounts for the attacks of severe headache and vomiting which occur.

In some cases the hypertension gives rise to cardiac failure with its associated symptoms, including œdema of cardiac type.

The retinal changes (*see* p. 145) which have so long been considered to be due to renal disease are now known to be related to the high blood-pressure. In advanced cases of retinitis vision becomes blurred and may fail completely. Temporary attacks of blindness (formerly known as uræmic amaurosis) may occur without obvious retinal changes. These are probably due to cerebral vascular spasm

c. Symptoms of Uræmia.—True uræmia is a state of chemical poisoning due to failure of the kidney to excrete toxic waste products of metabolism. In this state the patient develops nausea and anorexia, and later persistent vomiting. Loss of weight and dehydration are evident and acidosis may give rise to severe dyspnœa. Eventually drowsiness and coma, mental confusion, sometimes mania, supervene. There may be convulsions as a terminal phenomenon. The symptoms of uræmia may result from any gradually destructive bilateral disease of the kidneys.

These chronic cases are rarely associated with generalized œdema, though some œdema of the conjunctivæ and eyelids may be noted (*Fig.* 126). Such cases are nearly always accompanied by high blood-pressure, and it may be difficult or impossible without investigating the blood chemistry to decide whether symptoms such as headache and vomiting are due to hypertension or uræmia.

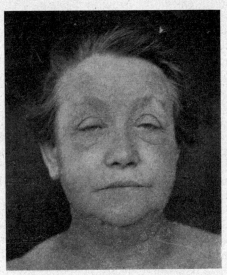

Fig. 126.—Chronic renal disease. Showing the characteristic puffy eyelids (œdema) and 'watery' conjunctivæ—the 'tear that never drops'.

PHYSICAL SIGNS : EXAMINATION OF THE URINARY SYSTEM

The examination of the urinary system comprises the following routine procedure :—

1. *General examination* of the patient, with particular attention to the cardio-vascular system, nervous system, and retinæ.

2. *Examination of the abdomen* to detect any enlargement of the kidneys or any tenderness over these or over the ureters or bladder. Occasionally it may be possible to palpate a thickened ureter or tumours arising from the bladder. The external genitalia should also be examined especially for evidence of tuberculous or syphilitic infiltration of the epididymis or testicle, and for present or past signs of gonorrhœa or syphilis.

3. *Examination of the pelvic organs* through the rectum or vagina.

4. *Examination of the urine* by chemical and microscopical methods.

1. GENERAL EXAMINATION

The presence or absence of *œdema* should be noted in every case. The colour of the patient is important, as anæmia is a common secondary effect of nephritis. Undue dryness of the skin and hæmorrhages should also be noted, as they are common in uræmia. In these cases the skin often has a dirty brownish appearance like fading sunburn. This is probably due to failure of excretion of urinary pigments.

In the examination of the *cardio-vascular system* it is necessary to look for arteriosclerosis, high blood-pressure, and cardiac enlargement, which are particularly common in certain types of nephritis.

The *nervous system* should be examined, especially for evidence of past vascular lesions.

Retinal Changes.—These occur only in types of nephritis associated with high blood-pressure, and are seen just as typically in severe cases of hypertension without renal disease. The more important *ophthalmoscopic* changes include exudates, hæmorrhages, vascular changes, and papillœdema.

a. Exudates.—' Cotton-wool ' patches and small dot-like exudates radiating from the macula—the ' star ' figure.

b. Hæmorrhages.—Seldom very large, usually flame-shaped, often radiating from the optic disk.

c. Vascular changes.—Sclerosis of the arteries ; tortuosity ; variation in calibre ; opacity at the crossing of the veins.

d. Papillœdema.—This may be indistinguishable from that seen in cerebral tumours, but is rarely greater than two dioptres. It usually connotes an unfavourable prognosis.

2. EXAMINATION OF THE ABDOMEN

The Kidneys.—*Palpation of the kidneys* is best carried out with the patient in the recumbent position and the head slightly raised. One hand (the right in the case of the left kidney) is placed under the loin with the

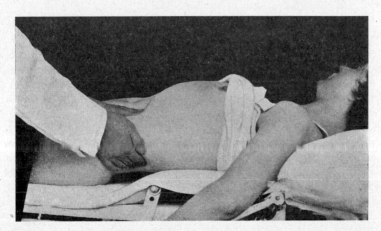

Fig. 127.—Palpation of the kidney. One hand is placed on the abdomen with the fingers pointing towards the costal margin, the other is pressed firmly against the loin. If the kidney is enlarged or mobile it moves downwards on inspiration and is sandwiched between the two hands.

10

tips of the fingers resting against the erector spinæ, whilst the other is placed flat on the abdomen with the fingers pointing upwards towards the costal margin (*Fig.* 127). The patient is then instructed to take a deep breath, and firm pressure is exerted by both hands, so that if the kidney is palpable it moves down into the space between the examining hands. When the organ can be felt in this way it is recognized as a swelling with a rounded lower pole, and if sufficient of it can be grasped between the hands the characteristic reniform shape with a medially placed notch (the hilum) can be recognized. The consistency of the swelling should be firm without hardness. It is *not uncommon to feel the right kidney in women owing to some degree of dropping of the organ* (nephroptosis), and in extreme cases both kidneys may be freely movable and can be manipulated into different parts of the abdomen (floating kidney).

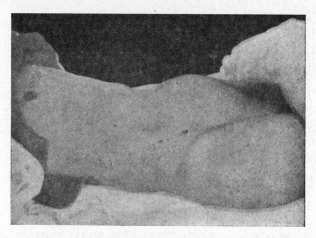

Fig. 128.—Distended bladder.

' *Tumours* ' of the kidney when of moderate size retain the characteristic kidney shape, but with experience can be recognized as larger than normal. Those commonly recognized on abdominal examination are hypernephromata and polycystic kidneys ; the former may be unduly hard and somewhat irregular, whilst in the latter cystic swellings may be palpable as characteristic bosses.

Inspection and percussion may confirm the presence of a renal swelling, and during inspection the *character of the skin in the loin should be noticed*, as redness and œdema may be present in perinephric infection.

The Ureter.—The ureter can only be examined by palpation if it is considerably thickened or if obstruction has led to its distension with urine. It is then palpated most easily in the lower abdomen about midway between the umbilicus and the anterior superior spine of the ilium.

The Bladder.—If distended with urine the bladder can be seen as a rounded swelling arising from the pelvis (*Fig.* 128) and extending upwards, sometimes as far as the umbilicus. Its outline is confirmed by palpation and percussion.

The External Genitalia.—The external genitalia may give important clues to the diagnosis. A pinhole meatus associated with phimosis may be a cause of urinary obstruction, particularly in infants, whilst thickening in the urethra may betray the presence of a stricture, which can be confirmed by the passage of bougies. Disease in the testicles (especially the epididymis) may be significant, especially in the case of tuberculosis, which may spread from the epididymis to the remainder of the urinary tract, and vice versa.

3. EXAMINATION OF THE PELVIC ORGANS : RECTAL AND VAGINAL EXAMINATION

Rectal examination is necessary in all cases of suspected urinary disease. It is convenient, especially in the male, to use the *knee-elbow*

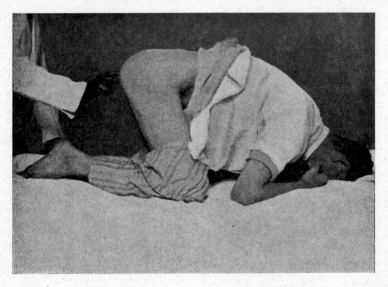

Fig. 129.—Rectal examination. The knee-elbow position.

position (*Fig.* 129), which gives better access to the organs lying round the base of the bladder.

The *prostate* can normally be felt as an elastic swelling with a median groove terminating in a notch at the top. Gross adenomatous enlargement of the gland makes it more difficult to feel the upper surface or the notch, though the consistency often remains the same. Irregularity and hardness in the prostate suggest malignant disease or occasionally prostatic calculi.

The *vesiculæ seminales* lie above the prostate, running upwards from its outer margins, but can only be felt if they are full. Thickening due to tuberculous infiltration is sometimes an important diagnostic point in suspected urinary tuberculosis.

Pelvic examination, rectal or vaginal, is also necessary to exclude disease of other pelvic organs, e.g., the uterus and appendages, the appendix, colon, etc., which may involve or irritate the bladder and cause urinary symptoms.

4. EXAMINATION OF THE URINE

Examination of the urine is pre-eminently the method by which the diagnosis of urinary diseases is established. The details of technique are dealt with in Chapter XIV, and only the significance of normal or abnormal constituents will be discussed in the present chapter.

Inspection.—Inspection shows the *colour* of the urine and any *deposit*.

Colour.—*Highly concentrated urine usually has a dark amber colour* inclining to orange. It frequently results from loss of fluid through other channels as by sweating or diarrhœa. It also occurs in heart failure and from the excessive excretion of urates which occurs in fevers and dyspeptic disorders. *Pale urine* on the contrary is found when the excretion of solids diminishes and the urine is of large amount and usually of low specific gravity. It therefore occurs after excessive intake of fluids and in certain types of chronic renal disease ; also in diabetes insipidus, in which the volume of urine is increased and its concentration diminished. A pale urine of high specific gravity (owing to the presence of sugar) occurs in diabetes mellitus.

Abnormal constituents may produce a complete change in the colour of the urine. *Bile* gives it a green or greenish-yellow appearance, *blood* a red or reddish-brown colour, and *melanin* and *alkapton* a very dark appearance, sometimes black. The possibility of excreted *drugs* modifying the colour of urine should also be borne in mind, especially such common ones as rhubarb, which gives an orange colour, and methylene blue (frequently contained in proprietary pills), which gives a green colour.

Deposit.—Fresh urine rarely has much deposit if it is normal, but on standing deposits of phosphates or urates may produce a cloudiness or even a thick heavy layer. *Phosphates* are usually white or light buff colour, whilst *urates* vary from a buff colour to a pink or brick-red. *These constituents have no pathological significance.* A fainter cloudiness may be produced by *bacteria,* giving the urine an opalescent or shimmering appearance. Pathological constituents such as *pus* and *blood* also produce turbidity, increasing in some cases to a thick deposit.

Specific Gravity.—The normal specific gravity of urine is generally about 1·015 to 1·025 (conveniently styled 1015 or 1025), but wide variations are found in health, according to the quantity of fluid ingested and the amount lost through the skin and bowels. A *persistently low specific gravity* (1010 *or rather less) is suggestive of chronic renal disease* if rarer causes such as diabetes insipidus can be excluded. Very *high specific gravities* (1030–1060) are rarely found except in the presence of large amounts of sugar in the urine in *diabetes mellitus*. When a specific gravity of over 1050 is found, the possibility of artefact must be excluded.

Reaction.—The urine may be acid or slightly alkaline in health. It is frequently alkaline for a short period during the digestion of food, the so-called 'alkaline tide'. Decomposition on standing and the liberation of free ammonia also renders it alkaline, especially when the urine is heavily charged with bacteria. The type of diet may also alter the reaction, vegetables and fruit tending to make it alkaline, meat acid.

Smell.—The student should familiarize himself with the characteristic smell of urine so that he can compare this with the strong ammoniacal smell frequently found in infants and after decomposition when the urine has been left standing.

Quantity.—The amount of urine passed in twenty-four hours should be recorded. In health it averages 50 oz.

ABNORMAL CHEMICAL CONSTITUENTS

The common abnormal constituents indicating the presence of urinary disease are albumin, blood, and pus.

Albuminuria.—The presence of albumin in the urine may vary from a trace to 10 g. per litre or more. Very small amounts may be derived accidentally from the urinary passages, particularly from the vagina and prepuce. Albumin derived from these sources is inconstant and has no pathological significance. Diseases of the pelvis of the kidney, the bladder, and the urethra, especially those in which pus or blood is produced, are also accompanied by albuminuria, and the possibility of these should be considered before attributing albuminuria to a renal origin.

Albumin excreted into the urine by the kidneys falls into two classes : (a) Functional albuminuria ; (b) Organic albuminuria. The distinction between these two is not always easy.

Functional Albuminuria.—This generally occurs in children or young adults, and the amount of albumin is usually small, though occasionally considerable. It appears in the urine under suggestive circumstances. Usually it is absent in the early morning specimen, but appears after the patient has been up for an hour or two ; sometimes it appears only after exercise. Various names have been applied to the different types of functional albuminuria, such as *orthostatic* or *postural* when it seems to be dependent upon change in posture of the individual, and *adolescent* because of its frequency at this period of life.

The cause of these functional types of albuminuria is still in dispute. Some authorities regard them as due to slight renal damage, i.e., a very mild and non-progressive type of nephritis ; whilst others think that they occur as a result of imperfect control of the kidney circulation, usually as one feature of a general vasomotor instability. *Repeated examination is often necessary before albuminuria can be called functional.* Its inconstancy is an important point, and also the fact that it is not accompanied by other evidence of nephritis—as shown by good response to the renal tolerance tests and the absence of casts (occasionally a few hyaline casts may occur) in the urine. Albumin may persist in appreciable quantities in the urine after an attack of nephritis when all other symptoms of this disease have gone. If the amount is only $\frac{1}{2}$ g. per litre or less, it may have no significance. Larger amounts are usually an indication of latent disease which may lead to chronic nephritis later.

Organic Albuminuria.—This is generally larger in amount, though in some types of chronic renal disease it is common only to find an inconstant cloud of albumin in the urine. The *persistent presence of more than* 1 g. *per litre of albumin* in the urine *generally indicates the presence of nephritis* unless blood or pus from surgical diseases of the urinary tract is responsible for it. The amount of albumin varies from a trace in sclerotic types of chronic renal disease to as much as 10 g. per litre in chronic glomerulonephritis and nephrosis. Cardiac failure may also produce small amounts of albumin in the urine without any real kidney disease, but this disappears quickly if treatment is successful. Toxic damage to the kidney as in eclampsia and sepsis is also a cause of moment. The slight toxæmia of febrile states only produces a transient albuminuria.

Hæmaturia.—Blood in the urine may vary in amount from large quantities visible to the naked eye to a few red corpuscles detectable only by microscopical examination. The blood may be derived from any part of the urinary tract—the kidneys, the ureters, the bladder, or the urethra. When *derived from the kidney* it has an opportunity to become *intimately mixed with the urine,* which is correspondingly reddish-brown in colour (' smoky '), but when derived from the bladder or urethra it may remain separate from the urine, and have the bright-red appearance of pure blood. *Blood from the urethra* may be dislodged by the urinary stream and thus *precedes the urine.* The reverse is the case *when the bleeding is taking place in the bladder,* for the *lighter urine is evacuated before the heavier blood.*

Hæmaturia may occur from traumatic, inflammatory, or neoplastic diseases of any part of the urinary tract, and its degree is often roughly proportionate to the severity of the lesion. The table on p. 151 shows the more common causes of hæmaturia.

Pyuria.—A few pus cells in the urine have little significance, especially in women, as they may be derived from the vagina. Larger quantities of pus usually indicate an inflammatory lesion of the urinary tract, and in most cases organisms are to be found on microscopical examination. In all cases in which pus is found, therefore, a specimen of urine collected aseptically is a necessity both to establish the presence and nature of the organisms and the fact that the pus has a urinary origin. In women a sterile specimen should be obtained by catheterization; in men it is sufficient to swab the meatus with a weak antiseptic and to allow the patient to pass urine into a sterile receptacle.

Cystitis, pyelitis, and suppuration in the kidney substance are important causes of pyuria, but smaller amounts of pus may occur from prostatitis and urethritis in men. Whilst albumin and blood are the usual abnormal

CAUSES OF HÆMATURIA

KIDNEY	URETER	BLADDER	URETHRA	CONSTITUTIONAL	EXTRA-URINARY
Injury	Calculus	Injury	Injury	*Blood diseases*, e.g., purpura, leukaemias, etc.	Menstruation
Calculus	Papilloma of renal pelvis	Calculus	Calculus	High blood-pressure, often in association with renal arteriosclerosis	Spread of inflammatory or neoplastic processes from neighbouring tissues, e.g., uterus or appendix
Infarction		Acute cystitis	Acute urethritis		
Acute nephritis		Tuberculosis	Stricture	Poisons, e.g., hexamine in large doses, cantharides	
Chronic nephritis (occasionally)		*Tumours*, especially papilloma and carcinoma, and *enlarged prostate* (adenoma and carcinoma)	Neoplasm		
Tuberculosis			(All causes rather rare)	Acute fevers, e.g., smallpox and yellow fever (rare)	
Neoplasm, especially hypernephromata. Polycystic disease		Parasites, especially bilharziasis		'Essential' hæmaturia, i.e., hæmaturia without obvious explanation	

constituents in cases of nephritis, a few pus cells are not uncommonly found. Pus may also be derived from extrinsic causes such as diverticulitis of the colon or the rupture of an appendix abscess into the bladder.

Pneumaturia.—Gas is rarely expelled with the urine, but pneumaturia may occasionally prove of considerable diagnostic value, suggesting a communication between the urinary tract (usually the bladder) and the alimentary tract (the colon). It is occasionally found, for example, in cases of diverticulosis in which the diverticulum has become adherent to the bladder.

MICROSCOPICAL EXAMINATION

The urine should always be examined microscopically. Apart from the presence of small numbers of red corpuscles and pus cells which may

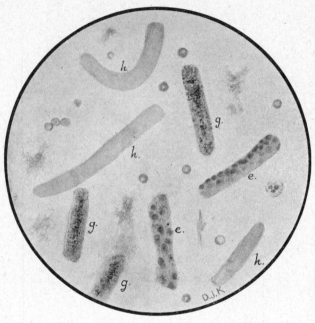

Fig. 130.—Casts in urine. *e*, Epithelial cast ; *h*, Hyaline cast ; *g*, Granular cast. A few red corpuscles are also seen, and one leucocyte on the right side of the field.

not be recognizable by chemical tests, microscopical examination may show the presence of casts, crystals, foreign bodies, and parasites.

Casts (*Fig.* 130) in appreciable numbers are most commonly found in cases of nephritis. In acute nephritis ' blood casts ', composed almost entirely of red corpuscles, may occur. They are merely clumps of corpuscles moulded into cylindrical shape by the renal tubules, but are not true casts, which are essentially composed of renal epithelium. When the renal epithelium is desquamated without material change occurring, *epithelial* casts are formed, and these are an important feature of acute nephritis. In

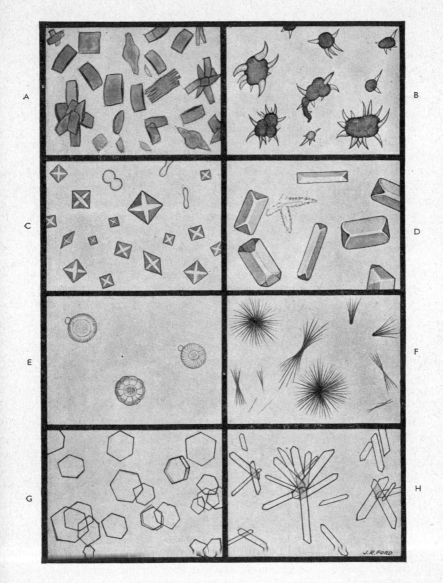

Fig. 131.—Crystalline deposits in urine. A, Uric acid; B, Ammonium urate; C, Calcium oxalate; D, Ammonio-magnesium phosphate; E, Leucine; F, Tyrosine; G, Cystine; H, Stellar phosphates. (From ' Pye's Surgical Handicraft '.)

the more chronic forms of nephritis the renal epithelium undergoes degenerative changes, which give rise to *hyaline* and *granular* casts.

Crystals are often found in the urine, but are rarely of diagnostic importance. Amongst the commonest are calcium oxalate, uric acid, and various types of phosphates. Calcium oxalate crystals are common in dyspepsias, and after eating rhubarb or strawberries. Cystine, leucine, and tyrosine crystals are present rarely, but when found are important. Cystinuria occurs only as a congenital metabolic defect ; leucine and tyrosine are diagnostic of acute yellow atrophy of the liver. The characters of the commoner crystals are seen in *Fig.* 131.

Many other bodies may be seen in urine, and some of these need experience for their recognition. They are rarely indicative of urinary or any other form of disease. They include vaginal epithelium, spermatozoa, amorphous debris or urates or phosphates, and all manner of foreign bodies.

Bacteria require stained preparations and sometimes culture for their recognition. They may be excreted in the urine apart from urinary disease, especially *B. coli*, and when found are more significant if pus is also present.

Parasites are rarely found in Great Britain. The most important is *Bilharzia hæmatobia*, the large ova of which are easily recognized under low magnification.

THE DIAGNOSIS OF URINARY DISEASES

Sometimes the symptoms already enumerated—frequency, dysuria, pain, œdema, and so forth—attract attention to the urinary system, but not infrequently, especially in cases of nephritis, the onset is insidious and silent, and routine examination of the urine may first throw light on the cause of a patient's poor health. This is one of a number of reasons for making the *examination of the urine a necessary part of every medical examination*, a measure often throwing unexpected light on an obscure case, and saving the examiner from making serious mistakes in diagnosis.

The more common diseases of the urinary system follow. Some of them fall more frequently within the province of the surgeon, but are mentioned briefly here as they sometimes overlap into that of the physician.

DISEASES OF THE KIDNEY

Acute Nephritis.—General malaise, with fever and *œdema* (*Fig.* 132), generally distinguish this disease at its onset, and the diagnosis is completed by urinary analysis, which shows the presence of *albumin* ($\frac{1}{2}$ to 10 g. per litre) and blood, with epithelial casts indicating the acute nature of the inflammatory process. The blood-pressure is generally raised, and gastrointestinal symptoms, especially vomiting, are common. The acute symptoms subside within a week or ten days, but albuminuria may persist for a long time afterwards, and in many cases denotes the transition to a chronic form of nephritis. Some cases of acute nephritis are distinguished by profuse hæmaturia without other symptoms. Pallor due to anæmia develops whether there is hæmorrhage or not, but is naturally greater if the hæmaturia is profuse.

Chronic Nephritis.—Many forms of chronic nephritis are described, according to the classification of various workers. It will suffice here to note that they are all characterized by persistent *albuminuria* in grades varying from a faint trace, not constantly present, to the permanent excretion of large amounts.

In certain types of chronic nephritis cardio-vascular changes are pronounced, e.g., high blood-pressure, cardiac hypertrophy, arteriosclerosis, and a tendency to congestive heart failure. In these, the albuminuria is usually slight but the kidneys show their failure of function by the secretion

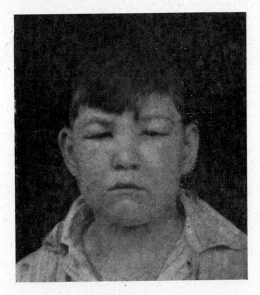

Fig. 132.—Acute nephritis. Note facial œdema, most pronounced around the eyes. Swelling of the eyelids and infra-orbital œdema narrows the palpebral fissures.

of large amounts of urine of low specific gravity. Granular and hyaline casts are generally found. These cases usually show considerable nitrogen retention as shown by increased non-protein nitrogen or urea in the blood. Retinal changes—arteriosclerosis, exudates, and hæmorrhages—are common. In other types of nephritis (subacute or early chronic nephritis and nephrosis) cardio-vascular changes are absent or slight, albuminuria is heavy, and œdema is usually a prominent symptom. Retention of nitrogen is rare, but blood-cholesterol values are often high.

Useful information can be obtained in chronic forms of nephritis, as regards the severity and probable course of the lesion, by the tests of renal efficiency already described.

Renal Calculus.—Stones may be present in the kidneys without symptoms. Sometimes a dull ache may occur, and if the stone becomes dislodged and passes down the ureter an attack of *renal colic* results (*see* PAIN, p. 142).

The traumatic effects of the stone, especially when in movement, often result in *hæmaturia*, and the urine should be examined microscopically for red corpuscles.

Calculi may lead to infection of the kidney, affecting the pelvis (pyelitis) or kidney substance (pyelonephritis).

Pyelonephritis.—This is an important and common disease, often referred to as pyelitis, urinary infection, or *B. coli* infection of the urinary tract. It may occur in an acute form with rigors, vomiting, and high temperature, or as a chronic illness. Pain in one or both loins is frequent—especially in acute cases.

The most important local symptom is frequency of micturition, as cystitis is part of the disease.

The diagnosis is made by the discovery of *pyuria* in the presence of these symptoms, and may be confirmed by tenderness over one or both kidneys, which may be palpable.

Renal Tuberculosis.—Renal tuberculosis may affect the pelvis (resembling other forms of pyelitis) or the kidney substance. It is often associated with tuberculous lesions in other parts of the urinary system, e.g., the bladder or epididymis.

The *constitutional symptoms* of tuberculosis—loss of weight, anorexia, fever, sweating—are generally present. Of the local symptoms, *frequency* of micturition is most important, though pain may occur. Pyuria is generally recognized if microscopical examination of the urine is made, but special methods of investigation, particularly examination for tubercle bacilli in the urine, and cystoscopy, may be necessary to establish the diagnosis. In doubtful cases inoculation of a guinea-pig with the urine may establish the diagnosis of tuberculosis.

Movable Kidney.—The right kidney is frequently mobile in women and yet produces no symptoms. This should be borne in mind when the student finds this abnormality and is tempted to explain vague symptoms by its presence. Extreme mobility may, however, lead to kinking of the ureter, resulting in renal colic or symptoms of hydronephrosis. A movable kidney is often a part of a general visceroptosis found in nervous and poorly nourished individuals who complain of manifold symptoms.

'Tumours' of the Kidney.—Kidney 'tumours' generally have the shape of the normal organ (*see* p. 146), but if very large may fill the whole loin or spread into other parts of the abdomen. They vary in consistency from that of normal renal tissue to the extreme hardness of some malignant growths. The more important tumours are hydronephrosis, polycystic disease, and hypernephroma.

Hydronephrosis is a ballooning of the kidney calices and pelvis by retained urine, due to *intermittent obstruction* in the ureter, in many cases of an unexplained nature, in some due to calculus. The kidney retains its normal shape, but is larger than normal, and may *vary in size* owing to the periodic release of the accumulated excretions which are voided by the patient.

Polycystic disease is characterized by the development of numerous cysts in the kidney which destroy its substance. The affection is generally bilateral, and the kidncys are palpable as large ' bossed ' reniform tumours. Other symptoms suggest the presence of chronic renal disease (polyuria, albuminuria, high blood-pressure, etc.) due to the limited kidney function. Hæmaturia is sometimes a symptom.

Hypernephroma, the commonest of malignant tumours of the kidney, is generally recognized by the presence of a renal tumour with hæmaturia.

DISEASES OF THE BLADDER

Cystitis.—Frequency of micturition and dysuria are the characteristic symptoms of cystitis. Fever is rarely marked. The diagnosis is completed by the finding of pyuria, by the discovery of some causal factor such as prostatic enlargement or vesical calculus, and sometimes by cystoscopic examination, which may be necessary to determine the essential nature of the cystitis.

Calculus.—Calculus in the bladder may cause dysuria and hæmaturia. Its presence generally requires instrumental (bougies, cystoscopy) or radiological methods for its recognition.

Tumours.—Tumours (papillomata and carcinomata) usually cause hæmaturia, and require cystoscopy for their diagnosis. Adenomatous or carcinomatous *enlargements of the prostate* may project as tumours into the bladder and cause urinary obstruction. This may be recognized by rectal examination. Enlargement of the prostate should always be considered as a cause of urinary symptoms in elderly men, especially when the symptoms resemble those of chronic renal disease (nocturnal polyuria, slight albuminuria, etc.).

CHAPTER VI

THE DIGESTIVE SYSTEM

THE digestive system comprises the alimentary tract and the accessory organs and tissues concerned in the digestion of food. It will be convenient to describe the symptoms and objective examination of each part separately, though certain general descriptions of symptoms common to all parts and the method of examining the abdomen as a whole will be necessary.

THE MOUTH*

SYMPTOMS

Soreness of the mucous membrane covering the mouth or tongue is found in the various forms of stomatitis, an inflammation of the buccal mucous membrane common in digestive disorders. Local soreness may arise from the irritation of carious teeth or from tumours of the tongue. The sore tongue of pernicious anæmia is one of the classical signs of that disease.

Toothache should call for an examination of the teeth, upon the integrity and proper use of which good digestion depends.

PHYSICAL SIGNS: EXAMINATION OF THE MOUTH

The examination of the mouth requires a good light and preferably the use of an electric torch.

The Teeth should be inspected and their number and condition noted. Deficient and carious teeth are an undoubted contributory cause in many forms of dyspepsia, and almost equally important in this respect is the presence of ill-fitting false teeth, which prevent the patient from chewing properly. A brownish deposit of indican in chronic intestinal putrefaction, and a yellowish easily removed deposit in diabetes, are occasionally observed.

The Gums.—The state of the gums should next be noted. A deep-red congestion is present when the gums are inflamed, *gingivitis*, and in *pyorrhœa* pus can be squeezed from the gum margins. Both in gingivitis and pyorrhœa the teeth are generally infected and are often loose and covered with a greenish-yellow exudate. Oral sepsis of this kind, whilst sometimes compatible with normal digestion, is a frequent aggravating factor in gastro-intestinal disease. The gums are *pale in anæmia*, and in lead poisoning a *blue line* may be seen at the

See also THE RESPIRATORY SYSTEM (Chapter III) and FEVER (Chapter X).

gum margin. The blue line is due to a deposit of lead sulphide in the gum tissues ; so it cannot be cleaned away with a pledget of cotton wool, and it is seen even better if the gum margins between the teeth are trans-illuminated from behind by a small electric torch.

The Tongue.—The condition of the tongue should always be recorded. In digestive troubles it is frequently covered with a fur consisting of proliferated epithelium, bacteria, and food debris. Furring also occurs in dehydration, severe fevers, and peritonitis. Slight degrees of furring, especially towards the back of the tongue, are not necessarily abnormal, and are commonly found in smokers. Dryness is common in mouth breathers and

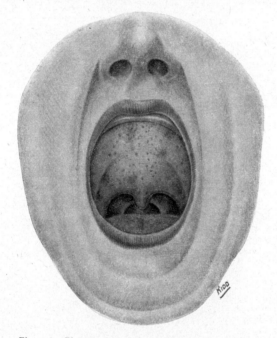

Fig. 133.—Pigmentation of the mouth in Addison's disease.

conditions causing diminished salivation. It may be a measure of dehydration, and in acute illness a useful guide to the necessity for fluids. When the tongue is dry and the fur becomes 'caked', it may be taken as a sign of grave import, occurring especially in serious abdominal catastrophes such as peritonitis and intestinal obstruction, and also in severe fevers such as typhoid.

Anæmia and jaundice may be evident in the tongue. In certain anæmias (pernicious anæmia and idiopathic hypochromic anæmias particularly) the tongue is depapillated, i.e., smooth and shiny, and sometimes sore. This is an important point in diagnosis.

The tongue is large in cretins and mongols, and in the latter often fissured. Allergy also causes a large flabby tongue.

Taste may be affected by alimentary disturbances, but not lost. Loss is due to lesions of the 7th and 9th nerves. Paralysis, atrophy, and tremors and abnormalities of movement of the tongue will be noted incidentally, but are referred to under the nervous system.

Anatomical peculiarities and the various forms of ulceration and other local disease (e.g., glossitis) will not be described here.

The Buccal Mucous Membrane.—It now remains to examine the mucous membrane of the rest of the mouth. This is normally of a pink colour and moistened by the mucus of the saliva. It is pale in anæmias and cyanosed in serious heart or lung diseases. Small *ulcers*

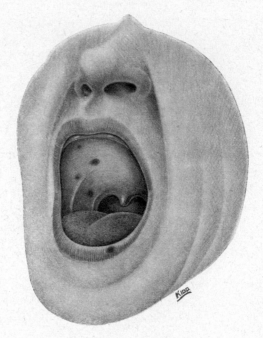

Fig. 134.—Purpuric spots in the mouth.

indicate the presence of stomatitis, and the more serious ulcers of syphilis and malignant disease should not be overlooked. The former tend to be central and the latter marginal. Tuberculous ulceration is associated with pulmonary infection and commonly involves the tip of the tongue. In Addison's disease brownish areas of *pigmentation* may be seen in the buccal mucous membrane, a useful confirmatory sign in doubtful cases (*Fig.* 133). Hæmorrhages are occasionally found in purpura (*Fig.* 134).

(*See also* KOPLIK'S SPOTS, p. 47.)

The Breath.—Lastly, the character of the breath should be noted. A slightly unpleasant odour is found in many forms of dyspepsia, but the breath can rarely be called *offensive* except when excessive fermentation is taking place in the gastro-intestinal tract, e.g., in gastric neoplasm. Offensiveness is more often due to dental sepsis or infection of the gums, tonsils, or nasopharynx. It is also pronounced in cases of bronchiectasis and gangrene or abscess of the lung. A *sweet smell* may be imparted to the breath by acetone in cases of diabetic coma and in acidosis, especially in children. The breath in uræmia sometimes has a uriniferous smell.

DIAGNOSIS AND DISEASES OF THE MOUTH

Most diseases of the mouth are within the province of surgical diagnosis and will not be described here. The one commonly seen in the medical wards is stomatitis.

Stomatitis.—An inflammation of the mucous membrane of the mouth may result, as already mentioned, from gastro-intestinal derangement or from the irritation of carious teeth. Numerous small ulcers are usually present in dyspeptic forms of stomatitis and are very painful to touch, causing considerable discomfort in eating. A similar form of stomatitis may arise from poisoning with mercury or bismuth. The presence of white patches in the mouth, in a child, should suggest the possibility of *thrush*, a specific form of stomatitis due to the *Oidium albicans*. Bacteriological examination may be necessary to determine the type of stomatitis. (*See also* SCURVY and AGRANULOCYTOSIS.)

THE ŒSOPHAGUS

SYMPTOMS

Dysphagia or difficulty in swallowing is the principal symptom of œsophageal disease. The difficulty is experienced at first only when the patient takes solid food, and he gets over it by chewing food until it is of fluid consistency, but as the obstruction becomes more complete he is unable to take even liquids with ease. Similar dysphagia results from obstruction at the cardiac end of the stomach. The patient complains that the food ' sticks ', and he may localize the obstruction fairly accurately either in the throat or more commonly at the lower end of the sternum. Dysphagia is found when the œsophagus is narrowed by any cause, functional or organic, or at times when the swallowing reflex is impaired, as in certain types of bulbar palsy. Neurotic persons frequently complain of a ' lump in the throat ', the so called ' globus hystericus ', which is not to be confused with dysphagia.

Pain may accompany dysphagia, especially when malignant disease is the cause of the obstruction. It is probably due to tension in the œsophagus above the obstruction. This is relieved by—

Regurgitation, and in malignant disease the regurgitated material is often foul.

Cardiospasm.—(*See* p. 162.)

11

PHYSICAL SIGNS: EXAMINATION OF THE ŒSOPHAGUS

The examination of the œsophagus is largely dependent on X rays (*see* Chapter XIII), but œsophagoscopy and the use of bougies have limited application. The clinician relies chiefly upon the history, but observes difficulties in swallowing and notes any glandular enlargement in the neck.

DIAGNOSIS OF DISEASES OF THE ŒSOPHAGUS

Œsophageal Obstruction.—Most cases of œsophageal obstruction are due to *malignant disease*. They show the characteristic dysphagia with pain and regurgitation of food. Loss of weight is pronounced owing to the site of the growth, which prevents the proper entry of food into the stomach. Simple strictures of the œsophagus (e.g., the result of corrosive liquids, or syphilis), the pressure of extrinsic tumours such as aneurysm or mediastinal growth, and the pressure of œsophageal diverticula filled with food, produce similar but less marked symptoms.

Cardiospasm (*Achalasia of the Cardia*).—In some cases of dysphagia it has been found that the food is held up at the cardiac sphincter, which becomes hypertrophied. It has been suggested that these cases are due to an inco-ordination between the longitudinal muscles of the œsophagus and the circular fibres of the cardiac sphincter, and when the waves of peristalsis propel the food against the cardiac sphincter they find this closed instead of open.

It will be seen that the diagnosis between the various forms of œsophageal obstruction requires not only an examination of the œsophagus itself but also of those structures which lie in contact with it, *especially the contents of the superior mediastinum.*

GENERAL SYMPTOMS OF ABDOMINAL DISEASE

ABDOMINAL PAIN

Before proceeding to the description of the symptoms and physical signs associated with individual abdominal viscera, it will be convenient to discuss in a more general fashion certain details concerning abdominal pain. This is a subject upon which much doubt still exists and the exact explanation of many types of abdominal pain is still obscure. The possibility that true *visceral pain* could not occur was first raised by the discovery that abdominal viscera, such as the stomach, intestine, and liver, and their covering visceral peritoneum, were insensitive to stimuli such as cutting, pricking, or burning. To explain pain over viscera certain theories of referred pain were developed and are chiefly associated with the name of Mackenzie. This author believed that most types of abdominal pain were experienced not in the viscus but at some point in the abdominal wall often remote from the actual position of the lesion. In the case of gastric ulcer he observed that the pain was felt by the patient in a different part of the epigastrium from the site of the ulcer as shown by operative or post-mortem findings. Similarly, in appendicitis, although the organ lay in the right iliac fossa, the pain was frequently experienced in the umbilical region. To explain this distribution of pain Mackenzie propounded the theory that stimulation of the splanchnic nerve-endings in a diseased viscus causes afferent impulses to pass to the spinal cord, where they produce a focus of irritability. Into the irritable segments of the cord, cerebrospinal nerve-fibres carry afferent impulses from the skin and deeper tissues of the abdominal wall, and as the viscus itself is insensitive the pain is referred by the patient to this area of the abdominal wall.

Tenderness on pressure is also explained as a *viscero-sensory reflex* in which the irritable focus in the spinal cord renders certain segments of the abdominal wall tender on pressure, whilst in some cases *muscular rigidity* is produced as a *viscero-motor reflex* through a similar mechanism. The stimulation of the afferent splanchnic fibres causes an irritable focus in the cord, from which efferent motor impulses are discharged to the muscles of the abdominal wall. As a result, the muscles go into reflex spasm over the area governed by the affected segment of the spinal cord.

By many authorities Mackenzie's views are considered an adequate explanation of most types of abdominal pain. Criticism, however, has been directed against them. It is pointed out that the theory necessitates a close connexion between afferent splanchnic fibres and afferent or efferent cerebrospinal fibres, a connexion which has never been demonstrated anatomically. Then in the case of gastric ulcer, the introduction of accurate radiological diagnosis has enabled the observer to localize the exact position of an ulcer and to determine the relationship of tenderness in the abdominal wall to this, and the evidence thus afforded does not support Mackenzie's views (held before radiology was so developed). Hurst, Morley, and others have shown that the area of tenderness corresponds quite accurately with the position of the ulcer, and Morley lays great emphasis on the fact that during palpation the ulcer is brought in contact with the exquisitely sensitive parietal peritoneum. He points out that the peritoneum and the area of abdominal wall over it are supplied by cerebrospinal nerves from the same segments of the cord. This would explain the close connexion between the sensitive area of the abdominal wall and the underlying gastric ulcer.

Hurst, Morley, and others believe, however, that true visceral pain exists in spite of the apparently insensitive character of the abdominal viscera. They point out that an adequate stimulus may be necessary, and just as the cerebrospinal nerve-endings in the skin are sensitive to cutting or pricking, and the retina is sensitive to light, so the correct stimulus to induce pain in a hollow muscular viscus is tension.

It is a familiar experience that a rapidly given large enema produces abdominal pain. Poulton has also shown that distension of the œsophagus by introduction of a balloon causes pain which is often relieved by the peristaltic waves above the site of obstruction. Yet in other instances it would appear that peristalsis of itself produces or aggravates pain. In intestinal colic the griping pains are definitely associated with increased peristalsis, which in cases of intestinal obstruction can be observed to coincide with the spasms of pain. *True visceral pain of this kind is not associated with tenderness or rigidity*—in fact, it is frequently relieved by manual pressure. Its localization is usually vague and deeply situated as compared with the referred pain of an inflammatory or irritative lesion of the peritoneum. The localization seems to depend upon developmental factors. Visceral pain arising from structures destined to form the foregut, biliary apparatus, and pancreas, is felt in the epigastrium.

Pain arising from the midgut loop is generally localized above the umbilicus in the midline, whilst the hindgut origin produces pain in the infra-umbilical region. *Somatic* or *referred* pain is transmitted through the cerebrospinal nerves to areas of the skin, which Mackenzie, Head, and others related to the diseased viscus, which was innervated from the same segments of the cord. Morley's conception, which receives other surgeons' support, is that the area of pain relates, not to the viscus, but to the region of the abdominal cavity where the pathological process is at work. This means that if a diseased viscus is in an unusual position, the pain will also be abnormally distributed—e.g., appendicular pain may not be in the right iliac fossa if the appendix is away from this region.

Further characteristics of pain arising from individual abdominal viscera will be described when dealing with these organs, but to sum up, it may be stated that abdominal pain of organic origin falls into two classes :—

1. *Visceral pain*, due to increased tension on the splanchnic nerve-endings in the muscular wall of the affected viscus. This pain, as mentioned, is vaguely and deeply localized, often colicky in type, and is found most commonly in obstructive lesions of the stomach, intestines, and bile-ducts. A similar pain is found in obstruction of other tubes, particularly the ureter in cases of renal colic.

2. *Referred pain*, probably due in many cases to the irritative effects of inflammatory, hæmorrhagic, or neoplastic diseases of the abdominal viscera upon the parietal peritoneum. The parietal peritoneum in contact with the viscus receives its cerebrospinal nerve-supply from the same segments of the spinal cord as the overlying parts of the abdominal wall. This explains why the pain and tenderness are experienced in many cases over the viscus, although the pain is referred. In other cases, as in the instance of shoulder-tip pain, the area of skin is situated remotely from the irritated peritoneum. Here irritation of the peritoneum (or pleura) covering the central portions of the diaphragm, which receives its nerve-supply from the phrenic nerve (4th cervical segment), causes the pain to be felt in an area supplied by other somatic nerves arising at the same level, namely, over the tip of the shoulder. *The pain of peritoneal irritation is usually associated with deep tenderness and often with muscular rigidity.* It is more constant than visceral pain, and is generally stabbing, cutting, or burning in character.

Special Features to be Noted.—An accurate description by the patient of his pain is of the greatest value in the diagnosis of digestive diseases. The following points should be ascertained in every case :—

1. *The Situation.*—From the preceding sections it follows that when pain is due to peritoneal irritation it is usually experienced over the affected viscus, but when truly visceral it may be more vaguely situated, and in the case of gastro-intestinal pain it is usually central. Visceral pain, as already pointed out, depends for its position on the embryological origin of the viscus. Fuller details are given in dealing with individual viscera.

2. *The Character.*—This includes the severity, which varies from the slight discomfort of gastric flatulence to the agonizing pain of a perforated gastric ulcer. The description of the type of pain—griping, gnawing, stabbing, cutting, and so forth—depends a good deal upon the intelligence and descriptive ability of the patient, and too much stress, therefore, cannot be laid upon it as a point in diagnosis. The distinction between visceral and somatic pain may be recognized from the patient's description.

3. *Conditions Aggravating the Pain.*—Abdominal pain so frequently arises from the stomach, intestines, or organs which modify the function of these that it naturally bears a close relationship to meals. Inquiry should be made whether the pain occurs after meals ; if so, how long ; and whether relief is afforded from the pain by taking more food. The patient should also be asked whether any particular kind of food disagrees with him and precipitates pain.

4. *Conditions Relieving the Pain.*—The effect of starvation should be ascertained, or whether abstention from particular articles of diet gives relief. Relief given by medicines, particularly alkalis, may also be a valuable diagnostic point. Comfort produced by evacuation of the bladder or rectum may suggest these organs as the seat of the pain.

5. *Duration.*—If the pain comes on after meals the patient should be asked whether it disappears before the next meal or whether it is continuous. In apparently continuous pain there are often spells in which the patient is comparatively comfortable. Intervals of freedom from the attacks of pain should also be noted. It is characteristic, for example, in gastric and duodenal ulcer to find periods of some weeks in which the patient is entirely free from discomfort. On the contrary, pain due to gastric and other visceral carcinomata often starts gradually, and becomes more severe and continuous as time goes on. Pain of short duration is more likely to be due to obstructive causes such as renal or biliary colic, for inflammatory and neoplastic affections cause pain of longer duration.

6. *Associated Phenomena.*—Indications of the severity of the pain and its reflex effects are often seen in the association of vomiting, sweating, and collapse. Bad pain especially due to peptic ulcer may wake the patient at night. It should be particularly noted whether vomiting gives relief from the pain, a common history in cases of gastric disease. The association of constipation or diarrhœa with abdominal pain should focus attention on the intestinal tract.

VOMITING

Vomiting is another symptom common to so many diseases of the digestive and other systems that it is convenient to describe it before proceeding further. It is a reflex act induced through the vomiting centre in the medulla, and may be caused by central or peripheral stimulation. Central stimulation of the vomiting centre may occur from psychical causes such as disgusting smells or sights, from increased intracranial pressure as in cerebral tumour, from toxæmias such as uræmia, or poisons such as apomorphine. It may arise reflexly from labyrinthine disturbances, e.g., in sea-sickness and Ménière's disease. It is also a fairly constant symptom in the early months of pregnancy. We are concerned in this chapter, however, chiefly with vomiting arising reflexly from irritation of the stomach mucous membrane. It is common as a result of indiscretions in diet, it may occur in organic disease of the stomach such as ulcer or cancer, or in reflex disturbance of the stomach from disease of the gall-bladder, appendix, or other viscera.

Vomiting must be distinguished from the regurgitation of small amounts of food into the mouth sometimes resulting from relaxation of the cardiac sphincter in healthy persons. *True vomiting implies the ejection of appreciable quantities of the stomach contents,* sometimes consisting of undigested food, sometimes of partially digested food to which the gastric secretions have been added. The association of vomiting with other symptoms of alimentary disease is presumptive evidence of an alimentary origin for the symptom.

Special Features to be Noted.—A careful note should be made of the following points :—

1. *The Relationship of the Vomiting to any Pain.*—Note whether the pain precedes or follows the vomiting and at what interval.

2. *The Time of Day at which Vomiting Occurs.*—In cases of pyloric stenosis each meal adds to the gastric contents, and vomiting may not occur until the latter part of the day when a large quantity has accumulated. The vomiting of pregnancy occurs characteristically in the mornings.

3. *The Presence or Absence of Nausea.*—Nausea generally precedes vomiting due to diseases of the digestive system, but in cases of increased intracranial pressure is often absent.

For details of the character of the vomitus, *see* p. 202.

SYMPTOMS ASSOCIATED WITH INDIVIDUAL VISCERA

THE STOMACH

Both pain and vomiting are common in gastric disease.

Pain.—Pain is generally of the visceral type, vaguely localized in the upper abdomen, and due in many cases to the peristaltic movements of the stomach. In gastric ulcer, in particular, the pain begins when the peristaltic movements of the stomach are most active, i.e., when digestion is well commenced *half an hour to an hour and a half after meals*. Although there is a considerable variation in different individuals with gastric ulcer, the same individual often shows a remarkable constancy in the relationship between pain and the ingestion of food. If the wall of the stomach is able to adapt its posture (tone) to its contents, pain is often relieved. Thus the administration of alkalis or food, by causing relaxation of the hypertonic stomach wall, often leads to a correct adaptation between the stomach and its contents, with the relief of pain. The pain of an ulcer is not entirely visceral, as it is frequently associated with localized tenderness on pressure and sometimes with muscular rigidity. It is possible that in such cases the ulcer has an irritant effect upon the parietal peritoneum with which it is in contact.

Gastric pain may also arise from hypertonus in the stomach wall plus pylorospasm reflexly produced by disease of other viscera, e.g., appendicitis and cholecystitis. In cancer of the stomach the pain is often more constant, and not so closely related to meals. Here other factors besides the tonus of the stomach wall, especially involvement of nerves and of the peritoneum, may be responsible for its production.

Short of actual pain, sensations of discomfort variously described as *fullness* or *pressure* may occur in functional or organic disease of the stomach, and are probably produced in the same way as actual pain, chiefly by alterations in tonus of the stomach wall and by increased peristaltic activity.

Vomiting.—This is a common but not invariable feature of organic disease of the stomach such as ulcer or neoplasm. Vomiting generally occurs after digestion has been in process for some time, often, also, when gastric pain is at its height. By relieving the tension on the hypertonic stomach wall it may diminish or abolish pain, and an intragastric cause may reasonably be suspected when abdominal pain is relieved by vomiting.

Hæmatemesis (*Vomiting of Blood*).—This is an important feature of gastric disease. It is most frequent in cases of gastric ulcer, and less commonly found in neoplasm of the stomach and in portal cirrhosis and Banti's disease (p. 225), in which the œsophageal and gastric veins are engorged and liable to rupture. Its occurrence in an otherwise doubtful case of gastric ulcer may clinch the diagnosis. The amount of blood vomited varies from a few ounces to several pints. The exact amount is difficult to estimate as the blood is usually mixed with the gastric contents, which alter its colour and sometimes give the vomit a ' coffee grounds ' appearance. If the loss of blood is great, the general signs of hæmorrhage will also be present.

These three symptoms, pain, vomiting, and hæmatemesis, are found usually in organic disease of the stomach, but pain and vomiting, like the symptoms now to be described, may also be found in reflex disturbances of the stomach function due to disease of other viscera, to faulty habits of life, especially of diet, and to psychological causes.

Nausea.—This is a sensation of sickness without actual vomiting, and is frequently accompanied by sweating and a feeling of faintness. It may be due to a relaxation of the tone of the gastro-intestinal musculature, and often results from psychic causes of an unpleasant nature, e.g., mental shocks and offensive smells. It is often present in organic disease of the gastro-intestinal tract and other abdominal viscera, especially in diseases like cancer of the stomach or chronic gastritis in which loss of tone in the gastric musculature is common. Vomiting of gastric origin is generally preceded by nausea.

Flatulence.—The stomach or intestines may be distended with gas, and the patient then complains of ' wind ' or ' flatulence ', or in America ' gas '. The wind may be belched through the mouth or passed per rectum ; the former is gastric flatulence, the latter intestinal. Flatulence is common in many types of digestive disorder, but even more in functional than in organic disease. The gas in the great majority of cases of gastric flatulence is probably mainly swallowed air, but both in the stomach and in the intestines excessive fermentation may be responsible for its accumulation.

Disturbances of Appetite.—Loss of appetite or *anorexia* is common as a temporary phenomenon and of little significance, but when it is persistent it is of great importance. It may then be caused by serious disease in many parts of the body, but is particularly common in local diseases of the stomach such as gastritis and carcinoma, in which the gastric musculature loses tone. General debilitating diseases such as tuberculosis and profound anæmias have a similar effect.

Excessive appetite, *bulimia*, is rare except in abnormal mental conditions, when the appetite is also frequently perverted.

Heartburn, Waterbrash, and Eructations.—These symptoms are often confused by the patient, who should, therefore, be asked to define clearly what he means by the terms.

Heartburn is a scalding or burning sensation experienced behind the sternum usually a little while after a meal. As a symptom of organic disease it has little importance.

Waterbrash consists in the regurgitation into the mouth of a watery fluid sometimes consisting of mucus, sometimes of saliva, or of both mixed. Like heartburn it has little significance.

Eructations of small amounts of the acid gastric contents are common both in functional and organic disease of the stomach.

THE INTESTINES

Pain, constipation, and *diarrhœa* are the most important symptoms caused by intestinal disease. Constipation and diarrhœa are even more common in temporary disturbances of health than in serious organic disease, yet it behoves the examiner to exclude the question of organic disease by all the means at his disposal. As in the case of most gastro-intestinal symptoms, the *persistence* of the symptom is a most significant point, for temporary constipation or diarrhœa rarely causes alarm except in acute abdominal disease.

Pain.—Pain is usually of the visceral type, vaguely localized and colicky in nature. It is almost certainly caused by increased tension on the intestinal musculature and exaggerated peristalsis. In gross intestinal obstruction where peristalsis is visible through the abdominal wall, the pain may be seen to coincide with the waves of peristalsis. Pain arising from the small intestine is generally situated in the centre of the abdomen. When the upper parts of the small intestine (jejunum) are affected, the pain is generally higher in the abdomen than when the lower parts are involved (ileum). Pain from the large intestine may also be experienced in the centre of the abdomen, but appears also to be common in the loins. Possibly the latter pain is not truly visceral but due to irritant effects upon the neighbouring parietal peritoneum.

Constipation.—In the average person evacuation of the bowels takes place once daily, but the event may occur twice daily or only once in two days in persons in quite good health. It is therefore of importance to inquire as to the normal habits of the individual over a period of some years. Most persons regard themselves as constipated if they do not have one action of the bowels in twenty-four hours. A sudden change in the habits is significant.

The degree of constipation should be ascertained. In all forms of *intestinal obstruction absolute constipation may take place*, that is, there is passage neither of fæces nor of gas. In partial intestinal obstruction incomplete constipation may occur. The patient finds he needs increasing quantities of purgatives, but the stools when passed are usually soft or fluid, and may be modified in shape—e.g., the ribbon-shaped stool—if the constricted area is in the rectum. There is as a rule no difficulty in the passage of flatus in partial intestinal obstruction.

Intestinal obstruction is the most serious cause of constipation but by no means the commonest. Constipation may arise from a great variety of factors, such as improper diet, insufficient exercise, *carelessness in habits*, and general ill health from disease in other parts of the body. It is important to distinguish between delay in the passage of fæces through the large bowel into the rectum and delay in emptying of the rectum itself. In persons of careless habits the fæces frequently pass normally through the colon into the rectum, but, owing to neglect of the call to defæcation, they accumulate and cause ballooning of the rectum with loss of tone in its walls. This condition is called *dyschezia*, and as a result of it a greater and greater amount of fæces is required to give the necessary sense of fullness which provokes the desire for defæcation.

Diarrhœa.—In diarrhœa the fæces are fluid in consistency and are evacuated more frequently than normal, usually several times a day, and in extreme cases almost continuously. Paradoxically, diarrhœa may occur in patients suffering from constipation ('pseudo-diarrhœa'), for a passage may be formed around a hard fæcal mass, allowing the fluid contents in the bowel above to pass by. This is not uncommonly the case in new growths of the large intestine, and also in spastic constipation, which by narrowing the lumen of the bowel cause fæcal impaction above.

Temporary diarrhœa is generally due to indiscretions in food or drink, and sometimes occurs with rapid changes in atmospheric temperature, and with many types of poisoning, especially with metallic poisons and those due to decomposing or infected food. It is a frequent manifestation of nervousness, occurring as a result of emotional causes.

Persistent diarrhœa is found in organic disease of the intestines (and sometimes of the stomach), e.g., neoplasm and tuberculosis, and in those bacterial infections which specifically attack the intestinal tract, e.g., typhoid, dysentery, and cholera.

The character of the motions in diarrhœa gives much useful information and is discussed under the examination of the stools (p. 203).

Tenesmus.—Tenesmus often accompanies diarrhœa, and consists in straining with a desire to empty the lower bowel without evacuation taking place.

THE BILIARY TRACT

The special symptoms which need consideration in connexion with the biliary tract are *pain* and *jaundice*, though many of the symptoms which have been described under the stomach may also be reflexly produced by disease in the gall-bladder or bile-ducts.

Pain.—A stone in the cystic duct affords the best example of the type of pain which results from obstruction in the biliary system. The pain is due to the violent peristaltic movements of the wall of the duct attempting to force onwards a hard foreign body. It is felt in the epigastrium and right hypochondrium, and is of such great intensity that the patient *rolls about in agony, sweats,* and *frequently vomits.* In many cases the pain radiates to the angle of the right scapula. It is essentially visceral, and lasts a few hours, but may be followed by a more localized pain in the right hypochondrium lasting several days. The latter is due to secondary cholecystitis and peritoneal involvement. This pain is associated with tenderness and rigidity on pressure.

Jaundice.—Jaundice is a yellow pigmentation of the skin and mucous membranes caused by the presence in the blood of an excess of bile-pigments.

Hæmolytic Jaundice.—It is now known that the bile-pigments are primarily formed by the breakdown of red blood-corpuscles in the reticulo-endothelial system (spleen, Kupffer cells of the liver, bone-marrow, etc.). The immature bilirubin thus produced, if present in the blood in excessive amounts, can cause a mild form of jaundice. This form is occasionally seen in the absorption of large hæmorrhagic exudates, and more frequently in blood diseases such as acholuric jaundice and pernicious anæmia where excessive amounts of hæmoglobin are set free in the circulation. It is known as hæmolytic jaundice.

Obstructive Jaundice.—Under normal circumstances the immature bilirubin passes to the liver, where it is modified by the polygonal cells into the normal bile pigments, which are secreted from the liver in combination with bile-salts and other constituents as the yellowish-green liquid known as bile. If obstruction occurs in any part of the biliary system, preventing the bile from flowing into the duodenum, it is dammed back into the liver and absorbed into the blood-stream. This is known as obstructive jaundice, and differs from hæmolytic jaundice principally in the fact that the circulating bile-pigments are fully formed, whereas in hæmolytic jaundice they are immature. Further, the bile-pigments do not reach the intestine, so that the stools lack bile-pigment derivatives (see below). Van den Bergh discovered that the two types of bile-pigment, mature and immature, reacted in a different way to Ehrlich's diazo reagent (a mixture of ammonia, sulphanilic acid, and sodium nitrite solutions), the immature pigments producing what is known as an indirect reaction (the pink colour developing only after addition of alcohol), the mature a direct reaction (a quickly produced violet coloration). It was this test, the van den Bergh reaction, which first threw light on the two types of bile-pigment responsible for the two principal forms of jaundice.

Hepatogenous Jaundice.—This includes those forms of jaundice in which the liver parenchyma is damaged by toxic agents such as trinitrotoluol, carbon tetrachloride, gold, arsenic, etc., by known infections such as yellow fever or Weil's disease, or by unknown infectious agents as in ' catarrhal jaundice ', or after administration of serum. The last group is commonly called infective hepatitis. The liver cells in hepatogenous jaundice are incapable of dealing adequately with the bilirubin presented to them for conversion into bile-pigment, and probably the exit of any formed bile is impeded by swelling of the liver cells.

In the present chapter we are more particularly concerned with obstructive jaundice, of which the best example is the obstruction produced by gall-stones.

Symptoms of Obstructive Jaundice.—Obstructive jaundice varies in intensity from a slight yellowish tinge in the skin and mucous membranes to a pronounced canary yellow, or, in long-standing cases, a greenish-yellow discoloration. It affects the skin of the whole body, but is most marked on the trunk and proximal portions of the limbs. Even before the skin is affected the yellowing is seen in the mucous membranes, and should be sought in the conjunctivæ and under surface of the tongue. Intolerable itching is common, and is probably due to bile-salts, as it may precede the actual pigmentation of the skin and mucosæ. The toxic action of the bile-salts on the sino-auricular node may also produce bradycardia. The excess of bile-pigments in the blood leads to their appearance in the urine, which may be visibly bile-stained or in which bile may be detected by special tests (see Chapter XIV). The lack of the normal flow of bile into the duodenum deprives the fæces of one of their colouring constituents, and further interferes with the digestion and absorption of fats. As a result, the fæces have a lighter colour than normal and are often clay-coloured. In complete obstruction urobilin is absent from the urine.

As the jaundice disappears, the bile disappears from the urine and the stools become coloured once more.

SUMMARY.—To summarize the differences between the three types of jaundice, it may be said that :—

Obstructive jaundice is usually deep yellow (*Fig.* 135), and associated

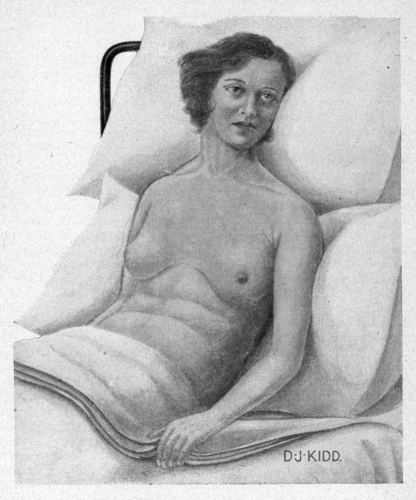

Fg. 135.—Obstructive jaundice. The yellow coloration is deep, and especially notice-able in the conjunctivæ ; the colour of the lips is normal, in fact it often appears redder by contrast with the jaundiced skin. Such a case would have clay-coloured stools and bile in the urine. Contrast with hæmolytic jaundice (*Fig.* 136).

with bile in the urine and a deficiency of bile in the stools causing them to be pale. The van den Bergh reaction shows a direct positive result.

Hæmolytic jaundice is a faint jaundice sometimes giving the classical lemon tint of pernicious anæmia (*Fig.* 136), in which there is no bile in the urine, but, on the other hand, urobilin is present in excess and the stools are normal in colour. The van den Bergh test shows an indirect positive reaction.

Toxic or infective jaundice, which may combine the features of the other two varieties, is rarely so deep as obstructive jaundice, although

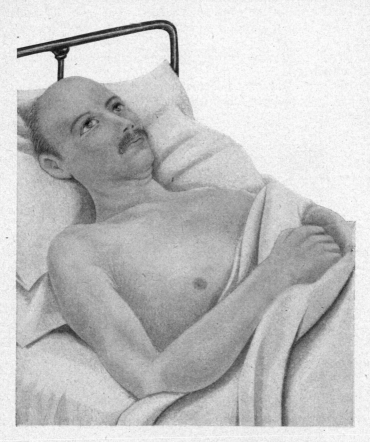

Fig. 136.—Hæmolytic jaundice (case of pernicious anæmia). The jaundice is comparatively pale; the conjunctivæ are a creamy yellow. Note the evidence of anæmia in the pallor of the lips. In such a case the stools would be normal in colour, the urine would contain no bile, but urobilin would be present in excess. Contrast with obstructive jaundice (*Fig.* 135).

inflammatory swelling of the bile-passages may add some degree of obstruction. Bile or urobilin or both may be found in the urine. The van den Bergh may show a biphasic reaction in which direct and indirect responses are obtained.

ANATOMICAL CONSIDERATIONS

Before proceeding to the detailed examination of the abdomen, certain anatomical facts may be recalled. It is customary for purposes of clinical description to divide the abdomen into nine regions by two vertical and two horizontal lines. Each vertical line may be taken as parallel with and midway between a vertical line from the episternal notch to the symphysis pubis and a vertical line passing through the anterior superior spine of the ilium. The upper horizontal line passes across the abdomen at the lowest point of the 10th costal arches. The lower horizontal line joins the two anterior superior spines of the ilia.* The ' regions ' thus marked out (*Fig.* 137) are :—

In the upper abdomen—the right hypochondrium, epigastrium, and left hypochondrium.

In the middle—the right lumbar, umbilical, left lumbar.

In the lower abdomen—the right iliac fossa, hypogastrium, and left iliac fossa.

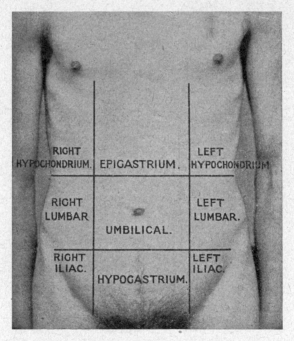

Fig. 137.—The regions of the abdomen.

It must be emphasized that the main value of the regions is to *describe the position of pain, tenderness, and rigidity, tumours, etc. Lists of viscera contained in these regions are fallacious.* The stomach, intestines, and kidneys (and other viscera to a lesser extent) are so mobile that they are

---

* Other lines are also in use, and it matters little which the student employs, as the division of the abdomen into regions is purely arbitrary, and is of more clinical than anatomical value.

not constantly found in the same regions, even in the same individual, and in different normal individuals differ widely in position (*Figs*. 138–141).

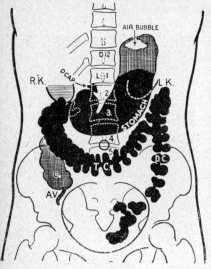

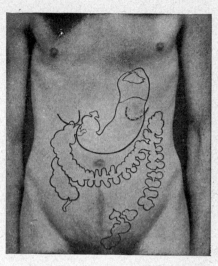

Fig. 138.Fig. 139.

Fig. 138.—Abdominal viscera. The position of the stomach, first part of the duodenum, large intestine, and kidneys is outlined in relation to the bony landmarks. Although constructed by superimposed radiographs from a sthenic individual, the position of these viscera is so variable that the results depicted must be taken as one type only (cf. *Figs*. 140-145). R.K., Right kidney; L.K., Left kidney; D, Duodenal cap; T.C., Transverse colon; D.C., Descending colon; A.V., Appendix vermiformis. (*Constructed with the help of Dr*. *P*. *H*. *Whitaker*.)

Fig. 139.—Abdominal viscera. The position of the same organs as in *Fig*. 138 in relation to the surface. (*Constructed from radiographs with the help of Dr*. *P*. *H*. *Whitaker*.)

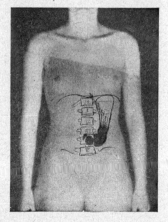

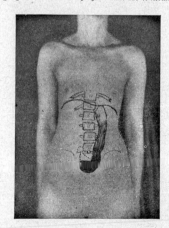

Fig. 140.Fig. 141.

Figs. 140, 141.—To show variation of position of stomach in different types—woman aged 27 and woman aged 55—with subject standing and at rest.

(*Figs*. 140, 141 *by kind permission from* Barclay's ' The Digestive Tract ', *Cambridge University Press*.)

Some organs, however, are more or less fixed. The gall-bladder is generally found in the right hypochondrium, the liver in the right hypochondrium and epigastrium, the spleen in the left hypochondrium. The hypogastrium contains the full bladder or pregnant uterus.

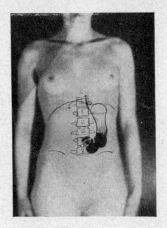

Fig. 142.

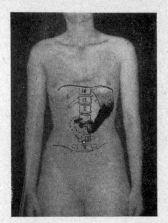

Fig. 143.

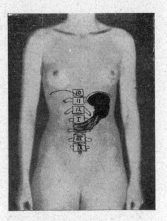

Fig. 144.

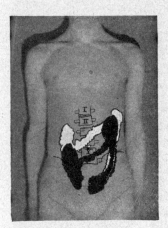

Fig. 145.

Figs. 142–144.—To show change of position of stomach with respiration and posture. Fig. 142 : Standing, full inspiration. Fig. 143 : Standing, full expiration. Fig. 144 : Lying supine at rest.

Fig. 145.—To show position of colon standing (black) and lying supine (white), taken in mid phase of respiration.

(Figs. 142–145 by kind permission from Barclay's ' The Digestive Tract ', Cambridge University Press.)

Posture and respiration have a profound effect on the position of the viscera (Figs. 142–145).

PHYSICAL SIGNS : EXAMINATION OF THE ABDOMEN

A careful history is most important in the diagnosis of diseases of the digestive system, and it is often disappointing that the symptoms are not corroborated by abnormal physical signs and that for a diagnosis the physician must frequently resort to special methods of investigation, such as radiology and chemical analysis. This admission, however, forms no excuse for the omission of the well-recognized clinical methods of examination. The examination of the mouth and œsophagus has already been considered. The examination of the abdominal viscera requires a knowledge of the method of examination of the abdomen in general, and certain special details concerning the individual viscera.

Examination of the abdomen should follow the routine described under the respiratory and cardio-vascular systems—inspection, palpation, percussion, and auscultation—though inspection and palpation are by far the most important methods of approach.

Inspection shows the condition of the abdominal wall, the size of the abdomen, and any irregularity in its contour caused by enlargement of viscera or the presence of abnormal swellings in the abdominal cavity. It also shows certain motile phenomena such as the movement of the abdominal wall with respiration, the presence of visible peristalsis in the stomach or intestines, and the pulsations of the aorta or an engorged liver.

Palpation determines the presence of superficial or deep tenderness, and of undue rigidity or laxity of the abdominal wall. It is the principal method by which enlargement of viscera such as the liver, spleen, and kidneys, and the presence of tumours, are detected.

Percussion may add confirmatory information in the case of enlarged viscera or tumours, and may help in recognizing the presence of free fluid in the peritoneal cavity. In cases of tympanites (gastro-intestinal distension) the note on percussion is drum-like.

Auscultation is rarely of value in the diagnosis of digestive disorders, but when X-ray examination is not available it may be used to determine the presence of œsophageal obstruction. It is also useful in distinguishing between paralytic ileus and other forms of intestinal obstruction.

INSPECTION

Inspection of the abdomen must be carried out in a good light and if possible with the patient both in the erect and recumbent postures.

Condition of the Abdominal Wall.—The *skin* of the abdomen should first be observed. When abdominal distension is present from any cause the skin is stretched, smooth, and shiny, and the umbilicus may be flattened or even everted. Undue laxity of the abdominal wall, causing wrinkling of the skin, is found when intra-abdominal pressure is suddenly decreased, as after childbirth (especially in multiparæ), and after removal of fluid from the peritoneal cavity. After repeated pregnancies

12

broad silvery lines known as *striæ gravidarum* are frequently seen on the abdominal wall.

Enlarged veins are useful evidence of obstruction in the vena cava and portal systems. The greater the distension and the more numerous the veins, the greater the obstruction is likely to be.

Obstruction in the inferior vena cava or common iliac veins usually causes veins to appear at the *sides* of the abdomen (*Fig.* 146), and when the veins are emptied by pressure with the fingers, they will be seen to fill again from below. The blood by-passes the inferior vena cava, travelling from the lower limbs (and certain viscera) to the thorax via the veins of the abdominal wall. These superficial veins are arranged longitudinally.

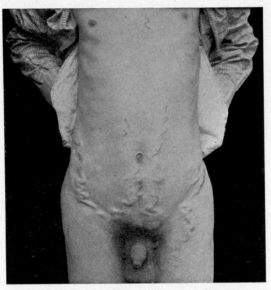

Fig. 146.—Enlarged abdominal veins.

Thrombosis of the inferior vena cava, owing to its completeness in obstructing the circulation, will cause the most pronounced collateral circulation to become apparent on the abdominal wall, but any increase in the intra-abdominal pressure (e.g., ascites) will have a similar though less striking result.

If the obstruction is in the portal system (cirrhosis of the liver, or more rarely thrombosis of the portal vein) the engorged veins are *centrally* placed, and may form a little cluster around the umbilicus (caput medusæ). The blood in these veins flows in all directions away from the umbilicus. The direction of the blood-flow should always be tested.

A section of vein can be emptied by 'milking' it with the fingers, and each end of the emptied part is sealed with the pressure of a finger. One finger can then be removed and the rate at which the vein fills is noted.

The performance is repeated, removing the finger at the other end. The blood enters more rapidly from the direction of the blood-flow.

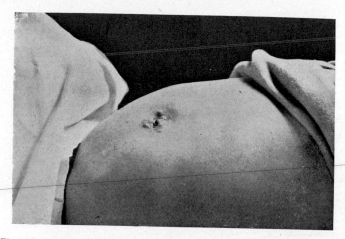

Fig. 147.—Secondary nodules at umbilicus associated with carcinoma of the bladder and secondary malignant liver.

Secondary nodules may be found in the skin in certain types of malignant disease (*Fig.* 147, *and see also Fig.* 19, p. 30). Œdema of the abdominal wall may be demonstrated by the usual phenomenon of pitting, and has the same origin as œdema elsewhere. It is not to be confused with the presence of dropsical fluid in the peritoneal cavity itself (*ascites*). Small herniæ due to extrusion of small pieces of extraperitoneal fat are not uncommonly seen in the midline of the upper abdomen (*Fig.* 148). They are usually symptomless. Larger herniæ may be seen at or near the umbilicus or protruding through abdominal scars.

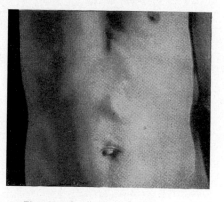

Fig. 148.—Small epigastric hernia. (By kind permission from de Quervain's 'Clinical Surgical Diagnosis', John Dale, Sons & Danielsson.)

Movements of the Abdominal Wall.—The movements of the abdominal wall should be carefully watched. In men with the abdominal type of respiration the movement should be free and equal on the two sides. In women the movement is often restricted owing to the costal type of breathing. An absolute *fixation* of the whole or greater part of the abdominal wall is a most important *sign of generalized peritonitis*, whilst in cases of localized peritonitis, e.g., due to appendix or gall-bladder infections, the segment of the abdominal wall lying over the affected viscus shows diminished movement.

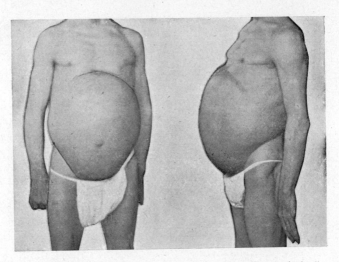

Fig. 149.—Abdominal distension. Great abdominal swelling due to colonic distension the result of fæcal impaction. (*Mr. C. A. Wells's case.*)

Contour of the Abdomen.—The contour of the abdomen should next be noted. When abnormal swelling is present it is important to observe whether it is uniform or asymmetrical. Uniform swelling may be caused by obesity, by distension of the abdomen by gas in the gastro-intestinal tract (*Fig.* 149), or by fluid in the peritoneal cavity (*Fig.* 150). Large abdominal tumours such as an over-filled bladder,

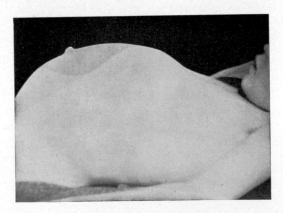

Fig. 150.—Abdominal swelling due to ascites (tuberculous peritonitis). Note the gentle curve extending from the pubis to the epigastrium only becoming steep where it joins with the ensiform cartilage. The umbilicus is everted.

pregnant uterus, or large ovarian cyst cause swelling of the abdomen which at a first glance may appear uniform, but which closer inspection shows to be limited to the contour of the enlarged viscus or tumour. In visceroptosis the lower abdomen bulges unduly when the patient stands (*Fig.* 151).

Irregularities in the contour of the abdomen may be caused by enlargement of viscera such as the liver (*Fig.* 152), spleen, kidneys, or gall-bladder, or by tumours arising from these and other organs, e.g., the stomach, intestines, pancreas, or peritoneum (*Fig.* 153). Distension of one portion of the alimentary tract may also produce irregularity in the abdominal contour, e.g., gastric

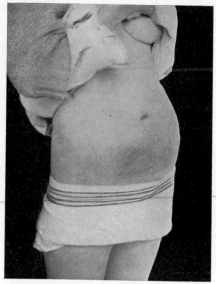

Fig. 151.—The visceroptotic abdomen. Note the protuberance of the lower abdomen, noticeable only when the patient is standing.

distension producing a bulge in the epigastrium or colonic distension causing a fullness in the flanks. The type and degree of irregularity

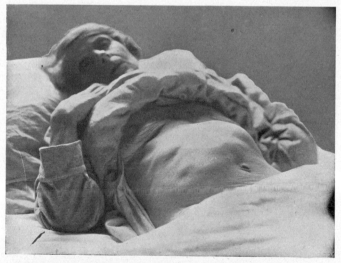

Fig. 152.—Malignant disease of liver. Enormous liver enlargement due to secondary growths from neoplasm of ovary. Note especially the nodular irregularity.

in the contour of the abdominal wall will depend upon the size, shape, and regularity of the underlying swelling.

Movements Beneath the Abdominal Wall.—Care should be taken to observe any movements occurring beneath the abdominal wall

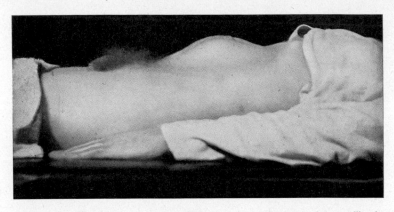

Fig. 153.—Abdominal swelling due to mesenteric cyst. The curve of the swelling has a fairly steep rise at the pubis and in the epigastrium, and obviously occupies chiefly the lower abdomen (cf. ascites, Fig. 150).

or communicated through it. *Visible pulsation of the abdominal aorta is frequent in nervous individuals, especially in those with a thin abdominal wall, and is of no moment.* It must be distinguished from aneurysm of the abdominal aorta. In this condition the pulsation is usually more marked, and it is generally possible by palpation to define the outline of an enlarged expansile arterial swelling. Often aortic pulsation is transmitted through an overlying viscus or tumour. For example, the aorta may cause pulsation of a carcinoma of the stomach, which must then be differentiated from aneurysm. In these cases of transmitted pulsation the pulsating tumour is usually irregular, and its pulsations may cease if the patient is examined in the knee-elbow position, so that the tumour falls away from the underlying aorta.

Peristalsis may be visible in cases of obstruction in the gastro-intestinal tube. Obstruction at the pylorus causes increased peristaltic movements of the stomach, seen through the abdominal wall as a slow wave moving from left to right across the upper abdomen (*Fig.* 154). Obstruction in the large intestine may also be accompanied by peristaltic waves in the upper abdomen, in this case moving from right to left. In obstruction of the small intestines the peristaltic waves may be seen in a ladder pattern down the centre of the abdomen.

PALPATION

Successful palpation needs much practice. The most favourable posture for the patient is lying flat on his back with the head slightly raised (one pillow), the arms to the side, and the knees well drawn up. In palpation of the lower abdomen it may be helpful to have the legs fully extended. The patient should be asked to breathe quietly and rather more deeply than normal, keeping the mouth open to encourage the abdominal type of respiration. When the examiner is satisfied that the abdomen is moving freely, palpation may be commenced, using the flat hand but exerting pressure with the fingers. The finger-tips should be used only after the flat hand has first been employed, and then only under special circumstances, as the discomfort caused by their use leads to reflex spasm of the abdominal wall which prevents satisfactory examination. The following points should be systematically observed :—

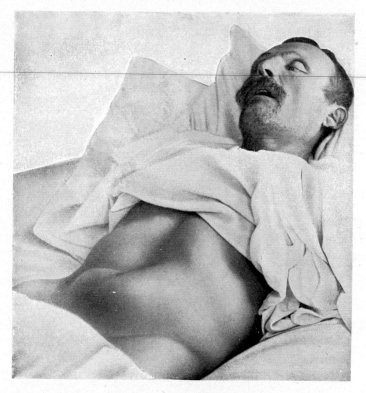

Fig. 154.—Stenosis of the pylorus due to cancer. An attack of gastric rigidity. (Stomach not artificially inflated.) (By kind permission from de Quervain's ' Clinical Surgical Diagnosis ', John Bale, Sons & Danielsson.)

1. **Tenderness.**—Tenderness means pain on pressure. It has already been stated that pain has been variously explained as a viscero-sensory reflex or a peritoneo-cutaneous reflex. Whatever the path may be in the nervous system, it is generally agreed that *deep tenderness* is most commonly found in inflammatory lesions of the viscera and their surrounding peritoneum. Tenderness, for example, in the right iliac fossa is most frequently found in appendicitis, tenderness in the right hypochondrium in cholecystitis, whilst purely visceral pain such as gastric or intestinal colic is not associated

with any tenderness. Occasionally pressure in one region of the abdomen may cause pain in another. For example, pressure in the left iliac fossa sometimes causes pain in the right, in cases of appendicitis. This is the exception rather than the rule, and is probably explained by transmission of the pressure to the right iliac fossa, e.g., through the colon. *Tenderness is usually found over the region where the inflamed viscus is lying.* If an area of tenderness is expected, the palpating hand should first be placed on the abdomen in some region distant from the suspected area. In appendicitis, for example, palpation should begin in the left iliac fossa, which, being normal, will form a contrast to the tenderness in the right iliac fossa.

Closely allied to deep tenderness are *cutaneous hyperæsthesia* and *tenderness in the superficial tissues* of the abdominal wall.

Hyperæsthesia may be detected by stroking the skin of the abdominal wall with the point of a pin. Over inflammatory lesions the sensation will be more acute than over the control area. The sign is not very constant and too much stress should not be laid upon it.

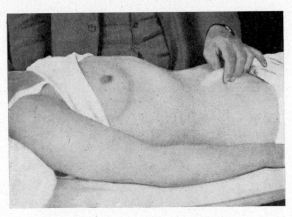

Fig. 155.—Ligat's tenderness. Hyperæsthesia of the subcutaneous tissues can be demonstrated by pinching them as shown, comparing a control area with the suspected one.

Superficial tenderness or *Ligat's tenderness* is elicited by pinching the skin and subcutaneous tissues between the fingers (*Fig.* 155). Like hyperæsthesia, it is often found in inflammatory abdominal lesions, but is also inconstant.

All forms of tenderness may be found in neurotic individuals who have no local abdominal disease, especially in patients with visceroptosis. As a temporary phenomenon *tympanites* (distension of the gastro-intestinal tract with gas) may also give rise to tenderness.

2. Rigidity.—Abdominal rigidity is due to muscular contraction, which often occurs reflexly as a part of a defence mechanism over an inflamed organ. This has already been discussed.

Many patients hold the abdominal wall so rigidly that examination is difficult or impossible, but in the majority, if the patient is put in a comfortable position and his mind set at rest by explaining that no undue pain will be caused by the examination, the abdominal muscles gradually relax. Nervous rigidity of this type generally affects the whole abdominal wall. *Localized rigidity is*, therefore, *more suggestive of disease.* The notable *exception* to this is the case of acute generalized peritonitis, where extreme and generalized abdominal rigidity occurs ('board-like rigidity'); but in this case other signs leave no doubt as to the significance of the rigidity.

As in the examination for tenderness, the palpating hand should *first test the rigidity of the abdominal muscles in some part away from the suspected lesion.* For example, if cholecystitis is suspected palpation should begin in the left hypochondrium, which then forms a standard of control to the rigidity in the right hypochondrium. The bellies of the rectus muscles sometimes cause difficulty in the examination of the abdomen. Portions of them may be so rigid as to simulate a lump beneath the abdominal wall, and it is important to compare carefully the two recti. If the rectus muscles are brought into use such a 'tumour' becomes more pronounced (*Fig.* 156). In some patients, on the other hand, the rectus muscles are

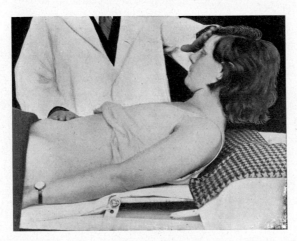

Fig. 156.—Method of bringing the rectus muscles into action. To determine whether a swelling is in or deep to the rectus abdominis muscles, the patient must bring these muscles into action whilst the observer's hand is placed over the swelling. This can be accomplished by instructing the patient to raise the head and shoulders against the slight resistance of pressure on the forehead.

so poorly developed and toneless that the hand can palpate through them with the same ease as through other portions of the abdominal wall. In perfectly healthy individuals it is not uncommon to find separation of the rectus muscles producing a wide gap in which the abdominal wall is so thin that the viscera beneath can be palpated more distinctly than normal.

3. Enlargement of Viscera.—

The Liver.—Palpation of the liver is made by resting the flat of one or both hands on the abdomen with the tips of the fingers gently inserted beneath the costal margin. To avoid overlooking *gross* enlargement it is advisable to *move the hand from the right iliac fossa gradually upwards* until any increased sense of resistance is noted. At this point the fingertips may be used to locate the liver edge accurately (*Fig.* 157). The enlarged viscus may project only half an inch below the costal margin, but in some conditions may extend well below the umbilicus.

The *character of the edge* should be recorded. When palpable in health it is sharp, firm, and regular, gradually passing upwards as it crosses the epigastrium into the left hypochondrium. In many normal persons it is not palpable, but may become so from slight displacement of the viscus without any other disease. Deformities of the chest as a result of kyphosis or rickets, and also tight lacing, are sometimes responsible

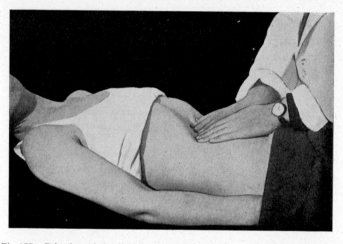

Fig. 157.—Palpation of the liver. Both hands are placed flat on the abdomen with the fingers directed towards the costal margin and gradually moved upwards until resistance is encountered. The patient then takes a deep breath and the edge of liver rides over the fingers.

for displacing the liver downwards so that it appears to be considerably enlarged. In infants also the liver is relatively enlarged and may be palpable in health.

An unusual tongue of liver substance, *Riedel's lobe*, may occasionally give rise to difficulty. It is sometimes freely mobile and may be mistaken for a movable kidney, or, if situated nearer the middle line, for a gallbladder swelling. It is almost invariably in the right upper quadrant of the abdomen.

When the liver is enlarged from fatty changes, its edge is soft and difficult to feel, especially in an obese person. Fortunately, this type of enlargement, though common, is rarely an important point in the diagnosis. In most other forms of liver enlargement the edge is firm or even harder than normal. Thus in passive congestion of the liver due to cardiac failure the edge is firmer than normal, whilst *in malignant disease* and gummatous infiltration it may be very *hard and irregular*.

The *surface of the liver* should next be palpated. In cancerous and gummatous infiltration it may be grossly irregular owing to the presence of large nodules. In malignant disease these nodules may have a characteristic depression in their centre called *umbilication*. In alcoholic cirrhosis of the liver the surface is finely irregular, but this cannot be determined with certainty on clinical examination. In most other forms of liver enlargement, e.g., chronic venous congestion, hepatic abscess, amyloid disease, fatty changes, and leukæmic infiltrations, the surface of the organ is quite smooth.

The *degree of enlargement* also gives useful information. In the congestion of heart failure, for example, the size of the liver is often roughly proportionate to the degree of cardiac failure, and its shrinkage is a useful indication of the response to treatment. In moderate cases of heart failure the liver edge extends two or three inches below the costal margin, and only in extreme failure does it reach the level of the umbilicus. Such gross enlargement of the liver is commoner in cancer, amyloid degeneration, tropical abscess, syphilis, and certain blood diseases. Moderate enlargement of the liver occurs in temporary obstruction to the common bile-duct, e.g., with gall-stones or catarrhal jaundice, in cirrhosis of the liver, and in other rarer conditions.

Finally, it should be noted whether the liver is *tender or painless* on palpation. Tenderness is often found in the congested liver of heart failure and in inflammatory lesions, e.g., hepatitis and liver abscess, whilst the gross enlargements of cancer, syphilis, and other diseases remain quite painless.

CAUSES OF HEPATIC ENLARGEMENT

TENDER ENLARGEMENT	PAINLESS ENLARGEMENT

Chronic venous congestion
  (e.g., from heart or lung disease)
Acute congestion
  (amœbic infection)
Hepatic abscess
  (portal pyæmia and tropical abscess)
Actinomycosis
	Obstruction to common bile-duct
	  (e.g., in catarrhal jaundice, gall-stones,
	  etc.)
	Cirrhosis
	  Alcoholic multilobular
	  Hanot's hypertrophic form
	  Banti's disease
	  Bronzed diabetes
	  Chronic perihepatitis
	Hæmopoietic diseases
	  Hodgkin's disease
	  Various forms of leukæmia
	Malignant disease
	  Primary carcinoma (rare)
	  Secondary carcinoma (common) and
	    sarcoma
	Syphilis
	  Gummatous masses
	  Syphilitic cirrhosis
	Degenerations and infiltrations
	  Amyloid disease (associated with
	    syphilis, tuberculosis, and chronic
	    suppuration)
	  Fatty liver

The Gall-bladder.—In obstruction of the cystic duct, commonly with stone, or of the common bile-duct, particularly by growth of the head of the pancreas, enlargement of the gall-bladder may be found. The organ is felt as a smooth tense swelling projecting beneath the right costal margin in the direction of the umbilicus. If the enlargement is great the swelling may be mistaken for another viscus—for example, an enlarged right kidney. Moderate degrees of enlargement may be obscured if the gall-bladder is covered by the liver. A distended gall-bladder in the presence of jaundice is due to some cause other than gall-stones (generally to carcinoma of the head of the pancreas). This is known as *Courvoisier's Law (Fig.* 158). It is explained by the fact that gall-stones, if present for a considerable time, cause fibrosis of the gall-bladder. Thus when a stone is later impacted in the common bile-duct, jaundice results, but the gall-bladder is unable to expand. Irregularity of a gall-bladder tumour

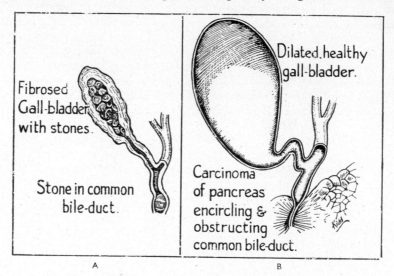

Fig. 158.—Courvoisier's Law. A, Jaundice caused by a gall-stone in the common duct. The gall-bladder cannot dilate as it is fibrosed from cholecystitis due to stones within it. B, Jaundice due to obstruction of the common bile-duct by carcinoma of the head of the pancreas. The gall-bladder is dilated owing to the back-pressure of the bile.

is found when the organ is filled with stones or is the seat of malignant disease.

The palpation of other enlarged abdominal viscera, e.g., the kidneys and spleen, not directly connected with the digestive tract, will be dealt with under the appropriate system.

4. Abdominal Tumour.—On detection of a tumour in the abdomen the following points should be observed.

Position.—An accurate description of the position often helps to decide the organ from which the tumour is growing, and when its outline has been defined the observer should consider what organs and tissues

lie in this region of the abdomen. The localization of tumours is sometimes difficult owing to the fact that only a small portion may present at
the abdominal wall, and the bulk of the tumour may be impalpable because
of its deep situation. When a tumour does not lie in the region of a
particular viscus, the possibility of a peritoneal origin should be
considered. Tuberculous masses may, for example, be distributed
irregularly in the omentum or mesentery, and in the latter cysts also
occur (*Fig.* 159). Care should be taken also to exclude the possibility of
the tumour arising from the abdominal wall. In this case modifications
of the shape and size of the tumour can be produced by making the
patient move the abdominal muscles.

Size.—The larger the tumour, the more difficult it is to determine
the tissue from which it is growing, but certain tumours by their very size
(e.g., an ovarian cyst, which forms a large round swelling in the lower
abdomen) give a valuable clue to their nature.

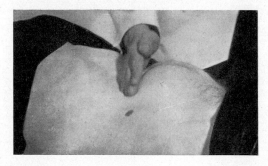

Fig. 159.—Abdominal swelling due to mesenteric cyst. Showing the hand placed so
as to define the upper border of the tumour. The upper limit of a pregnant uterus or
distended bladder may be similarly defined.

Consistency.—Some organs and tissues, e.g., the stomach, intestines,
and bladder, are normally impalpable unless they are distended respectively by gas, intestinal contents, or urine. If a tumour is found in the
region of these organs its consistency is, therefore, generally easy to
recognize. The consistency of organs such as the liver and spleen may
help to distinguish a simple enlargement of these viscera from enlargement
due to neoplastic infiltration. Most *malignant tumours are hard and
irregular*, though degeneration in them may lead to areas of softening.
Cystic tumours, e.g., pancreatic, peritoneal, or ovarian cysts, have a jelly-
like consistency.

Shape.—In the early stages a tumour may correspond in shape with
the viscus from which it is arising. This is especially so in the case of
the kidney and spleen. As the tumour grows larger the characteristic
shape is often lost and therefore gives no information as to its origin.

Mobility.—Tumours of the stomach, transverse colon, liver, gall-
bladder, kidneys, and spleen generally move downwards with inspiration

owing to the depressing effect of the diaphragm, but tumours of the pancreas, a relatively fixed organ, and of the viscera in the lower abdomen (bladder, uterus, etc.), upon which respiratory movements have little effect, are frequently immobile.

5. **Fluid in the Peritoneal Cavity.**—When free fluid is present in the peritoneal cavity (*Fig.* 160), palpation of enlarged viscera is difficult, but the edge of the enlarged organ, e.g., the liver or spleen, may be felt by ' *dipping* '. This method of palpation is performed by a quick pressure

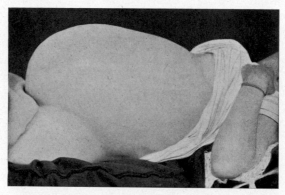

Fig. 160.—Ascites, probably due to tuberculous peritonitis.

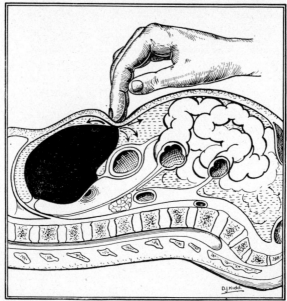

Fig. 161.—' Dipping ' for enlarged liver. Enlarged organs cannot be palpated easily in the presence of ascites. ' Dipping ' may, however, be employed with success. The palpating fingers prod sharply over the expected enlarged viscus, the fluid is displaced as shown by the arrows, and the fingers strike the surface or edge of the organ. Note also the gas-containing intestines which float to the surface and give a central area of resonance on percussion.

of the tips of the fingers over the region where the edge of the viscus is expected. The pressure displaces the fluid temporarily and allows the fingers to come in contact with the enlarged viscus (*Fig.* 161).

The *fluid thrill* is also used to detect the presence of free fluid. The observer places one hand flat on one flank and with the fingers of the other hand gives a sharp tap in the opposite flank. This produces a wave in the fluid which is detectable by the palpating hand. A similar sensation may be obtained if the abdominal wall is very fat, and to avoid this a second observer should place the edge of his hand along the linea alba, exerting firm pressure so as to damp out any vibrations in the abdominal wall itself (*Fig.* 162).

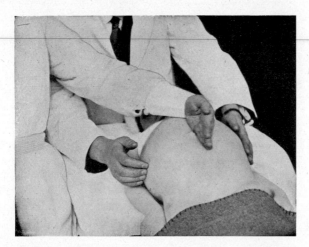

Fig. 162.—The fluid thrill. The nurse's hand is placed firmly along the linea alba. The observer places one hand flat on the flank, whilst the fingers of the other percuss on the opposite flank.

6. The Hernial Ring.—Apart from epigastric and umbilical herniæ the external abdominal rings should be carefully examined in every case. This is particularly necessary in any case suggestive of intestinal obstruction, of which strangulation of an inguinal or femoral hernia is quite a common cause. In the case of a male the patient should stand upright and the finger should be inserted through the invaginated scrotum into the external abdominal ring and the patient told to cough. Small herniæ can be detected in this way as they give a forcible impulse to the palpating finger.

Rectal Examination.—Digital examination of the rectum is employed for many purposes, and is mentioned elsewhere in dealing with other systems. In the examination of the digestive tract it is used to determine the tone of the anal sphincter, the presence of any hæmorrhoids, the condition of emptiness or fullness of the rectum, and above all the *presence of any new growth* in the rectum itself or any tumour of the surrounding tissues which may press on or obstruct the rectum. ' Ballooning ' of the rectum suggests obstruction at the pelvi-rectal junction. Under ordinary circumstances the examination should be made with the patient in the left lateral position with the knees well drawn up towards the chin. The finger should be inserted gently with an adequate amount of lubricant, and exploration of all parts of the wall of the rectum and of the surrounding structures may then be made. It is sometimes easier, especially in fat persons and when examining the anterior wall of the rectum or tissues lying in contact with it, to make a rectal examination with the patient in the knee-elbow position. In this position the patient rests on the knees and elbows, with the thighs vertical (see Fig. 129).

PERCUSSION

Percussion has only a limited use in the examination of the alimentary system. Light percussion as a rule gives more information than heavy, and is of most value in helping to elucidate the cause of abdominal enlargement. Uniform enlargement caused by gastro-intestinal distension with *gas yields a tympanitic note*, whilst a similar enlargement caused by *fluid yields a dull note*, which may be present all over the abdomen if the fluid is large in amount, or only in the flanks if the fluid is insufficient to cover the centrally placed coils of intestine. When fluid is suspected, percussion should be performed firstly with the patient lying on his back and then lying alternately on each side. This movement will lead to a displacement of the fluid into the flank nearest the bed, over which a dull note will be obtained, whilst the empty upper flank will yield a tympanitic note. This phenomenon is known as *shifting dullness*.

Percussion may be used as an accessory method to palpation in defining the outline of enlarged viscera or abdominal tumours. The nearer the viscus or tumour lies to the abdominal wall, the more definite will the results of percussion be.

(*See also* LIVER, p. 198.)

AUSCULTATION

Auscultation is rarely a method of much interest in the examination of the digestive system, as most of the information it gives is more accurately obtained by radiological and laboratory methods. Occasionally in œsophageal obstruction auscultation over the lower part of the chest may give some indication of the delay in the passage of fluid from the pharynx to the cardiac end of the stomach. The patient should hold the fluid in his mouth until instructed to swallow, and the observer should listen for two sounds, firstly as the fluid goes from the pharynx into the œsophagus, and secondly as it passes from the œsophagus through the cardiac sphincter. Between these two sounds there is usually an interval of five to ten seconds, and considerable delay may occur in œsophageal obstruction, or the second sound may be entirely absent.

In cases of *peritonitis*, the *absence* of the normal sounds due to peristaltic activity may be a suggestive sign ; the sounds disappear first in the neighbourhood of the lesion. On the other hand, in *obstructive lesions* of the gastro-intestinal tract the sounds may be greatly *exaggerated*.

PHYSICAL SIGNS : EXAMINATION OF INDIVIDUAL VISCERA

After the general abdominal examination which has been described the observer turns his attention to the particular viscus which the symptomatology of the case places under suspicion.

THE STOMACH

Clinical examination of the stomach is often disappointing.

Inspection may show the outline of the organ when it is distended with gas or food, and may show irregularities in contour due to the presence of neoplasms. Visible peristalsis and the outline of a large stomach may be seen in cases of pyloric obstruction.

Palpation determines the presence of any tenderness or rigidity such as may be found in the abdominal wall over an ulcer or neoplasm. It is the main method employed for detecting the presence of new growths, but unless the growth is of moderate size it may be overlooked even after careful palpation.

Percussion is of most value in marking out the limits of solid tumours arising from the stomach. It is sometimes used to determine the size and position of the stomach, but this is so much more accurately accomplished by X rays that it is no longer a method of importance.

The absence of any definite signs on examination of the stomach frequently makes special investigations necessary.

The *special investigations* include radiology, and fractional test-meal (*see* Chapters XIII and XIV).

DIAGNOSIS OF DISEASES OF THE STOMACH

When the symptoms suggest a lesion of the stomach it is to be remembered that the organic lesions of this organ are few. The more important are :—

1. **Gastritis.**—In its *acute* form this occurs as a temporary phenomenon (normally after dietetic errors or alcoholic excess), characterized by pain, vomiting, and fever, with tenderness in the epigastrium. In a *chronic* form, gastritis occurs as a chronic catarrhal inflammation in which anorexia, nausea, and vomiting of mucus are the dominant features. There are usually no abnormal physical signs, and the diagnosis is made from the symptoms, together with a history of repeated dietetic errors or of those illnesses such as cirrhosis of the liver and cancer of the stomach which cause a chronic gastritis. Chronic suppuration or infection of the nasal sinuses, or in the mouth and fauces, should receive attention as a

13

possible cause. *Gastritis with hyperchlorhydria* may exist without symptoms unless an ulcer is also present, but in some cases symptoms similar to those of ulcer apparently occur.

2. Ulcer.—This may occur in the body of the stomach or on either side (gastric or duodenal) of the pylorus. Regular attacks of pain, usually of a visceral type, and related specifically to meals ; vomiting, with relief of pain ; hæmorrhage ; and tenderness on pressure are the diagnostic features. In most cases these symptoms show characteristic *remissions* for months at a time. Sometimes the diagnosis is clear-cut, but at others it can only be completed by the special methods already mentioned.

3. Neoplasm.—Cancer of the stomach causes symptoms similar to those of ulceration, but less regular, and associated with loss of weight, cachexia, and in some instances with a palpable lump in the epigastrium. There are no remissions as in the case of simple ulcer, and the *appetite is lost.* X rays, gastric analyses, and tests for occult blood are necessary to prove the diagnosis in early cases.

4. Mechanical Deformities.—These often result from ulcer or neoplasm. The most important is *pyloric stenosis*, an obstruction at the pylorus interfering with the normal onward passage of the chyme. The digesting food is retained in the stomach and periodically vomited in large quantities. Pyloric stenosis may also be congenital, manifesting itself early in infancy.

A less common deformity is the *hour-glass stomach*, usually resulting from a chronic gastric ulcer. The deformity results from a constricting band which divides the stomach into two portions. The symptoms are similar to those of pyloric stenosis, and the diagnosis is generally made by radiological examination.

Such are the common organic diseases of the stomach. The symptoms and signs may take such definite shape as to make diagnosis easy, but on the other hand may be simulated by so many other organic and functional diseases that the special methods of radiology, biochemistry, and pathology must frequently be invoked. If these organic diseases can be excluded, attention is next directed to certain *reflex dyspepsias* in which an organic lesion of some other tissue is responsible for derangement of the stomach function. Appendicitis, cholecystitis, and pancreatic disease are examples of diseases in this category, but the reflex cause is not always to be found in a lesion of the abdominal viscera. Familiar examples of remote causes are pulmonary tuberculosis and cerebral tumour.

Lastly, there remain many cases of *indigestion* or *dyspepsia of a functional nature*, that is, in which no organic lesion is to be found in the stomach or other related organ. For these some cause will usually be found if the general health and habits of the patient are carefully considered. Examples of such causes are worry, dietetic indiscretions, toxæmias, and anæmias.

THE INTESTINES

Inspection may show the coils of intestine through a thin abdominal wall, and in cases of obstruction of the bowel visible peristalsis may be seen ;

also, distension of a uniform or localized type may be observed, varying in position with the site of obstruction. Tumours arising from the large intestine are also sometimes visible.

Palpation may be used to excite visible peristalsis. It is of most value in the detection of new growths in the large intestine. The palpating fingers should examine in turn the cæcum, transverse colon, descending colon, and pelvic colon, and particular attention should be directed to the flexures. Carcinoma of the cæcum, ascending colon, or transverse colon is often palpable as a mass, but malignant disease of the descending colon usually takes the form of a stricture, which is frequently impalpable. The transverse colon when loaded with fæces is often palpable in health as a sausage-like tumour lying across the upper abdomen. In the left iliac fossa it is also common to feel the pelvic colon when its walls are in a state of contraction (spastic colon). Tenderness may be present in intestinal diseases, e.g., typhoid or ulcerative colitis, but it is difficult to know how far this sign is peritoneal in origin rather than due to the actual intestinal lesion. In diseases such as appendicitis or diverticulitis the tenderness is chiefly peritoneal and usually accompanied by rigidity.

Percussion, by yielding a drum-like note, may demonstrate the presence of distension of the small intestine. This may be a sign of intestinal obstruction, or of temporary intestinal paresis such as occurs after operations and in severe intestinal diseases such as typhoid fever. Abdominal distension of this type is called *meteorism* or *tympanites*. In distension of the large intestine due to obstruction low in the colon, a tympanitic note is obtained in the flanks.

Auscultation is of limited value in intestinal diseases (*see* p. 192).

The value of *rectal examination* has already been considered.

The *special investigations* include radiology, gastroscopy, duodenal intubation, and sigmoidoscopy (*see* Chapters XII and XIII).

DIAGNOSIS OF DISEASES OF THE INTESTINES

Apart from duodenal ulcer (*see* GASTRIC ULCER, p. 194), diseases of the intestine are generally characterized by diarrhœa, constipation, or both. These symptoms have already been described, and it remains to add that when they are persistent, full investigation of the fæces, bacteriological and biochemical, X rays, and sigmoidoscopy may be necessary to make a diagnosis. These investigations are the more necessary because the symptoms and physical signs of intestinal disease are few, and common to many varieties. Four types may be mentioned :—

1. **Enteritis.**—Whether due to food poisoning, cholera, or tuberculosis, to mention only three of many possible causes, all forms of enteritis (inflammation of the intestine) have colic and diarrhœa as their cardinal symptoms, with few or no physical signs. The term *colic*, as applied to the intestine, means a pain of griping or twisting character lasting only a few seconds at a time and corresponding with waves of peristalsis. Bacteriological examination of the stools is necessary for a complete diagnosis.

Typhoid fever deserves special mention as an example of an enteritis, affecting chiefly the ileum. In addition to local symptoms such as diarrhœa (pea-soup stools) or constipation, there are well-developed constitutional symptoms and signs due to the blood-stream infection. Notable points are the pyrexia (*see* Chapter X), the splenic enlargement and positive blood-culture, the rash, and positive agglutination reactions (Widal).

2. **New Growth.**—Neoplasm of the large bowel or rectum is also associated with diarrhœa or constipation, and frequently with hæmorrhage, but unless the mass is palpable per rectum or on abdominal examination, the diagnosis must rest on the special methods of investigation.

3. **Intestinal Obstruction.**—Here again, constipation and colic are the initial symptoms. Soon, however, vomiting follows as a distinguishing feature in cases of acute obstruction. At first the vomitus consists of the stomach contents, later of bile regurgitated from the duodenum, and later still of the fæculent contents of the small intestine. In chronic cases of obstruction this characteristic vomiting is not present and the diagnosis must depend upon the history of constipation and colic and the special methods of examination. In obstruction of the large intestine excessive oral flatulence is common and the flatus may be offensive. It must be emphasized again that the symptoms assume a special importance when they are persistent, for colic may arise from trivial disorders such as irritant food or temporary constipation, but as a rule passes away in such cases within a few days.

4. **Appendicitis.**—This common condition is representative of acute inflammatory disease affecting a localized portion of the intestine. The onset is comparatively sudden, with generalized abdominal pain of a colicky type. Later the pain becomes more localized in the right iliac fossa and is accompanied in most cases by tenderness and rigidity. A mass may be palpable if *abscess formation* takes place. Although the signs are usually maximal in the right iliac fossa, they may be found in other places, e.g., the right loin or right hypochondrium, according to the position of the appendix. A pelvic appendix when inflamed may fail to produce localizing signs. Vomiting is common, but seldom occurs more than once or twice. The temperature and pulse-rate are raised, but present no constant features. Leucocytosis is usual. Constipation is the rule, but diarrhœa may occur, and this or other anomalous symptoms such as frequency of micturition require careful consideration. Rectal examination, advisable always, is of particular value in such cases, and tenderness in the rectovesical pouch may be noticeable.

Appendicular colic is a term usually applied to abdominal colic associated with tenderness and rigidity in the right iliac fossa, but without inflammatory reactions such as pyrexia and increased pulse-rate.

Appendicular dyspepsia may imitate a duodenal ulcer in symptomatology, but the diagnosis is suspected by tenderness and rigidity in the right iliac fossa. The condition must be distinguished from *recurrent appendicitis,* in which the symptoms are essentially those of appendicitis as already described.

Appendicitis has many manifestations, which are described more fully in surgical text-books. In doubtful chronic cases X-ray examination is sometimes useful in revealing constrictions or concretions in the appendix.

THE PERITONEUM

It is convenient to consider the peritoneum at this stage in view of its close association with the alimentary tract. In the description of abdominal pain it has already been pointed out that the peritoneum plays a great part in the production of pain in disease of individual viscera, and it is preferable to envisage such diseases as appendicitis and cholecystitis as diseases affecting the appendix and gall-bladder with their enveloping visceral and neighbouring parietal peritoneum.

In some instances the involvement of the peritoneum is the most important aspect of the case. This is so (1) in acute generalized peritonitis, and (2) in certain forms of chronic peritonitis.

DIAGNOSIS OF DISEASES OF THE PERITONEUM

1. Acute Generalized Peritonitis.—The examination of the ' acute abdomen ' more frequently falls to the surgeon than to the physician, but acute abdominal accidents are not infrequent in medical wards, and the condition, therefore, warrants some attention here. The *symptoms are similar whatever the cause* of the acute peritonitis (e.g., perforated gastric ulcer, ruptured appendix abscess, acute pancreatitis). Intense, agonizing abdominal pain, and collapse are the notable features. Many finer points of distinction are familiar to the surgeon, such as the less severe pain of a perforation into the lesser sac of the peritoneum, and the relative absence of rigidity in acute pancreatitis, but only general features will be described here.

Inspection shows the abdomen to be fixed, exhibiting little if any movement with respiration. Breathing is of a thoracic type. The anxious distressed facies leaves no doubt as to the severity of the symptoms.

Palpation shows extreme abdominal tenderness and board-like rigidity of the abdominal muscles. The tenderness is often accompanied by hyperæsthesia of the skin.

Percussion—which, if employed, should be practised gently—may demonstrate tympanites due to the paresis of the intestinal musculature and the accumulation of gas in the intestines. Free gas may also be present in the peritoneal cavity, and may cause tympany in place of the usual liver dullness.

Several non-surgical conditions may simulate peritonitis quite closely, and when the signs are at all indefinite particular care should be taken to examine the cardio-vascular, respiratory, and nervous systems. Severe abdominal pain may be caused by coronary thrombosis, by aneurysm, by pleurisy, by nerve-root irritation, and by tabes dorsalis, to mention only the more important lesions. If signs of disease are found in another system they must receive due consideration, but it is equally important that if they are trivial they should not be allowed to weigh against a correct diagnosis of peritonitis.

2. Chronic Peritonitis.—Several types of chronic peritonitis are described, but the most important and commonest is the *tuberculous form.*

The symptoms are indefinite, and depend more upon mechanical interference with the stomach and intestines than upon the disease of the peritoneum itself. Thus colic, constipation, and diarrhœa may occur. Constitutional symptoms of the causative disease are added, e.g., loss of weight, anæmia, fever, etc., in tuberculosis.

Inspection may show enlargement of the abdomen due to the presence of *ascites* or of infiltrating *masses* in the peritoneum. The signs of ascites have been described. Peritoneal masses are most commonly seen in the upper abdomen lying in a transverse manner so that they may resemble an enlarged liver or a loaded transverse colon. Their contour, however, is more irregular and does not conform to the shape and size expected from these viscera.

Palpation helps to define a ' rolled omentum ' of this kind from the liver and transverse colon.

THE LIVER

Inspection may show a bulge in the right hypochondrium and epigastrium in cases of liver enlargement, and irregularities may be noticed, especially in malignant disease.

Palpation, however, is the most satisfactory method of demonstrating liver enlargement, and has already been discussed.

Percussion is an accessory method of examination useful in detecting enlargement which is principally upwards. Percussion over the chest wall normally shows a change of note due to the liver at the fifth intercostal space in the mid-clavicular line, at the seventh to eighth rib in the mid-axillary line, and at the ninth to tenth rib in the mid-scapular line. Extension upwards of these limits of dullness suggests enlargement of the liver unless the sign can be accounted for by other conditions. It is rare, however, for the liver to be enlarged upwards without some degree of downward enlargement. More accurate impressions of the size of the liver are gained by X-ray examination.

The *special investigations* include the lævulose test, the van den Bergh reaction, and tests for urobilinuria (*see* Chapter XIV).

DIAGNOSIS OF DISEASES OF THE LIVER

Diagnosis of diseases of the liver is often very difficult, as the symptoms and physical signs are equivocal and the special methods of examination somewhat unreliable. *Serious disease of the organ may be present without abnormal physical signs*, as quite a small amount of liver tissue appears able to carry on the functions of the diseased portions.

A suspicion of liver disease may be aroused by *enlargement of the organ* (*see* p. 185), or conversely by *diminution* in its size.

Pain over the right lower ribs or right hypochondrium, *jaundice* (*see* p. 170), toxæmia, or signs of portal obstruction may also point to liver damage, but very careful consideration of these symptoms is necessary before they can be attributed to liver disease.

Many of the causes of liver enlargement and jaundice are not primarily those of liver disease, and necessitate the examination of other systems for the discovery of their cause (*see* pp. 170, 171, 187).

Three primary diseases of the liver need mention, namely : (1) Acute yellow atrophy ; (2) Cirrhosis ; (3) Abscess.

1. **Acute Yellow Atrophy.**—The initial symptoms of this disease are similar to those of catarrhal jaundice, but the symptoms of a profound toxæmia soon follow. The diagnosis is made by the gravity of the patient's general condition, by diminution in the size of the liver as shown by percussion, and by the presence of unusual constituents in the urine. The more important of these are albumin, bile, urobilin, ketone bodies, and leucin and tyrosin crystals.

2. **Cirrhosis of the Liver.**—The usual form of this disease is the *multilobular cirrhosis* generally caused by chronic alcoholism. The early symptoms are often those of chronic gastritis, also due to the alcoholism. The diagnosis is usually made by discovery of enlargement of the liver in the early stages, or shrinkage in the later stages. The surface of the organ may be finely granular on palpation. Slight jaundice appears later, and the development of ascites may call attention to the presence of portal obstruction. A confirmatory sign is the enlargement of the spleen.

Other types of cirrhosis are rare. The variety known as *Hanot's hypertrophic biliary cirrhosis* is characterized by recurrent jaundice, and enlargement of the liver and spleen.

Syphilitic cirrhosis may resemble the multilobular type.

3. **Liver Abscess.**—*Multiple abscesses* of the liver may result from systemic infection, but, more commonly, from spread of suppurative processes through the portal system from some other part of the alimentary tract—e.g., the appendix. The latter condition is known as *portal pyæmia* and the liver symptoms are essentially secondary.

Amœbic abscess of the liver, although strictly speaking secondary to amœbic infection of the intestine, forms such a separate entity that it is considered here as a primary disease of the liver. Pain over the liver due to hepatitis, toxæmia, and fever are the characteristic symptoms. The diagnosis is completed by the discovery of enlargement of the liver, usually upwards and downwards. There is often tenderness over the liver edge, and irregularities in the surface of the organ are occasionally found. Examination of the stools may show the presence of *Entamœba histolytica*, and a puncture of the liver itself through the abdominal wall or intercostal space enables the typical ' anchovy sauce ' pus to be withdrawn.

A rarer cause of liver abscess is *actinomycosis*, which is secondary to a focus elsewhere in the alimentary tract, usually in the ileocæcal region.

THE GALL-BLADDER AND BILE-DUCTS

Examination of the biliary passages is made by inspection and palpation, especially the latter. Obstruction to the cystic duct and sometimes to the common bile-duct may cause *enlargement of the gall-bladder*. The organ may produce a tumour, occasionally visible through a thin abdominal wall, but more often only *palpable*. (For the characters of a gall-bladder tumour, *see* p. 188.)

The chief *special investigation* is X-ray examination (*see* Chapter XIII).

DIAGNOSIS OF DISEASES OF THE BILIARY PASSAGES

1. **Cholecystitis.**—Inflammation of the gall-bladder commonly results from gall-stones, and its symptoms are often combined with those due to calculi. Certain cases may occur independently of stones, especially the cholecystitis occurring during infections—e.g., typhoid fever.

Pain in the right hypochondrium and at the angle of the right scapula is common. Irregular dyspeptic symptoms, especially flatulence, may also result, and the possibility of cholecystitis should always be considered when these symptoms are not explicable by any gastric lesion. The diagnosis is usually established by a radiograph by Graham's method.

2. **Gall-stones.**—These may merely produce the symptoms of cholecystitis just described. If a stone lodges in the neck of the gall-bladder or passes into the cystic or common bile-duct a characteristic attack of *biliary colic* results (*see* p. 170). Obstruction of the common bile-duct further gives rise to jaundice (*see* p. 170). The diagnosis of calculus is completed by X-ray examination.

THE PANCREAS

The pancreas is a difficult organ to investigate. The symptoms arising when it is diseased are by no means characteristic, and are often erroneously attributed to disease of other viscera. Epigastric pain and dyspeptic symptoms may be present. Jaundice occurs in tumours of the pancreas obstructing the common bile-duct. (*Fig.* 163.)

Examination of the organ is singularly difficult, as it lies deep in the upper abdomen and cannot be successfully palpated.

Tumours of the pancreas, especially cysts, may form rounded swellings in the upper abdomen which may occasionally be both visible and palpable. Cancer may occasionally be detected by the presence of a hard irregular mass in the upper abdomen which is most easily palpated with the patient in the knee-elbow position.

The *special investigations* include tests for steatorrhœa and creatorrhœa, and estimation of blood and urinary diastase and of the blood and urinary sugar content (*see* Chapter XIV).

DIAGNOSIS OF DISEASES OF THE PANCREAS

Two lesions may be mentioned as illustrative types of pancreatic disease :—

1. **Acute Pancreatitis.**—The symptoms of this condition are more dependent upon the intense irritation of the surrounding peritoneum by extravasation of blood and pancreatic juices than upon the loss of pancreatic function.

Intense agonizing pain in the upper abdomen with severe collapse occurs. The degree of tenderness and muscular rigidity which might be expected in such an abdominal catastrophe is not found, as the parietal peritoneum against the anterior abdominal wall is not involved to any great extent. If the patient survives long enough for investigations to be made, signs of pancreatic insufficiency are usually found.

2. **Cancer of the Pancreas.**—By contrast with acute pancreatitis, cancer is a chronic disease of the pancreas. The early symptoms are those common to many dyspepsias, pain, loss of appetite, flatulence, etc. There are superadded the symptoms of malignant disease, namely, loss of weight,

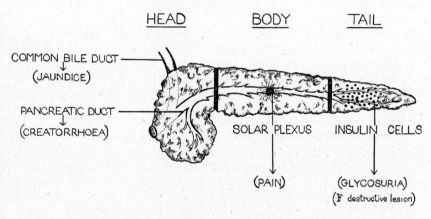

Fig. 163.—Symptomatology of pancreatic disease. The diagram, suggested by Dr. Robert Coope, indicates the common symptoms and signs arising from affections situated in different parts of the pancreas.

loss of strength, and the development of cachexia. An important symptom when present is *jaundice* of a persistent and increasing nature, due to the increasing constriction of the common bile-duct by the growth. The tumour may be palpable (*see* p. 189). Signs of pancreatic insufficiency are often only slight until the late stages of the disease, and in many cases sufficient pancreatic tissue is left to carry on the functions of the organ fairly well although the patient is dying from other effects of the malignant growth.

EXAMINATION OF THE GASTRO-INTESTINAL CONTENTS

The naked-eye inspection of vomited material or of the gastric contents removed by the stomach tube, and of the stools, often gives invaluable help in the diagnosis of gastro-intestinal diseases. The more detailed analyses of the gastric contents by fractional test-meals, and of the fæces by microscopical and chemical tests, generally require the skill of the pathologist, and will, therefore, only receive a brief description in this book.

VOMITUS

Instruction should be given to the nurse or whoever is in charge of the patient to save any vomited material. This should be examined for its *quantity, odour, colour,* and *reaction,* and for the *presence of normal and abnormal constituents.*

Quantity.—The vomit may be large in quantity if there is delay in the passage of the food through the pylorus, especially when this is due to pyloric carcinoma, and the gastric contents increase throughout the day to be vomited in the afternoon or evening. In organic lesions causing pyloric obstruction the food is frequently *undigested,* and the nature of the last meal should always be ascertained so that undigested articles of diet may be recognized.

Odour.—Most vomit possesses a sour odour due to the acid present, but offensiveness usually indicates serious disease. It occurs late in intestinal obstruction, when the vomit may have a *fæculent odour.* Excessive fermentation occurring in malignant disease of the pylorus may also cause an offensive smell.

Colour and Constituents.—The colour of the vomit varies considerably with the length of time the food has been in the stomach, with the amount of duodenal regurgitation, and with the presence of abnormal constituents. *Blood* may give it a bright-red appearance if vomiting occurs soon after the hæmorrhage, but usually the blood remains in the stomach sufficiently long to be altered to a dark brown colour—' coffee-grounds ' (*see* HÆMATEMESIS, p. 167). *Bile* is a normal constituent, giving a yellowish or greenish appearance to the vomit, but it may be excessive in disease. In certain phases of intestinal obstruction the vomit may consist very largely of bile, later being replaced by a thin brownish fluid derived from the small intestine and recognized only by a fæculent odour. *Mucus* is identified by its jelly-like appearance and is present in small amounts in most vomit. In large amounts it suggests a catarrhal inflammation of the gastric mucosa—chronic gastritis. Rarer constituents of vomit are *pus,* which may be swallowed or derived from some extrinsic abscess ; pieces of new growth ; and various parasites and ova. These constituents usually require microscopy for their recognition.

Reaction.—The reaction of the stomach contents may be tested with litmus, and the presence of free hydrochloric acid can be shown with Günzburg's reagent (*see* Chapter XIV).

THE FÆCES

A simple examination of the stools should never be omitted when the patient has symptoms of alimentary disease.

The fæces are made up of voluminous soap gels, residues of intestinal secretions, excretions, and innumerable bacteria, many of them dead. Normally the only food residues are remnants of muscle fibre and the rough débris of vegetables, for practically all the food is digested and absorbed by the time it reaches the ileocæcal valve.

The *quantity, odour, colour, consistency,* and *presence or absence of abnormal constituents* should be systematically noted.

Quantity.—This varies considerably in different individuals and according to the type of diet, but is usually about 3 to 4 oz. daily in one or two motions. It may be considerably increased by undigested food, as in the bulky stools of certain types of pancreatic disease or of gastrocolic fistula.

Odour.—A certain degree of offensiveness is normal, due to the presence of indol and skatol, constituents which are more plentiful when the diet contains much meat. When offensiveness is excessive some derangement of digestion or absorption should be suspected, though it may only be temporary and have no serious significance. The odour is often persistently offensive in marked constipation. Putrefaction of protein, such as may occur in pancreatic disease, gives a musty smell; carbohydrate fermentation produces "acids of fermentation" and the rancid smell of butyric acid.

Colour.—The colour also varies with the type of diet. In persons on a *milk diet the stools are canary yellow in colour*; in those taking *much meat they are dark*. In an average mixed diet the stools are usually of a light brown colour. Certain articles of diet, such as wines and fruit, may cause *darkening of the stools*, as may medicinal preparations, especially those containing iron or bismuth. These points should be borne in mind before attributing any pathological significance to an alteration in the colour of the stools. When peristalsis is excessive and the intestinal contents are hurried downwards, bile gives a greenish or yellowish-green appearance to the fæces. When bile pigments do not reach the intestine, the stools become *clay coloured. Blood* is found in the stools in two forms; firstly, bright-red blood in small or large amounts derived from the large intestine, especially in its lower parts (e.g., hæmorrhoids, cancer, and polyps of the lower bowel); secondly, altered blood originating from the stomach or small intestine and partially digested on its way down, so that it gives the stool a *dark tarry appearance—melæna* (e.g., from gastric and duodenal ulcer). Small amounts of altered blood may not be visible on inspection but can be shown by tests for occult blood (*see* Chapter XIV). Similarly, unaltered blood in small amounts may only be detected by microscopical examination.

Consistency.—The normal stool has a pultaceous consistency. It should be sufficiently soft for it to be moulded by the intestinal tube, the shape of which it retains. If too soft it may have the fluid or semi-fluid consistency of a diarrhœic stool (*see* DIARRHŒA, p. 169). If the stool is unusually hard it may form rounded masses called *scybala*. In extreme cases of constipation these scybalous masses may be very dry owing to the great absorption of water from them during their prolonged stay in the large intestine.

Abnormal Constituents.—Many of these are more easily recognized by microscopical examination, and may cause considerable difficulty to the inexperienced observer.

Fæces may be abnormal either because normal constituents are absent (stercobilin, derived from bile pigmentation) or because abnormal constituents are present (undigested food constituents, blood, serum, pus, mucus, parasites). *Mucus* occurs in two forms : as small flakes, intimately mixed with the fæces (usually due to inflammation or catarrh), and as jelly-like masses either coating the surface of a hard fæcal mass (constipation), or appearing separately as a cast or membrane (spastic constipation or muco-membranous spasm of the colon). The recognition of *blood* has already been mentioned in describing the colour of the stools, but unaltered blood may be passed without any fæcal material. Excess of translucent *starch granules*, which stain blue with iodine, suggests failure of carbohydrate digestion. Excess of *fats* is recognized by the light, greasy nature of the stool, and generally indicates failure of fat digestion through insufficiency of bile or pancreatic secretion. Failure of protein digestion may lead to the presence of undigested *meat fibres*, which, though generally recognized through the microscope, may appear as light brown threads in the stool. *Pus* may appear in masses separate from the fæces, especially when it is derived from an extrinsic abscess bursting into the intestine. It is more intimately mixed with the stool in ulcerative conditions of the bowel such as malignant disease and ulcerative colitis.

Foreign constituents such as gall-stones, enteroliths, and many varieties of worms and ova may establish or give valuable clues to the diagnosis.

CHAPTER VII

THE HÆMOPOIETIC SYSTEM

UNDER this heading are included the blood and those tissues concerned in its production or destruction, namely, the bone-marrow, the lymphatic glands, and the spleen and liver. Changes in these organs and tissues usually occur concurrently, and attention may be drawn in the first place to disease affecting them by such external signs as enlarged lymphatic glands or pallor, or by the discovery, on systematic examination, of enlargement of the spleen or liver, or of significant changes in the blood-count.

SYMPTOMS AND SIGNS OF DISEASE OF THE HÆMOPOIETIC SYSTEM

The symptoms and signs of hæmopoietic disease include :—
1. Symptoms and signs of anæmia.
2. Symptoms and signs of the hæmorrhagic diathesis.
3. Enlargement of lymphatic glands.
4. Enlargement of the liver and spleen.
5. Retinal changes.

These symptoms and signs are rarely sufficient for a diagnosis without microscopic and macroscopic examination of the blood itself.

Anæmia.—This term means a deficiency in the quantity or quality of the blood, generally in both. The symptoms which result from it are often independent of its cause and are due chiefly to the reduction in the iron-containing pigment hæmoglobin, which is responsible for the normal pink coloration of the mucous membranes and skin, and which carries the necessary oxygen to all organs and tissues of the body. The more important signs and symptoms resulting from this deficiency are : (1) Pallor of the skin and mucous membranes ; (2) Symptoms of oxygen deficiency.

Pallor of the Skin and Mucous Membranes.—Pallor of the skin without a corresponding loss of colour in the lips, tongue, and buccal cavity, can frequently be disregarded, as many persons normally have a pallid complexion. In true anæmia, pallor occurs both in the skin and in the mucous membranes, and varies in grade from a slight loss of colour only appreciable to the experienced eye, to the extreme *waxy appearance of profound hæmorrhagic anæmias* or *the lemon yellow tint of pernicious anæmia.* In anæmias due to malignant disease an *earthy pallor* is often seen, and in infective endocarditis the skin colour has been likened to *café au lait.* The degree of pallor in the mucous membranes is a rough guide to the severity of the anæmia, but should always be corroborated by a blood-count. It is important not to rely solely on the conjunctivæ for evidence of anæmia in the mucous membranes, as injection of the former from other causes not uncommonly gives a false redness, which is belied by the pallid appearance of other mucosæ.

Symptoms of Oxygen Deficiency.—*Dyspnœa* is one of the earliest manifestations of anæmia, and directly results from the lowered oxygen-carrying power of the blood. In extreme cases the dyspnœa may be as severe as in certain forms of heart or lung disease, though the patient is *rarely breathless except on effort.* To ensure an adequate oxygen supply to the tissues *respiration is more rapid during exertion* and the heart beats more quickly. The rapid action of the heart is appreciable to the patient in the form of *palpitation.* The impoverished quality of the blood also affects adversely most of the organs and tissues of the body. The patient complains of general *lassitude* and inability for physical or mental work. Sleep is deranged and the poor blood supplied to the brain may result in *mental disturbance.* The gastro-intestinal tract suffers, and *loss of appetite, nausea,* and *constipation* are common symptoms. Perhaps owing to malnutrition of the capillary endothelium or altered osmotic relationships of blood and tissue fluids, increased transudation of plasma takes place into the tissues and moderate degrees of *œdema* result in the dependent parts of the body. If the anæmia is at all prolonged the viscera may be seriously affected. Dilatation of the heart may increase the breathlessness, and is recognized by cardiac enlargement and the development of systolic murmurs at the base and apex. The kidney function may be impaired and *albuminuria* result.

Certain special symptoms of pernicious anæmia will be considered in describing that disease.

Hæmorrhagic Diathesis.—This is a manifestation of the familial disease hæmophilia, and of various forms of purpura. Hæmorrhagic manifestations are also common in scurvy (vitamin C deficiency) and in severe anæmias and leukæmias.

Hæmophilia is essentially an hereditary disease, affecting males but transmitted by the female, in which the individual bleeds seriously from such minor causes as cuts, tooth extraction, etc. (*See also* HÆMOPHILIA, p. 222.)

Purpura rarely has a familial or hereditary basis. It is characterized by extravasation of blood into the skin and mucous membranes, causing purple spots varying in size from a pin-head (petechiæ) (*Fig.* 164) to large bruises (ecchymoses), associated with mucous membrane hæmorrhages; there is often spontaneous loss of considerable quantities of blood.

Enlarged Lymphatic Glands.—Sometimes the enlargement of the lymphatic glands is so great as to be the most striking physical sign, but in all cases of suspected blood disease or malignant disease and in fevers a systematic search should be made for glandular enlargement in the neck, axillæ, groins, and abdomen. Enlargement of one group of glands only, e.g., the axillary glands on one side, should throw a suspicion of sepsis or malignant disease upon the area drained by those glands. More generalized enlargement (*Fig.* 165) is suggestive of generalized infection, e.g., syphilis, tuberculosis, and plague, especially when accompanied by fever, or

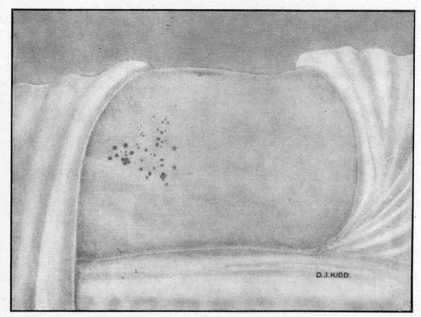

Fig. 164—Purpura. From a case of leukæmia in its terminal stages.

of one of the diseases of the hæmopoietic tissues which lead to infiltration of the glands, e.g., lymphadenoma (Hodgkin's disease) and the leukæmias. Lymphosarcoma may cause rapid enlargement of many groups of glands, soon followed by malignant cachexia.

The points which should be noted in the examination of enlarged lymphatic glands follow.

1. *The Group or Groups of Glands Affected.*—The student should examine the area which these glands drain.

2. *The Consistency.*—A stony hardness, especially when accompanied by irregularity, usually suggests malignancy, rarely hæmopoietic disease. Glands of moderate firmness are found in tuberculosis and other chronic infections, also in lymphosarcoma and in the infiltrations of leukæmia and Hodgkin's disease. Lymphadenomatous enlargements frequently have a springy elastic character, though this may be imitated by tuberculous glands. The ' breaking-down ' processes due to abscess formation in septic glands, or to secondary infection in tuberculous glands, produce an area of softness usually on the surface, and characteristic ' fluctuation ' may be demonstrable.

3. *The Attachments of the Glands.*—If the glands are small they tend to remain discrete, but with further enlargement usually fuse together.

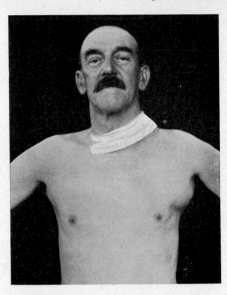

Fig. 165.—Enlarged glands. The axillary masses can be seen. A gland in the neck has been removed for section.

Notable exceptions to this are found in *lymphadenoma and leukæmia, where the glands may be quite large and yet discrete.* Inflammatory changes such as sepsis or tuberculosis generally result in adherence of the glands to the skin and subcutaneous tissues, which can no longer be moved freely over them. Malignant disease may also lead to attachment of the glands to the subcutaneous tissues, but even more important is the infiltration which anchors the glands to the deeper structures.

4. *The Presence of Tenderness.*—Tenderness usually accompanies acute inflammatory changes in the glands, especially those due to coccal infections. In these infections the superficial lymphatic vessels can frequently be seen as red streaks on the skin between the inflamed glands and the original focus of infection (*lymphangitis*).

Enlargement of the Spleen.—This organ may attain such huge dimensions that it causes a sense of weight and discomfort in the abdomen, of which the patient complains. More often the enlargement is moderate and only detected upon abdominal examination. Pain due to perisplenitis may also occasionally lead to examination for a splenic tumour. It is experienced in the left hypochondrium and over the left lower ribs, but is sometimes referred to the tip of the left shoulder (*see* ABDOMINAL PAIN, p. 162.)

If a splenic tumour is large it may be seen on inspection occupying the left hypochondrium and in extreme cases extending into the left iliac fossa (*Fig.* 166) and across the middle line of the abdomen.

Palpation is the most successful method of determining splenic enlargement (*Fig.* 167). The patient should be in the recumbent posture with the head slightly raised and the knees drawn up. Palpation should commence well away from the tumour and the fingers be gradually brought upwards until they encounter the sharp margin of the enlarged organ. Two of the most distinctive features of a splenic tumour are that it is *sharp-edged* and *superficial*, and the fingers need not be sunk deeply into the abdomen

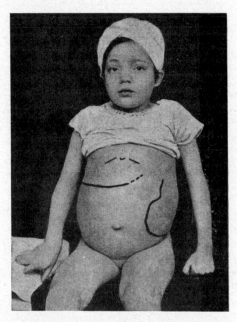

Fig 166.—Myeloid leukæmia. The splenic enlargement is greater than the liver enlargement.

to palpate it. The edge should be defined and its medial border followed until the *notch* can be felt, another diagnostic feature. The *consistency* of the organ should be noted, firmness being the usual characteristic in most hæmopoietic diseases. In infections the spleen is frequently soft and sometimes difficult to feel. Small degrees of splenic enlargement may not be detectable, as the organ must be considerably enlarged before it is palpable below the costal margin. The enlarged organ may be pressed forwards to some extent by placing the right hand on the loin, as in palpating a kidney tumour. When very large it may resemble the latter in filling the left loin, but can generally be distinguished by the sharp edge and the notch. During palpation a note should be made of any friction present, generally denoting the presence of perisplenitis. In these cases a friction rub is also to be heard.

Percussion may help to outline the borders of the spleen, especially when this is enlarged upwards. Normally, dullness is found between the

14

ninth and eleventh ribs in the mid-axillary line, but may be found as high as the eighth or seventh rib in cases of great splenic enlargement. Percussion, however, is an unsatisfactory method of determining enlargement of the spleen as compared with palpation. It is perhaps of most use when doubt exists as to the nature of a large tumour in the left hypochondrium which also fills the loin. If the tumour is of renal origin, dullness may be obtained by percussion over the loin, but not usually with splenic tumours.

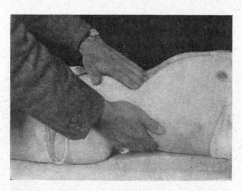

Fig. 167.—Palpation of the spleen. The fingers of one hand are pressed under the costal margin and the patient asked to take a deep breath. With the other hand the loin is pressed forwards as in palpation of the kidney. This helps to bring an enlarged spleen in contact with the examining fingers.

The commoner causes of enlargement of the spleen will be seen in the accompanying table.

CAUSES OF ENLARGED SPLEEN

GREAT ENLARGEMENT	MODERATE ENLARGEMENT	PALPABLE
Myeloid leukæmia	Lymphatic leukæmia*	Septicæmias
Chronic malaria $\left\{\begin{array}{l}\text{rare in}\\ \text{Great}\\ \text{Britain}\end{array}\right.$ Kala-azar	Splenic anæmia*	Enteric infections
	Acholuric jaundice	Undulant fever
Gaucher's disease (rare)	Polycythæmia vera*	Typhus
	Portal cirrhosis (and other types of portal obstruction)	Malaria (acute)
		Also occasionally in many other infections
	Lymphadenoma	Pernicious and hypochromic anæmias
	Syphilis (congenital; acquired—tertiary stage)	
	Rickets	
	Amyloid disease	
	Tuberculosis	
	Infarction	
	Tumours $\left.\begin{array}{l}\\ \\ \end{array}\right\}$ rare Hydatid cysts	

* Occasionally causes great enlargement. The classification of splenomegaly according to size is, of course, arbitrary, as occasionally enormous spleens are found in the diseases mentioned in the second column, whilst great enlargement in any disease is only attained after passing through intermediate stages, in any of which the patient may chance to be examined.

Enlargement of the Liver.—This physical sign has already been considered under the digestive system. Liver enlargement in diseases of the blood and blood-forming organs is generally of secondary moment to that of enlargement of the spleen ; but as the liver contains a part of the reticulo-endothelial system, of which the spleen is the principal member, it becomes enlarged under similar circumstances—for example, in pernicious anæmia, splenic anæmia, and leukæmias (*Fig.* 168).

Retinal Changes.—Examination with the ophthalmoscope not infrequently gives useful information in blood diseases.

Pernicious Anæmia.—The fundus and disk are paler than normal and the retinal vessels somewhat engorged. Small flame-shaped hæmorrhages,

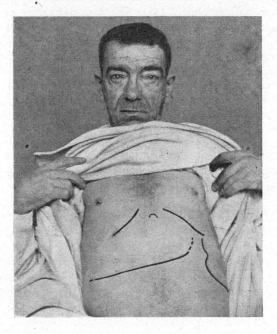

Fig. 168.—Lymphatic leukæmia. Showing outline of enlarged liver and spleen.

or circular hæmorrhages, often with pale centres, occur when the red cell count is down to about 30 per cent.

Leukæmia.—The fundus is frequently of a light brick-red or orange colour. The disk margins are blurred from œdema in the later stages. The retinal veins and arteries are engorged, and both sets of vessels become strikingly light-coloured and the difference in colour between the veins and arteries is abolished. Hæmorrhages may be very extensive, and are flame-shaped, diamond-shaped with pale centres, or, if in the deeper layers of the retina, circular.

EXAMINATION OF THE BLOOD

The symptoms and signs which have been described are rarely sufficient to establish a diagnosis. For this an examination of the blood itself is necessary. The technical details of this examination will be found in Chapter XIV, and in the present chapter the significance of various abnormalities will be discussed.

NAKED-EYE EXAMINATION

Certain rough observations may be made by observing the character of the blood as it flows when the finger is pricked. It may be obviously thinner and paler than normal, suggesting a deficiency in red cells and their contained hæmoglobin. This would indicate the presence of an anæmia without giving any clue as to its nature. More rarely an increased viscosity might be recognized, suggesting polycythæmia, an increase in the number of red corpuscles. A buff or cream-coloured blood of consistency normal or thicker than normal is present in leukæmias when the white cells are greatly increased.

If the blood is allowed to stand, the *serum* may be inspected. In pernicious anæmia and other conditions in which excessive blood destruction takes place, it may be a deeper yellow than normal. The clot in cases of purpura fails to retract, so that there is no expressed serum. Other observations on the blood serum may be important but bear no direct relationship to the diagnosis of blood diseases : for example, the serum may be tinted pink by the presence of free hæmoglobin in cases of paroxysmal hæmoglobinuria, may be milky in lipæmia due to diabetes or excessive ingestion of fats, and may be brown in methæmoglobinæmia.

The length of bleeding time and clotting time may also be roughly noted (*see* Chapter XIV).

MICROSCOPIC EXAMINATION

Under the microscope the numbers, form, and staining characteristics of the red and white corpuscles and blood-platelets may be studied (*Figs.* 169, 170). The data so obtained are frequently referred to as the ' blood picture '. This term generally includes the red- and white-cell counts, hæmoglobin estimate, and the differential white-cell count.

The Blood-film.—

RED CORPUSCLES.—An *unstained film* may be used to measure the size of the red cells by means of a halometer or a Price-Jones curve, though for the latter a stained film is often used, and is essential for other observations.

In the *stained film*, the size and shape of the cells may be noted. Small cells are known as *microcytes*, abnormally large cells as *megalocytes*. When there is much variation, the phenomenon is known as *anisocytosis*.

Variation in shape is known as *poikilocytosis*, the cells appearing oval, pear-shaped, dumb-bell-shaped, or grossly irregular.

The recognition of *nucleated* cells is very important. Cells of normal size with a nucleus are known as *normoblasts*. The precursors of these are the larger nucleated erythroblasts, the nuclear chromatin granules of which are arranged in a rosette-like manner. *Megaloblasts* are large nucleated erythroblastic cells precociously hæmoglobinized and commonly found in pernicious and allied anæmias. Nucleated red cells are the precursors of normal erythrocytes, and are therefore found when the bone-marrow is highly active. Intermediate in position between normal erythrocytes and these primitive cells are some without nucleus but closely related.

These cells may be stained blue with the methylene blue of Leishman's stain, either uniformly—*polychromasia*—or with a fine blue stippling, known as *punctate basophilia*. If these cells are stained intravitally with cresyl blue, the basophilic material appears as a network or skein within the cell, which is known as a *reticulocyte*.

The phenomena of polychromasia, punctate basophilia, and reticulocytosis are seen in anæmias (punctate basophilia especially in the anæmia of lead poisoning), but above all *when active regeneration of red corpuscles is taking place in the bone-marrow*.

The pink coloration of the normal red cells is a criterion of the amount of hæmoglobin they contain. When this is deficient the red corpuscles may appear as colourless disks, defined only by a thin pink rim (*hypochromic cells or achromasia*).

WHITE CORPUSCLES.—The various types of white cell are recorded as a *differential count*. This is made by staining a blood-film and examining the leucocytes with a high magnification. One or two hundred white cells are counted and the number of each variety recorded as a percentage. The individual characteristics of each type will best be seen from *Fig.* 170 and its accompanying legend. The cells are of two main types—granular and non-granular.

Granular Cells.—These cells, the granulocytes, include the *polymorphonuclear, eosinophil*, and *basophil leucocytes*, which respectively contain fine pink granules, coarse red granules, and coarse blue granules. The nuclei are usually multilobulated.

Non-granular Cells.—These include the large and small lymphocytes and the monocytes. The small lymphocyte has a darkly staining nucleus, with a narrow rim of cytoplasm. The large lymphocyte has a much broader rim of cytoplasm which often stains less deeply. Monocytes (large hyaline mononuclears), often twice the size of a lymphocyte, have a lightly staining reticular and indented nucleus, and a variable amount of powder blue cytoplasm. Monocytes are the largest cells present in normal blood and are few in number. They are derived from the reticulo-endothelial system and must not be confused with immature cells. Although lymphocytes are not granular in the same sense as leucocytes they often contain (particularly the large lymphocytes) a small number of brightly staining red (azurophil) granules, and the monocytes similarly exhibit a dusty pseudo-granular appearance.

Degenerate forms of white cell are not uncommon. Polymorphonuclear leucocytes may be swollen and œdematous and lose the clear definition of their nuclear protoplasm; in lymphocytes vacuoles may appear.

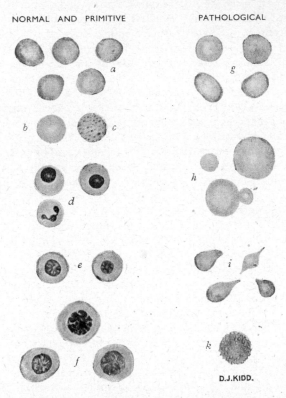

NORMAL AND PRIMITIVE   PATHOLOGICAL

D.J.KIDD.

Fig. 169.—NORMAL, PRIMITIVE, AND PATHOLOGICAL RED CORPUSCLES.—*a*, A group of normal red corpuscles ; note uniformity of shape and size ; average size 7.21 μ ; standard deviation 0.45 μ (Price-Jones); well filled with hæmoglobin, with slightly more at the edges, leaving comparatively pale area in the centre. *b*, Cell showing polychromasia. *c*, Cell showing punctate basophilia, which is closely allied to polychromasia, shown in *b*. *d*, Three normoblasts, one showing early fragmentation of its nucleus. Note the size, shape, and colour of cells are normal, but they contain small contact nuclei staining deeply, with a pale area in the centre. *e*, Earlier forms ; note the bluish cytoplasm with larger and less compact faceted nuclei ; cells slightly larger than the normoblast. *f*, Primitive erythroblasts ; note large size and rosette-like arrangement of the chromatin of the nuclei. (*Note* : The cells from below upward are grouped in progressive stages as they emerge from the primitive megaloblasts of the bone-marrow to the fully-formed normal red corpuscles.) *g*, Hypochromic or achromasic red corpuscles ; normal size and often normal shape ; pale owing to deficiency of hæmoglobin associated with low colour index. *h*, Group of red cells from case of pernicious anæmia ; show great variation in size (anisocytosis) ; limits from 3·75 to 13 μ. *i*, Variation in shape of red corpuscles (poikilocytosis), some showing polychromasia. *k*, Red corpuscle showing crenation. (*Leishman's stain.*)

Immature White Cells.—In the examination of a stained blood-film, the presence of abnormal, immature white cells is especially significant, and, when these are abundant, generally indicates the presence of a leukæmia. The classification of these cells by different workers varies somewhat, but the more minute points of distinction are of academic rather than of clinical interest. All these immature cells are larger than leucocytes, many two or three times so. The chief varieties are the myeloblast and the myelocyte.

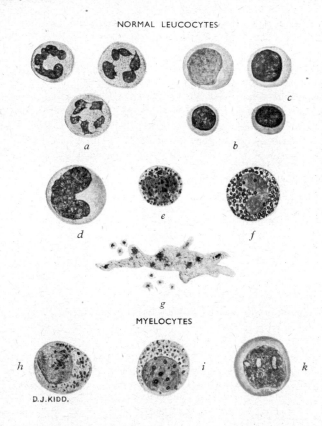

Fig. 170.—NORMAL LEUCOCYTES AND MYELOCYTES.—a, Polymorphonuclear leucocytes ; average size 10 to 12 μ, showing nuclei with 1 to 5 lobes. b, Large and small lymphocytes ; note bright blue cytoplasm ; the smaller have dark and dense nuclei, while the larger nuclei are paler and more loosely knit ; some exhibit deep blue cytoplasm (Türk cells, c). d, Monocyte, 12 to 20 μ ; note grey-blue cytoplasm and less dense nucleus. e, Basophil or mast cell ; nucleus obscured by coarse basophil granules ; indistinguishable from basophil myelocyte. f, Eosinophil ; average size 13 to 15 μ ; tightly packed coarse granules of brilliant red colour (eosinophilia) ; almost never obscure the nucleus ; usually two lobes, sometimes three. g, Group of blood-platelets. h, A neutrophil myelocyte, 18 to 20 μ ; fine granular appearance in nucleus and cytoplasm. i, Eosinophil myelocyte. k, Myeloblast ; vacuoles and nucleoli shown ; no nuclear membrane ; the lymphoblast is almost indistinguishable from the myeloblast. (Leishman's stain.)

The transition of cells is probably as follows :—

Myeloblast   Lymphoblast
↓   ↓
Myelocyte   Lymphocyte
↓
Normal leucocyte

The lymphoblast is practically indistinguishable from the myeloblast, but if immature cells of this type are found associated with many granular cells, it is reasonable to assume they are myeloblasts ; if they are associated with an excess of lymphocytes they are probably lymphoblasts.

Intermediate stages are of course well recognized, but for a description of these the student should consult a text-book of pathology or medicine.

The myeloblast is a large cell with a large nucleus containing nucleoli and a zone of deep blue cytoplasm *free from granules.*

The myelocyte is also a large cell, with a smaller nucleus and a zone of cytoplasm *containing granules*—neutrophil, eosinophil, or basophil, according to the type of leucocyte of which it is to be the precursor.

Blood-counts.—An average normal blood-count is as follows :—

Red blood-corpuscles ... $\begin{cases} 5,000,000 \text{ to } 6,500,000 \text{ per c.mm. (men)} \\ 4,000,000 \text{ to } 6,000,000 \quad,, \quad,, \quad \text{(women)} \end{cases}$

(adapted from Price-Jones's figures)

White blood-corpuscles   5,000 to   8,000 ,,   ,,
Blood-platelets ...   ...   250,000 to 350,000 ,,   ,,

These are estimated in the Thoma-Zeiss hæmacytometer (*see* Chapter XIV).

The Differential White-cell Count.—The differential count of the white blood-corpuscles is represented by the following average normal figures :—

Polymorphonuclear leucocytes   ...   ...   50 to 70 per cent
Lymphocytes ...   .   25 to 30 ,,   ,,
Monocytes   ...   .   6 to 8   ,,   ,,
Eosinophil leucocytes ...   .   1 to 3   ,,   ,,
Basophil leucocytes   ...   . $\frac{1}{2}$,,   ,,

These *figures are arbitrary,* and considerable individual variation may be found in health. When the total number of white cells is reduced (leucopenia—*see* p. 217) the relative proportions of the various types of cell are disturbed. This commonly results in a decrease in the percentage of polymorphonuclear leucocytes and an increase in the percentage of lymphocytes, which *must not be confused with a true lymphocytosis,* in which not only is the lymphocyte percentage high, but the absolute number of lymphocytes is increased. This relative lymphocytosis occurs in certain infections and in some anæmias.

The Arneth Count.—The number of lobes to the nucleus of the neutrophil polymorphs is counted in 100 cells. Normally the percentages are as follows (Piney) :—

One lobe   ...   .   5 per cent
Two lobes   ...   .   35 ,,   ,,
Three lobes ...   .   41 ,,   ,,
Four lobes   ...   .   17 ,,   ,,
Five lobes   ...   .   2 ,,   ,,

Simplification of the nucleus is known as a " shift to the left "; an increase in the number of cells containing multilobed nuclei a " shift to the right ". A shift to the left occurs in severe infections, especially septicæmias and acute forms of tuberculosis. A shift to the right is rarely seen save in pernicious anæmia.

Pathological Variations of the Red-cell Count.—The red blood-corpuscles may be *increased* to eight, ten, or more million cells per cubic millimetre in various types of polycythæmia. This condition may occur as a primary blood disorder or may be secondary to deficient oxygenation, e.g., in congenital heart disease and in persons dwelling at a high altitude. To some extent it may occur in severe dehydration and in certain intoxications (carbon monoxide, aniline derivatives, etc.). The primary type, *polycythæmia vera*, is associated with splenic enlargement and a brick-red colour changing to cyanosis in cold weather. A *decrease* of red cells occurs in all types of anæmia, whether these be idiopathic, e.g., pernicious anæmia and idiopathic hypochromic anæmias, or secondary to hæmorrhage and the many constitutional diseases which will be discussed later. In moderate anæmias the count may vary between three and four million, but in extreme cases, especially in pernicious anæmia, it may fall as low as half a million.

Pathological Variations of the Total White-cell Count.—Allowance must be made in the interpretation of the white-cell count for the diurnal variation which frequently occurs and may appear to be related to meals. Physiological leucocytosis may also occur during pregnancy. These variations are not usually more than 2000 to 3000.

Increase in the number of granular white cells (*leucocytosis*), as a pathological phenomenon, appears most frequently in *sepsis* (coccal infection) if the body is capable of making a good defensive reaction. The count may rise to between 15,000 and 30,000 per c.mm. Leucocytosis of this grade is frequently seen in such septic conditions as cellulitis, pneumonia, and erysipelas, and where pus has actually been formed, e.g., in empyema, the count attains the higher levels. A similar leucocytosis, but less marked, is often found in cachectic conditions, such as carcinoma and certain intoxications. In *grave infections leucocytosis is often slight* or absent owing to the profound toxæmia, which impairs the function of the bone-marrow. Non-suppurative bacillary and protozoal infections are usually accompanied by an absolute lymphocytosis. In *leukæmias*, especially of the myeloid type (splenomedullary leukæmia), the number of white cells may be enormous, varying between 25,000 and 1,000,000, though usually averaging 300,000 to 400,000 per c.mm. The greater part of these are immature.

The number of white cells may be *diminished* (*leucopenia*), not only where the body is incapable of an appropriate defensive reaction against infection, but also in certain specific diseases, such as typhoid, influenza, and measles. Further, various types of anæmia are characterized by leucopenia—e.g., the splenic anæmias, pernicious and aplastic anæmia. In the rare disease called *agranulocytosis*, the leucopenia affects the granular cells, and is severe. The disease is usually characterized by ulceration of the fauces, and generally ends fatally. Some drugs, especially those of the amidopyrine and sulphonamide groups, acting on susceptible persons, are frequently found to be the basis for this condition, and it should be suspected in cases in which throat symptoms are found in a patient who is disproportionately ill.

Pathological Variations in the Differential Count.—Leucocytosis frequently disturbs the normal numerical relationship between the different types of white cell. In *sepsis* there is not only an absolute increase in the number of leucocytes, but a relative increase in the percentage of the polymorphonuclear variety (75 to 90 per cent).

In *leukæmias* there is generally a large excess of white cells, usually of an immature type (lymphoblasts, myeloblasts, myelocytes), though occasionally the predominating cell is of a mature type. The distinction between simple leucocytosis and leukæmia is occasionally difficult, as the numerical increase may be similar in the two conditions, but is generally decided by the presence of large numbers of abnormal cells in the case of leukæmia.

The Blood-platelets (Thrombocytes).—The platelets are small bodies present in circulating blood. In health they usually number 250,000 to 350,000 per c.mm. They are *increased* in certain phases of diseases in which spontaneous clotting of blood is present—e.g., in various types of phlebitis, and in predisposing conditions such as pregnancy and sepsis. Platelets also increase in early stages of splenomedullary leukæmia. They are *diminished* (*thrombocytopenia*) in diseases characterized by bleeding, such as purpura and some types of splenomegaly with anæmia, and also in pernicious anæmia.

The Hæmoglobin Content.—Hæmoglobin is usually estimated by colorimetric methods (*see* Chapter XIV). The absolute amount is not usually calculated for ordinary clinical purposes, but in its place an arbitrary figure of 100 per cent is taken to be the standard colorimetric response, and is equivalent to 14·5 g. per 100 c.c. of blood. Many healthy persons have less than this full percentage, though figures of less than 80 per cent should probably be regarded as abnormal. In most diseases the variation in hæmoglobin runs parallel with that of the red corpuscles. In polycythæmia of all types the hæmoglobin content is higher than normal (120 to 130 per cent), whilst in anæmias it falls in accordance with the degree of anæmia and may reach figures as low as 20 per cent. But although there is usually a parallelism between the hæmoglobin content and the red-cell count, the one may be reduced to a greater extent than the other. This is shown by variations of the *colour index* (C.I.), which is normally taken as unity. For purposes of calculating the colour index, the normal hæmoglobin content is taken as 100 per cent and a red-corpuscular count of 5,000,000 is taken as 100 per cent normal. The formula for the calculation then reads in a normal individual :—

$$\text{C.I.} = \frac{\text{Percentage hæmoglobin}}{\text{Percentage erythrocytes}} = \frac{100}{100} = 1$$

In many anæmias the hæmoglobin is reduced to a greater extent than the number of red corpuscles, and the hæmoglobin index is therefore less than 1 (0·8 or less). In chlorosis or other types of hypochromic anæmia (e.g., idiopathic hypochromic anæmia), in which there appears to be a primary failure in the production of hæmoglobin, the colour index may be very low (0·5 or less). Pernicious anæmia virtually stands alone *among the common anæmias* in having a high colour index. This is due to rapid reduction in the red cells without a corresponding decrease in their hæmoglobin content. The hæmoglobin remains relatively high because the corpuscles are, in the mean, larger and contain more. On the other hand the low colour index of hypochromic anæmias is due to the fall in the mean corpuscular hæmoglobin concentration.

SPECIAL INVESTIGATIONS

The special investigations include estimation of the clotting and bleeding time, and of the fragility and sedimentation rate of the red corpuscles (*see* Chapter XIV).

THE DIAGNOSIS OF HÆMOPOIETIC DISEASES

DISEASES WITH ANÆMIA AS THE PRINCIPAL SYMPTOM

When a patient presents the symptoms of anæmia which have been described, it is necessary to ascertain : (1) If any cause can be found for the anæmia ; (2) What changes are present in the blood picture.

The Cause.—In many anæmias it is possible to find a definite cause such as hæmorrhage, neoplasm, or severe infection. In others, so called idiopathic anæmias, no such cause can be found and in these cases the diagnosis often depends upon the blood picture. In every case it is necessary to make a comprehensive medical examination to exclude systematic disease and to search for signs such as glandular and visceral enlargement which may be associated with anæmias.

The Blood Picture.—In some anæmias, the best example of which is pernicious anæmia, the blood picture is practically diagnostic ; in others the changes are not characteristic and must be considered in conjunction with other physical signs before a diagnosis can be made.

The majority of anæmias fall into three main groups : (1) Those due to loss of blood ; (2) Those due to defective blood formation ; (3) Those due to excessive intra-vascular destruction. Of these three the commonest is those due to loss of blood.

It is not possible here to describe all the anæmias, but some of the commoner examples in each group have been picked out to illustrate the general method of diagnosis and to call attention to the commonest forms of anæmia.

Post-hæmorrhagic Anæmias.—The most apparent cause for anæmia is *hæmorrhage*, and where it is from obvious sources, e.g., wounds, hæmoptysis, or epistaxis, it is unlikely to escape notice. This is particularly so in cases of acute hæmorrhage. Chronic bleeding is more liable to be overlooked, and where no information is volunteered by the patient special questions should be directed towards the possibility of small losses of blood from piles, menorrhagia, or melæna. Severe anæmias may also result from the hæmorrhages of ankylostomiasis, hæmophilia, and purpura. The loss of blood by *profuse hæmorrhage* causes symptoms of shock, referable to the sudden decrease in blood volume (collapse, low blood-pressure, feeble action of the heart, thirst, etc.). These symptoms due to decreased blood volume are not to be confused with those of anæmia, which may be of a severe grade without such symptoms if the loss of blood is gradual.

The possibility of concealed hæmorrhage must not be overlooked as a cause of rapidly produced anæmia, and when symptoms of hæmorrhage occur without obvious cause, such contingencies as melæna, hæmorrhage into tumours and serous spaces, or ruptured ectopic gestation should be considered. The blood picture in post-hæmorrhagic anæmias shows a reduction in corpuscles and hæmoglobin, the latter to a greater extent, though not so disproportionately, as in idiopathic hypochromic anæmias. The colour index is rarely below 0·8.

Dyshæmopoietic Anæmias (Anæmias due to Defective Blood Formation).—Some of the anæmias in this group are attributable to very different causes. Though allied from a pathological standpoint their clinical features may be diverse, and illustrate the necessity for consideration of the blood picture in conjunction with other abnormal clinical signs.

Often the blood picture is the most important diagnostic sign, e.g., in pernicious anæmia, but unless the whole clinical picture is considered, rarer diseases causing similar changes in the blood may be overlooked.

The subdivision of the dyshæmopoietic anæmias used here is essentially a pathological concept, but the more important associated clinical signs have been emphasized.

a. ANÆMIAS DUE TO IRON DEFICIENCY.—These include idiopathic hypochromic anæmia, chlorosis, and the anæmias resulting from certain gastro-intestinal lesions which interfere with the proper absorption of iron.

The blood picture is characterized by the low hæmoglobin content of the corpuscles, giving a colour index below that commonly found in post-hæmorrhagic anæmias, often as low as 0·5.

Idiopathic hypochromic anæmia is the commonest example. The patient is usually a woman between 20 and 50 years and the symptoms of anæmia are severe. Achlorhydria is common and the disease is sometimes called *achlorhydric anæmia*; it is also referred to as *microcytic anæmia* because of the abundance of small red corpuscles. The nails may be spoon-shaped (koilonychia), and occasionally stomatitis and dysphagia may be present (Plummer-Vinson syndrome). Enlargement of the spleen is slight to moderate. Doubts in diagnosis are often dispelled by the remarkable therapeutic response to iron.

Chlorosis is now rarely seen, but had many of the characteristic features of idiopathic hypochromic anæmia. It was common in younger persons, usually adolescent girls living under poor circumstances as regards diet and fresh air. The colour of the skin had a greenish cast which gave the name to the disease.

Alimentary diseases which lead to failure of iron absorption may also result in a hypochromic anæmia, e.g., malignant disease of the alimentary tract, dysentery, and so forth.

b. ANÆMIAS DUE TO DEFICIENCY IN SPECIFIC HÆMOPOIETIC PRINCIPLE. —The main and only important member of this group is pernicious anæmia, which has distinctive blood changes. These may be closely simulated, though rarely, by sprue, bothriocephalus infestation, and certain gastro-intestinal lesions. These diseases must be borne in mind especially in tropical countries when fatty diarrhœa and stomatitis may suggest sprue, or examination of the stools may discover the *Bothriocephalus latus*, or its ova. Similar macrocytic anæmias occasionally occur in cirrhosis and other diseases of the liver, in serious ulceration or resection of the stomach or small intestine, and in cœliac and pancreatic disease.

Pernicious Anæmia.—This disease occurs in both sexes, but is commoner in the male. Persons over 50 are usually affected but it may occur earlier.

The usual symptoms of anæmia are exhibited in a pronounced form, especially asthenia, but certain special features are helpful in diagnosis, notably the sore tongue, achlorhydria, slight icterus, nervous signs, and splenic enlargement.

The *sore tongue* is due to glossitis, recognizable by the smooth depapillated tongue.

Anacidity is complete, i.e., both free HCl and organic acids are absent, a useful point in distinguishing pernicious anæmia from carcinoma of the stomach. Anorexia and nausea are common accompanying clinical features.

Icterus is of the hæmolytic variety, i.e., slight and not accompanied by pale stools or dark urine, though the latter may contain an excess of urobilin. In classical cases the patient may be lemon yellow.

The *nervous signs* are due to the common occurrence of *subacute combined degeneration of the cord* (*see* p. 274), in which paræsthesiæ, loss of tendon reflexes and vibration sense, with a Babinski sign, may be found.

The degree of *splenic enlargement* is slight.

c. ANÆMIAS DUE TO OTHER FACTORS AFFECTING HÆMOPOIESIS.—These include the following :—

1. *Scurvy* (vitamin C deficiency).—The possibility of this disease will be considered when the diet is inadequate or unbalanced. Spongy bleeding gums often excite suspicion first.

2. *Myxœdema* (thyroid deficiency).—The coarse skin, dry scanty hair, increasing weight, and sluggish cerebration give grounds for the diagnosis.

3. *Nephritis.*—Both acute and chronic forms of nephritis are usually associated with anæmia. Œdema, albuminuria, and cardio-vascular changes establish the diagnosis.

4. *Physical and Chemical Agencies.*—These must be suspected if the patient's work demands exposure to X rays, radium, or chemical poisons such as benzol, T.N.T., or lead.

5. *Sepsis and Infections.*—The possibility of concealed sepsis, e.g., osteomyelitis or internal abscesses, must not be overlooked. Both acute and chronic infections interfere with hæmopoiesis, e.g., acute rheumatism and tuberculosis.

6. *Carcinomatosis.*—Most forms of malignant diseases are associated with some degree of anæmia. Loss of weight and localizing signs will lead to a correct diagnosis.

7. *Diseases affecting the Bone-marrow.*—Leukæmia and myelomatosis, for example, also interfere with the formation of red cells.

8. *Aplastic Anæmia.*—Toxic causes are probably at work in this disease—sometimes known, more often unknown, but producing a profound anæmia with failure of the bone-marrow to respond to treatment, as indicated by a complete absence of reticulocytosis.

Anæmias due to Excessive Blood Destruction (Hæmolytic Anæmias).—These include some of the rarer causes of anæmia.

Acholuric Familial Jaundice.—This disease should be considered if slight icterus and anæmia are present. Splenic enlargement, icterus, increased fragility of the red cells, and a family history are the diagnostic features.

Hæmolytic Poisons.—These may be responsible for anæmia, as in arseniuretted hydrogen or chronic lead poisoning, certain snake bites, and the hæmolytic effects of certain bacteria, notably streptococci. Occupational exposure to poisons and the presence of septicæmic signs are especially important.

Hæmoglobinuria.—Dark reddish urine (port-wine colour) generally draws attention to this condition, which is due to various hæmolytic poisons and occurs also in paroxysmal hæmoglobinuria and in malaria (blackwater fever). The urine shows positive chemical tests for blood, but under the microscope there are few or no red corpuscles.

Anæmia of Uncertain Origin.—The main disease falling under this heading is *splenic anæmia*, characterized by considerable or great splenic enlargement, associated with a reduction of red and white cells and of hæmoglobin. It is not uncommonly combined with the signs of cirrhosis of the liver (Banti's disease), and may be aggravated by the associated hæmatemesis.

HÆMORRHAGIC DISEASES

When bleeding is the principal symptom the possibility of three diseases should first be considered, namely, *hæmophilia*, *purpura*, and *scurvy*, but it must not be overlooked that bleeding may also result from severe anæmias and leukæmias, and a full blood examination is necessary in every case.

Hæmophilia.—This disease has been well defined as "an inherited tendency in males to bleed." It is entirely unknown in woman, although transmitted through the mother, but it must also be noted that a hæmophilic male transmits the carrier state to all his daughters, who in turn can produce actively hæmophilic sons (50 per cent). A careful family history must therefore be taken in a bleeding disease.

The diagnosis of hæmophilia is usually made, after the occurrence of profuse hæmorrhage from trivial causes, by the discovery that the *clotting time is greatly prolonged*, sometimes as long as half an hour. Spontaneous hæmorrhage into the joints may occur ; slight trauma as the precipitating factor cannot easily be excluded.

Purpura.—As a manifestation of the bleeding diathesis this disease is best exemplified in the type known as *purpura hæmorrhagica*, in which profuse bleeding may take place from almost any mucous membrane in the body, e.g., epistaxis, gastro-intestinal and uterine hæmorrhage. The diagnosis of purpura generally depends on the presence of hæmorrhages into the skin (petechiæ or ecchymoses), but purpura hæmorrhagica is an exception in that hæmorrhage may take place from the mucosæ without hæmorrhages into the skin. It is usually associated with thrombocytopenia. The *bleeding time is greatly prolonged, but the clotting time is not appreciably altered* (cf. hæmophilia).

Another type of purpura—sometimes known as anaphylactoid purpura, of which one variety is Henoch's—is not associated with thrombocytopenia, but is characterized by a tendency to visceral hæmorrhage (gastro-intestinal tract and kidneys) and serous effusions into the skin and joints. The joint manifestations have given rise to the name purpura rheumatica when they predominate, and to some extent they are noticeable in all forms of anaphylactoid purpura.

These points apply to the *idiopathic* forms of purpura, but like anæmia purpura is frequently *symptomatic* of other conditions, e.g., septicæmia, hæmorrhagic forms of the exanthemata, cachexia from neoplasms and Bright's disease, grave blood diseases such as the anæmias and the leukæmias, and the effect of various poisons.

The tendency to purpura may sometimes be demonstrated by application of a tourniquet round the arm, when a crop of purpuric spots will appear below the constriction. The test is useful if the history suggests purpura and there are no objective manifestations present.

Scurvy.—This disease, both in the adult and the infantile forms, is due to a deficiency of vitamin C in the diet, which apparently causes increased permeability and fragility of the capillaries. Hæmorrhages from any mucous membrane may take place, but are most commonly seen in the mouth, where the *spongy bleeding gums* are always a suggestive feature in a patient who has been undernourished or incorrectly fed. Leukæmias and uræmia may produce similar changes in the gums, but other signs of these diseases are present, and the necessary dietetic history of the scorbutic patient is lacking.

The bleeding in all types of hæmorrhagic diathesis leads to a posthæmorrhagic anæmia with the corresponding symptoms and blood picture.

HÆMOPOIETIC DISEASES WITH ENLARGED LYMPHATIC GLANDS

The presence of 'lumps' in the neck, axillæ, or groins may be the first symptom noticed by the patient, and calls for a full blood examination. In other cases the symptoms of anæmia may appear first and the enlarged lymphatic glands are only discovered on examination. Some of the characteristics used in distinguishing one type of glandular enlargement from another have already been described, but reference may again be made to lymphadenoma and the leukæmias.

Lymphadenoma (Hodgkin's Disease) (*Fig.* 171).—Lymphadenoma is the most important and commonest type of a large group of apparently neoplastic overgrowths of the reticulo-endothelial elements of lymph-glands,

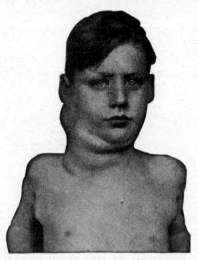

Fig. 171.—Lymphadenoma. Masses of glands in the neck forming the so-called 'lymphadenomatous collar'. Axillary masses are also visible.

spleen, and marrow. These are collectively known as 'reticuloses'. Some are very slowly progressive, others have the features of malignancy; some show a uniformity of cellular structure, others a marked degree of pleomorphism. Hodgkin's disease is an example of this last type. Groups of lymphatic glands are enlarged and may attain a considerable size without losing their individual shape. These *discrete glands* are no adherent to the skin, have a peculiar elastic character on palpation, and may involve any of the superficial or deeply placed lymphatic groups Lymphadenoma is commonest in young persons, and in its later stages i accompanied by a profound anæmia. Eosinophilia is occasionally found Fever may occur, in certain cases exhibiting the *Pel-Ebstein phenomenon* in which the temperature remains raised for a number of days (10 to 14 and then falls for an equal length of time (*see Fig.* 259). This cycle may b repeated for some months. The diagnosis from tuberculous lymphadenitis is not always easy, but in the latter the glands tend to adhere to one another, thus losing their individual shape, and to become attached to the skin and deeper structures. Constitutional signs of tuberculosis may also be present, and the secondary anæmia is rarely of the grade seen in advanced lymphadenoma.

Leukæmia.—The leukæmias, especially the lymphatic variety, also cause glandular enlargement, similar in many of its characteristics to that of lymphadenoma, but a blood-count and a blood-film show the correct diagnosis.

Lymphosarcoma.—As in lymphadenoma and the leukæmias, the superficial groups of glands in the neck are most frequently involved by lymphosarcoma. Rapidly growing masses occur, fusing together and sometimes ulcerating. The course is much shorter than that of lymphadenoma, death occurring within a few weeks to months, though it may be temporarily influenced by X-ray treatment. Occasionally the blood picture may bear some resemblance to a leukæmia, particularly in chloroma.

The non-hæmopoietic causes of glandular enlargement are dealt with elsewhere (p. 206).

HÆMOPOIETIC DISEASES WITH SPLENOMEGALY

Diseases under this heading are as yet ill understood. Three, however, deserve attention—namely, splenic anæmia, acholuric family jaundice, and leukæmia.

Splenic Anæmia.—It may well be shown in the course of time that this name applies to a *group* of diseases having the symptoms of anæmia and splenomegaly in common. In the present state of our knowledge the term is applied to cases presenting the blood picture of a *hypochromic anæmia, with leucopenia and enlargement of the spleen* usually two or three inches below the costal margin. *Hæmorrhages* from mucous membranes are also common (particularly hæmatemesis), especially in those cases in which thrombocytopenia occurs. In a certain number of cases, especially in children, cirrhosis of the liver develops during the course of the disease, and to this syndrome the term *Banti's disease* is applied.

Acholuric Familial Jaundice.—This disease has already received attention as a form of hæmolytic anæmia (p. 222). In some ways it resembles splenic anæmia, as in both there is splenic enlargement with a hypochromic type of anæmia. The distinguishing features are the presence of a variable degree of jaundice of the hæmolytic type, an *increased fragility* of the red corpuscles, microcytosis and spherocytosis of the red cells, and the constant presence of very large numbers of reticulocytes (10 to 20 per cent or even more). The reticulocytosis represents the intense activity with which the marrow replaces the red cells which are continually being hæmolysed. The disease may be hereditary and familial or be acquired during adult life. The jaundice is often slight and of the hæmolytic variety, but the

15

obstructive form may occur when pigment calculi block the common bile-duct. Their presence is not uncommon, and may be associated with biliary colic.

Leukæmia.—The possibility of a leukæmia is often considered first after the discovery of splenic enlargement, especially when a profound anæmia is also present. In myeloid (splenomedullary) types of leukæmia enormous enlargement of the spleen occurs, and the organ may occupy the greater part of the abdomen. In chronic lymphatic and in the acute forms of leukæmia splenic enlargement is generally moderate. The diagnosis is established by the blood-count, which usually shows a great excess of white corpuscles, varying with the type of leukæmia—myelocytes and myeloblasts in the myeloid forms, lymphocytes in the lymphatic types. In the acute forms hæmorrhagic symptoms are pronounced, e.g., epistaxis, spongy bleeding gums, gastro-intestinal hæmorrhage, and purpura, anæmia, and œdema. The acute forms are distinguished more by the constitutional symptoms than by the blood picture. Monocytic leukæmia also runs a short course and there is little splenic or liver enlargement. Gingivitis and angina are common features, and hæmorrhages from the buccal mucosæ are frequent. In all forms of leukæmia a secondary anæmia develops with varying degrees of rapidity, and the symptoms are chiefly due to this anæmia.

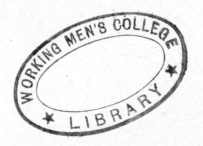

CHAPTER VIII

THE NERVOUS SYSTEM

THE diagnosis of nervous diseases offers an excellent example of the importance of grouping symptoms and signs together so as to present a picture of the underlying pathological processes. This should be the physician's aim and should not be obscured by a mere name such as chorea, paralysis agitans, etc., unless these names are qualified by full details of the cause and extent of the disease. For example, in the case of paralysis agitans, the symptom-group is often that of Parkinsonism, and it is essential to know the origin of this—e.g., post-encephalitic, arteriosclerotic, toxic, and so forth.

In arriving at a full diagnosis, careful history-taking is of great moment as in other systems ; age, sex incidence, and time relationships play a great part in deciding the pathological nature of the lesion. The anatomical diagnosis, as will be explained, depends upon careful assessment of changes in motor power and sensation, alteration in reflexes, and disturbances of the special functions of the brain, cranial nerves, and spinal cord. Some of the signs are due to paralysis of function in the damaged areas and are likely to be permanent, as are the various 'release' phenomena due to loss of control of one part of the nervous system over another. Others are temporary in character, e.g., irritative fits or abolition of function due to shock to the brain or spinal cord, but they are none the less valuable evidence of the anatomical site of the lesion.

THE MOTOR SYSTEM

One of the most common and obvious symptoms of nervous disease is loss of power—paralysis—and it is convenient to begin this description of the nervous system with an account of the motor system.

ANATOMICAL AND PHYSIOLOGICAL CONSIDERATIONS

The neurones responsible for voluntary motor action run in two relays. The first extends from the cortical cells in the motor area, which covers a wide region of the ascending frontal convolution, and the area just in front of it, to different parts of the spinal cord, there to terminate in the grey matter of the ventral horns. The second relay begins in the anterior-horn cells and ends in the individual branches of the nerves as they enter the voluntary muscles. To the first relay the name *upper motor neurone* is given ; to the second *lower motor neurone* (*Fig.* 172).

All forms of organic paralysis, except those due to uncommon primary muscular diseases and mechanical fixation from bone, joint, or muscle disease, are due to an interruption in one of these neurones. The clinical

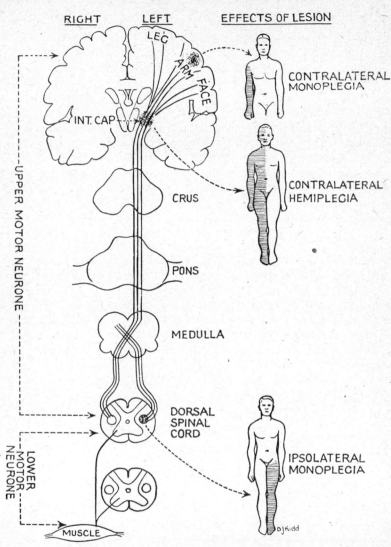

Fig. 172.—Diagram to show the extent of the upper and lower motor neurones, and the effects of a lesion in different parts of the motor system. Only the common positions for a lesion have been illustrated.

signs are similar in every upper neurone lesion and again in every lesion of the lower neurone, but the contrast between the physical signs of upper and lower motor neurone affections is so pronounced that the examiner is at once able to localize the lesion to one or the other. The differences in these signs are briefly discussed on p. 233.

The Upper Motor Neurone.—The upper motor neurone starts in the pre-Rolandic area in groups of cells which control movements rather than individual muscles. These cells are arranged in a fashion which has been proved experimentally, and is shown on the accompanying diagrams (*Figs.* 173, 174). It will be observed that the motor area covers a considerable region of the cortex, and it follows that a small lesion may pick out only a small part of the motor area, e.g., that governing movements of the hand,

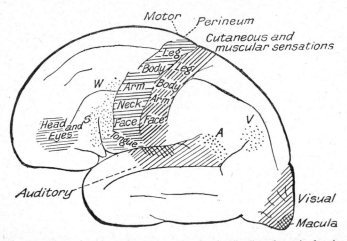

Fig. 173.—External surface of cerebrum showing localization of certain functions in definite areas of the cortex. Those areas from which only muscular movements have been evoked are marked by horizontal lines, while those which are believed to be associated with special afferent impulses are marked by oblique lines. Where a receiving area has been demarcated into a sensory and psychic region the sensory area is cross-hatched. Parts of the cortex concerned with language are shown stippled: V, Visual for the written word; A, Auditory for the spoken word; W, For writing; S, Muscles for speech. (*From Roaf's* '*Text-book of Physiology*', *Edward Arnold & Co.*)

and lead to a strictly limited paralysis. Left-sided cortical lesions are sometimes associated with aphasia in right-handed persons. In left-handed people the speech centres are on the right side of the brain, and aphasia may occur in lesions of this side. (*See* APHASIA, p. 308.)

From these cortical cells projection fibres known as the *pyramidal tract* pass through the substance of the brain in the *corona radiata*, converging towards the *internal capsule*, where they are densely packed. The result of quite a small lesion in this region will be an extensive paralysis—usually the face, arm, and leg on the contralateral side. The position of the fibres in the anterior two-thirds of the posterior limb, in the genu, and in a small part of the anterior limb of the internal capsule, is shown in *Fig.* 175. The relative position of the motor fibres for different parts of the body is not the same as in the motor cortex. (Cf. *Figs.* 173 and 175.)

Sensory fibres and visual paths in the capsule may be involved simultaneously with the motor fibres.

From the internal capsule the fibres pass through the *crus* and *pons* to the *medulla*, where the bulk of them decussate and travel down the lateral

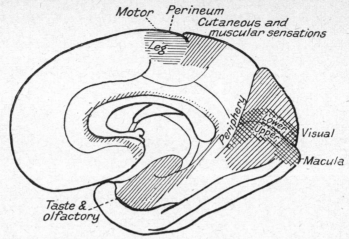

Fig. 174.—Mesial surface of cerebrum showing localization of certain functions in definite areas of the cortex. The hatching has the same significance as in *Fig.* 173. (*From Roaf's* ' *Text-book of Physiology* ', *Edward Arnold & Co.*)

columns of the *spinal cord* as the crossed pyramidal tract. The few fibres which do not decussate, but form the direct pyramidal tract, have little clinical importance.

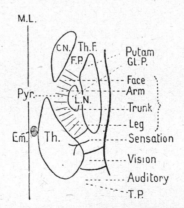

Fig. 175.—Horizontal section through the base of the brain to show the basal ganglia and the internal capsule (diagrammatic). M.L., Middle line; Pyr., Pyramidal tract; Em., Path for emotional expression; C.N., Caudate nucleus; Th., Thalamus; Th.F,. Thalamo-frontal tract; F.P., Fronto-pontine fibres; Putam, Putamen; Gl.P., Globus pallidus; L.N., Lenticular nucleus; T.P., Temporo-pontine fibres. (*From Samson Wright's* ' *Applied Physiology* ', *by kind permission of the Oxford University Press.*)

In the crus and pons some of the fibres terminate in relationship with the nuclei of the cranial nerves. They form the upper neurones of these nerves, the lower neurones starting from each cranial nerve nucleus.

As in the internal capsule, the dense aggregation of pyramidal tract fibres in the crus, pons, and medulla renders a lesion in these parts unusually disastrous in its results. Paralysis is often extensive and bilateral, and other brain-stem structures (sensory fibres, cranial nerve nuclei, etc.) may be damaged.

The fibres of the pyramidal tracts pass along the spinal cord for a varying distance, some ending in the upper and some in the lower segments of the cord in close proximity to the posterior-horn cells. Between the terminations of the pyramidal fibres and the anterior-cornual cells there appear to be short connecting fibres.

The results of pyramidal tract destruction will vary with the level at which the tract is interrupted : for example, if in the cervical regions both arms and legs will be paralysed ; if in the lower dorsal region, only the legs. Certain movements, notably of the upper part of the face, the jaw, and the larynx, are bilaterally represented in the cortex and are therefore little affected by lesions of the pyramidal system. In the frontal lobes eupraxic centres also exist which exercise the highest control over motor power, namely, the *will* to movement. Sometimes movements are performed without the patient realizing it, which indicates that the pyramidal system is intact, yet if the patient consciously wishes to make the same movements he is unable to do so. This is known as *motor apraxia*.

The Lower Motor Neurone.—From the anterior-horn cells, fibres pass out as the anterior nerve-roots to become eventually the peripheral nerves, in many of which sensory fibres are present. The motor fibres end in the voluntary muscles. This lower neurone may be interrupted by lesions in the anterior horns, in the nerve-roots, or in the peripheral nerves. The results will differ in the distribution of the paralysis, and the effects of a lesion of the anterior-horn cells or nerve-roots will be entirely motor ; in peripheral-nerve damage sensory changes often occur.

The lower motor neurone is influenced by the upper neurone and also by the extra-pyramidal system, and modifications of muscle tone result when the correct balance between these neurones is lost (*see* DISTINCTIONS BETWEEN UPPER AND LOWER MOTOR NEURONE LESIONS, p. 232). Reflexes through the lower neurone are also modified by the upper.

It appears also that the lower motor neurone is responsible for maintaining nutrition of the voluntary muscles and skin.

The Extra-pyramidal System.—Much obscurity still exists concerning the exact connexions and functions of this system. It includes the strio-spinal fibres from the striatum and subthalamic nuclei, the vestibulo-spinal tract descending from Deiter's nucleus, the rubro-spinal tract from the red nucleus, the tecto-spinal tract from the mid-brain, and the reticulo-spinal tract from the grey matter of the brain stem. These tracts bring the spinal cord, especially the anterior-horn cells, under the influence of the cerebellum and subcortical nuclei.

Lesions involving the extra-pyramidal system do not result in paralysis comparable with those of the pyramidal tracts, but some degree of weakness is common. More important is the interference with that delicate precision which characterizes perfect movement. Such interference is manifested in *rigidity* and *tremors*.

Both the extra-pyramidal and cerebellar systems exert considerable influence on posture, the cerebellar system working under control of the pyramidal system.

CLINICAL DISTINCTIONS BETWEEN UPPER AND LOWER MOTOR NEURONE LESIONS

UPPER NEURONE	LOWER NEURONE
Paralysis affects movements rather than muscles	Individual muscles or groups of muscles affected
Wasting only from disuse, therefore slight	Wasting pronounced
Rigidity of ' clasp-knife ' type. Muscles hypertonic	Flaccidity. Muscles hypotonic
No trophic changes in skin (exceptions in infantile hemiplegia)	Skin often cold, blue, and shiny. Ulceration may result
Tendon reflexes increased (*see* p. 276). Clonus often present	Tendon reflexes diminished or absent
Superficial reflexes diminished or modified (*see* p. 282). Note especially absent abdominal reflexes and Babinski's sign	Superficial reflexes unaltered
Associated movements sometimes present (*see* p. 241)	No associated movements. Fibrillations and myotatic irritability often present
Electrical reactions unchanged	Reaction of degeneration, partial or complete (*see* p. 390)

SYMPTOMS OF DISEASE OF THE MOTOR NEURONES

The two outstanding symptoms are (1) *paralysis*, and (2) *fits*. Paralysis is due to loss of function in motor neurones, fits to irritative effects causing disordered function.

Paralysis.—The patient may complain merely of weakness in a limb or other part of the body. To this the name *paresis* is given. When the part is immovable or almost so the term *paralysis* is applied. A paralysis affecting one side of the body is known as *hemiplegia*; if it is confined to one limb, *monoplegia*; if it affects both legs, or both arms and both legs, without involvement of the face, *paraplegia*. When both arms and both legs are paralysed the term *diplegia* is also used. Paralysis is as obvious to the patient as to the doctor ; paresis may only be discovered on examination. In upper neurone lesions paralysis is, to some extent, selective. The limbs are affected more than the trunk, and smaller and more precise movements of the hands are usually interfered with more than the grosser movements, e.g., of the shoulders.

In the lower limb dorsiflexion of the toes and feet is usually affected and also flexion at the knee and elbow, whilst extension at the knee and hip is little affected.

Paralysis arising from lower neurone lesions affects individual muscles or groups of muscles controlled by spinal segments of the cord. Knowledge of the segmental control is of localizing value, e.g., in spinal cord compression, and the accompanying table indicates the motor distribution of the main spinal segments.

SEGMENTAL REPRESENTATION OF MUSCLES

C.4.—Scaleni, trapezius, levator anguli scapulæ, diaphragm
C.5.—Levator anguli scapulæ, scaleni, supraspinatus, rhomboids, infraspinatus, teres minor, biceps, brachialis anticus, deltoid, supinator longus, serratus magnus, pectoralis major (clavicular part)
C.6.—Subscapularis, pronators, teres major, latissimus dorsi, serratus magnus, pectoralis major
C.7.—Triceps, extensors and flexors of wrist and digits

C.8.—Small hand muscles
Th.1.—Interossei and small hand muscles
Th.1 to 10.—Intercostals
Th.5 to 11.—Abdominal muscles
L.1.—Quadratus lumborum
L.3.—Sartorius, adductors of hip, iliopsoas
L.4.—Quadriceps extensor femoris, abductors of hip
L.5.—Flexors of knee
S.1.—Calf muscles
S.2.—Small foot muscles
S.3, 4.—Pelvic muscles

Fits.—In the case of the irritative phenomena known as fits, convulsions, or epilepsy, the patient's history is of paramount importance, as it may not be possible to see him during an attack. Fits may be *localized* or *generalized*. From a topographical diagnostic point of view localized fits are of great importance in lesions of the motor system.

LOCALIZED CONVULSIONS.—These are commonly due to irritation of the motor cells of the cortex, as, for example, by a tumour or depressed fracture of the skull, which causes an uncontrollable discharge of impulses to the groups of muscles which the cells govern. The same group of cells is irritated on each occasion and the *convulsive movements start in the same group of muscles* each time. The irritability may later extend in a definite order to other cortical cells and the convulsion becomes more generalized. Thus, twitchings may be observed in the right hand, followed by movements of the arm and shoulder-girdle, and then by movements of the whole of the right side, sometimes even spreading to the left. Unless the convulsion becomes generalized there is *no loss of consciousness*. This type of localized fit without loss of consciousness is called *Jacksonian epilepsy*, after the pioneer neurologist, Hughlings Jackson. Following the fit, *weakness* of the muscles affected is usually to be observed. Focal fits are not confined to the motor area, but may involve other brain centres, producing visual, auditory, and sensory phenomena. Although the main value of such fits is in suggesting a structural local change, sometimes no such change is found. This fact is important as it indicates that Jacksonian attacks may merely be a form of idiopathic epilepsy.

GENERALIZED CONVULSIONS.—In *adults* generalized convulsions may result from diseases which have a direct or indirect irritative or toxic effect on the brain substance, or interfere with its blood-supply. They occur, for example, in certain cases of cerebral tumour, traumatic lesions of the brain, general paralysis of the insane, and cerebral vascular lesions, in which the brain or its meninges are directly affected. They may also result from the indirect effects of poisons and toxins and of vascular disturbances, as in uræmia, lead poisoning, alcoholism, anæmia, and eclampsia. These are examples of *symptomatic epilepsy*. Their clinical form is similar to that described under *idiopathic epilepsy*, in which no such underlying cause is found.

Generalized convulsions *in childhood* have not the same serious import as in adult life. They represent the response of a yet unstable nervous system to comparatively slight degrees of irritation or toxæmia. They are common, for example, in acute fevers such as pneumonia or the exanthemata, and may occur from dietetic errors, teething, phimosis, etc. If the convulsions are persistent, however, the possibility of more serious causes similar to those mentioned in adults must be considered.

Idiopathic Epilepsy.—The fits of epilepsy follow, in classical cases, such a definite sequence of events as to make their recognition easy. The events are : (1) The aura ; (2) The cry ; (3) The tonic stage ; (4) The clonic stage ; (5) Post-epileptic phenomena.

1. *The aura* : This is a warning occurring a short time before the fit. It usually takes the form of a peculiar subjective phenomenon, e.g., tingling in one hand, queer sensations in the epigastrium, sense of constriction round the leg, visual or auditory sensations, etc. The aura is generally constant for the same individual. It is important, though difficult, to distinguish an aura of motor character (trivial twitchings followed by other phenomena) from true Jacksonian epilepsy.

2. *The cry* : As the patient falls to the ground the respiratory muscles are in a state of tonic spasm and a grunting cry is emitted. The patient is unaware of this as he falls unconscious.

3. *The tonic stage* : The muscles of the whole body are in tonic contraction. The body is therefore rigid, the hands and jaws clenched. The cessation of respiratory movements causes cyanosis and engorgement of veins in the neck. Occasionally the muscular involvement is unequal, twisting the body to one side. This stage lasts about half a minute and passes into—

4. *The clonic stage* : Clonic movements affect the whole body almost instantaneously. The limbs are alternately flexed and extended, and the movements rapidly increase in excursion and then diminish in intensity and frequency. The convulsions last about three minutes. During them the patient may injure himself by the champing movements of the jaw (laceration of the tongue ; injury to the teeth) or by contact with surrounding hard or dangerous objects. The presence of repeated injuries is always an important argument for the organic nature of the attacks. During the clonic stage another symptom usually indicative of organic disease may be present, viz., *incontinence* of urine and sometimes of fæces.

5. *Post-epileptic phenomena* : Following the clonic stage coma of short duration occurs during which the tendon reflexes are abolished and the plantar responses extensor. The pupils are dilated and the corneal reflexes absent. Usually the patient passes from coma into a natural *sleep* which lasts for several hours. More rarely *post-epileptic automatism* results : the patient may perform acts (e.g., undressing or walking) of which he afterwards has

no recollection. This automatism is, however, commoner in petit mal. The pronounced psychic changes of petit mal are rare after grand mal.

Petit Mal.—The term petit mal is given to epileptic attacks in which there is momentary loss of consciousness without convulsions. The patient may suddenly cease his conversation, drop something he is holding, pale or flush, or in more severe cases fall to the ground. In some cases ' psychic equivalents ' of epilepsy may be found—e.g., complete change in personality and habits, and liability to criminal acts of which the patient later has no knowledge.

THE HISTORY IN CASES OF FITS.—No opportunity must be lost of seeing the patient during a fit if this is possible. If not, the history obtained from the patient and from anyone who has observed an attack is of the greatest moment. As far as the patient is concerned he should be asked if he has any aura, whether he has injured himself during an attack, whether there has been incontinence, and what his condition is after the attack (sleep, headache, mental confusion, etc.). The relatives or other observers should be asked about the type and distribution of the convulsive movements and the duration of unconsciousness. It should be stressed that idiopathic epileptic attacks recur at intervals for a considerable period of life in most cases, and tend to take the same forms.

The electro-encephalogram may prove useful in the diagnosis of doubtful cases (*see* p. 389).

PHYSICAL SIGNS: EXAMINATION OF THE MOTOR SYSTEM

The prime function of the motor neurones is to permit precise and well-ordered *voluntary movement* of the muscles. The examination of the motor system is firstly concerned, therefore, with testing this movement. Many incidental observations are made, however, which have a direct or indirect bearing on the integrity of the motor neurones. Briefly these fall under the following headings : *Atrophy or hypertrophy of muscles; trophic changes; muscle tone (hypertonia or hypotonia); fibrillations and myotatic irritability; contractions and contractures; involuntary movements; abnormal postures;* and *gaits.* Inspection is the chief method by which these physical signs are elicited, and they are often noted before *muscular power* is tested. In the interpretation of these abnormal signs, the integrity of the sensory system and reflex arcs must be taken into account (*see later*), but the signs are more conveniently described in the present section.

Atrophy and Hypertrophy.—The contour and size of the muscles should be noted.

Atrophy is a characteristic of lower motor neurone lesions, but also occurs in muscular dystrophies (*Figs.* 176–178), and to a lesser extent from disuse. The limb loses its normal rounded contour.

For accuracy the circumference may be measured and compared with the normal side when possible. Each limb must be measured at the same level. In the case of the legs, for example, the measurement may be made 6 in. below the lower border of the patella with the limbs extended.

Hypertrophy is more difficult to recognize. Slight grades may result from increased occupational use of certain groups of muscles, or occasionally as a developmental defect (*Figs.* 179, 180). Without such cause, the presence of apparent muscular hypertrophy usually suggests muscular

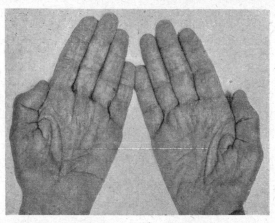

Fig. 176.—Wasting of the small muscles of the hand. From a case of progressive muscular atrophy. Note especially the flattened thenar eminences.

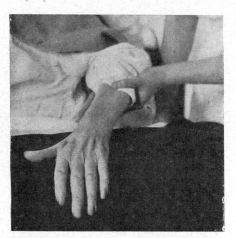

Fig. 177.—Wasting of interosseous muscles. Case of progressive muscular atrophy.

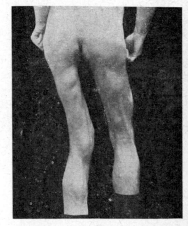

Fig. 178.—Muscular dystrophy. Shows atrophy of thigh muscles and buttocks and apparent hypertrophy of calf muscles.
(*Professor John Hay's case.*)

dystrophies. In the pseudo-hypertrophic form of muscular paralysis the relatively enormous calves and buttocks stand out in marked contrast with the atrophic flexor muscles of the thighs (*Fig.* 181).

Trophic Changes.—The colour and temperature of the skin should be recorded and the presence of any ulceration. In certain lower neurone lesions, especially infantile paralysis, the skin is blue, shiny, and cold. These signs may result from involvement of the vasomotor fibres. Trophic ulcers are more frequently seen when the sensory tracts are involved, e.g., bed-sores in myelitis.

Muscle Tone.—*Hypertonicity* occurs in upper neurone lesions and lesions of the extra-pyramidal system. The muscles are firm to the touch, though this is not a reliable sign. When the limb is passively moved, involuntary resistance is encountered, known as *rigidity* or *spasticity*. In

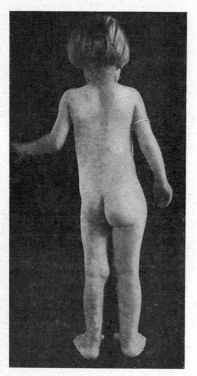
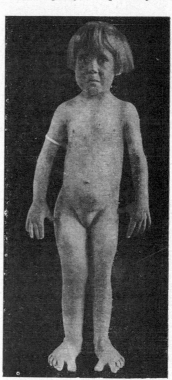

Figs. 179, 180.—Hemi-hypertrophy. (*Prof. Henry Cohen's case.*)

upper neurone lesions this is of the ' clasp-knife ' type—that is, when the limb is moved the maximum resistance is noticed almost at once, but it gives way suddenly after some effort on the part of the examiner, and allows the limb to be moved with comparative ease. The ' cog-wheel ' type of rigidity occurs in extra-pyramidal lesions. Here the resistance to passive movement diminishes in jerky steps, said to be due to the combination of rigidity and tremor. Some cases without tremor give ' lead pipe ' rigidity.

In lower neurone and cerebellar lesions and in states of profound debility, the muscles are *hypotonic* or *atonic*. To the palpating fingers they are soft and flabby. Passive movement is freely accomplished, often through a greater range than normal. This is well seen in the flail-like limbs of infantile palsy, and in tabes dorsalis (*Fig.* 182). Muscle tone depends on the 'stretch reflex', i.e., the increased tension produced by stimulation of sensory end-organs in the muscle, when it is passively stretched. Tendon reflexes and clonus are both produced by evoking this stretch reflex, the former by a single stimulus, the latter by repeated stimuli.

Fibrillations and Myotatic Irritability.—*Fibrillary tremors* are not uncommonly seen in chronic degenerative lesions of the anterior-horn

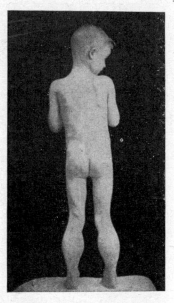

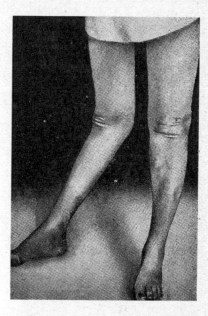

Fig. 181. — Pseudo - hypertrophic muscular paralysis, exhibiting the Hercules type of pseudo-hypertrophy of the calves. (*Dr. Patterson's case.*) (*From French's 'Index of Diagnosis'.*)

Fig. 182.—Severe hypotonia in tabes dorsalis causing genu recurvatum. (*From Dr. Roy R. Grinker's 'Neurology', by courtesy of Charles C. Thomas, Publisher.*)

cells, particularly progressive muscular atrophy and amyotrophic lateral sclerosis; more rarely syringomyelia. The muscle-fibres produce a quivering of the skin by their slow irregular contractions. The muscles affected are usually those which are seriously wasted.

These organic fibrillations are not to be confused with the quivering occasionally noticed in debility and neurosis, which affects chiefly the orbicularis palpebrarum, but may be found in larger muscles. This is known as *myokymia* ('live flesh'), and is never so persistent or widely distributed as true fibrillary tremors. Equally it must be recognized that even widespread fibrillations may occur in health, and unless accompanied by other neurological signs have no special significance.

In wasting muscles a quick tap will often start a contraction. This *myotatic irritability* is found in wasting due to lower neurone paralysis, but is often seen also in wasting diseases such as phthisis. Sometimes the muscle-fibres on contraction produce a localized swelling lasting for a few moments, a phenomenon known as *myoidema*. In muscles whose nerve has been severed a tap with a knee-jerk hammer will produce a slow wave of contraction like that elicited with the galvanic current. This clinical test gives much the same information as electrical reactions.

Contractions and Contractures.—When a group of muscles is paralysed the action of unopposed groups causes the limb to assume an abnormal position. This happens by virtue of *muscular contraction*. In time fibrotic changes take place in the paralysed muscles and their tendons, resulting in true *contractures* (*Fig.* 183), which are of a permanent and progressive nature. The effects of contraction (*see* MUSCLE TONE—Rigidity,

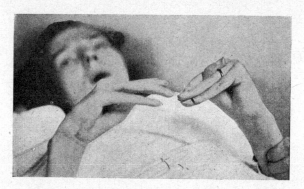

Fig. 183.—Contractures following encephalitis lethargica.

p. 237) can be overcome by passive movement, but this is not possible with contractures unless considerable force is used.

In upper neurone lesions affecting the pyramidal tracts alone, e.g., cerebral hemiplegia and spinal paraplegia, the limbs are in an extended position; but if the lesion also involves the extra-pyramidal tracts, an attitude of flexion in the limbs results. *Paraplegia in flexion* (*Fig.* 184) is thus indicative of a more severe lesion of the spinal cord than *paraplegia in extension*.

The attitude resulting from these types of paralysis may become permanent if contractures are allowed to ensue.

Involuntary Movements.—If movements of the limbs, face, or trunk are observed, their exact distribution and type must be recorded. Factors aggravating or diminishing the movements should also be noted, especially the effect of voluntary movement, sleep, and emotion.

Choreiform Movements.—Choreiform movements are irregular and spontaneous. They are quick and apparently purposeless, and may occur anywhere in the body, but particularly affect the larger joints. Emotion and voluntary effort usually increase them, but during sleep they disappear.

A familiar example is seen in *rheumatic chorea*, popularly called St. Vitus's dance. Children are most frequently affected, and the involuntary movements cause the child to drop things and to 'pull faces'. Chorea

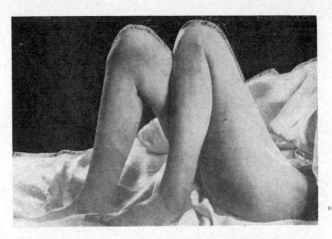

Fig. 184.—Paraplegia in flexion. From an extreme case of disseminated sclerosis. The limbs are permanently contracted into this position.

frequently affects one side of the body more than the other, *hemichorea.* Weakness of the affected side is common, and may be so extreme as to be called paralytic chorea. Particular signs such as the Jack-in-box tongue, a rapid protrusion and withdrawal of the tongue, depend upon the inability to perform sustained voluntary movements. Such choreiform manifestations are probably due to cortical excitation.

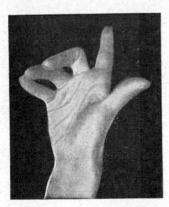

Fig. 185.—The hand in athetosis. (*From French's ' Index of Diagnosis '.)*

In *Huntington's chorea* similar involuntary movements are seen, but as this disease is familial, and occurs in the fourth and fifth decades and is associated with progressive dementia, no difficulty is found in distinguishing it from rheumatic chorea. Moreover the movements are slower. Unlike the movements of rheumatic chorea they are probably a release symptom due to a lesion of the basal ganglia.

Athetosis.—In cases of hemiplegia of long duration, especially infantile hemiplegia, peculiar slow 'snake charming' movements may be seen, known as athetosis. They chiefly affect the hands, and consist of alternate flexion and extension at the wrist and fingers, with spreading of the latter (*Fig.* 185).

Athetosis is only seen when some degree of voluntary movement i retained by the paralysed limb. Occasionally the movements occur in the feet (hyper-extension of the big toe), and great facial contortion may result if the affection is bilateral. The phenomenon is thought to arise from a lesion in the extra-pyramidal system and is sometimes found without upper neurone signs. It is in the nature of a release symptom.

Spasms and Tics.—Some difficulty may be experienced by the junior student in distinguishing choreiform movements from the more *purposive* movements seen in habits, spasms, and tics. These are of many different types. Some are very simple, such as shrugging the shoulders or blinking the eyes ; others are highly complex, affecting many groups of muscles and perhaps associated with verbal abnormalities such as the frequent uncontrollable repetition of the same word or sentence.

The most important point of distinction from chorea is the *repetition of the same movements*, though a new movement may replace an old one. The movements may go on for much longer than chorea, e.g., months, without much variation in intensity. Habits, spasms, and tics have a psychogenic origin. The patient is of an unstable nervous temperament, but some physical cause may originally sow the seed of a habit. Disease of the eyelids may, for example, cause blepharospasm, which normally passes away when the local cause is cured, but may persist in the psychopathic patient.

Although spasms are generally of a psychogenic functional nature, it is important to remember that they may be sequelæ of encephalitis lethargica.

Tremors.—Tremors are most easily demonstrated by asking the patient to extend the arms and separate the fingers. They may then be seen, and in many cases felt by touching the patient's fingers lightly.

Fine tremors are common in states of exhaustion and toxæmia, in neurasthenia, and in hyperthyroidism. The tremor is rapid, and, although most obvious in the fingers, affects the whole body. The toxic tremor of alcoholism and the tremor in general paralysis of the insane are noticeable also in the lips and tongue.

Coarse tremors often have a rhythmic character. In paralysis agitans the typical ' pill-rolling ' movements affect the hand, but the tremor eventually extends to the whole of one side. A similar tremor occurs in post-encephalitic Parkinsonism and in senility.

The tremor of disseminated sclerosis is exaggerated by voluntary effort, and is known as ' *intention* ' tremor. It is a manifestation of cerebellar ataxia due to a defect in postural fixation (tone). The usual way of eliciting this sign is to ask the patient to touch the tip of the nose accurately with the tip of the index finger, when the excursion of the involuntary movement will be seen to increase as the finger approaches the nose (*see Fig. 204, p. 267*).

Tremors affecting the head are seen in the ' head rolling ' of infants and in senility.

Associated Movements.—These are sometimes noticed in upper motor neurone lesions, and are in the nature of reflexes, similar to those observed

16

in decerebrate animals. They are really changes in posture rather than movements. Four examples may be given :—

1. When an attempt is made to raise one leg whilst the patient is recumbent, the other leg is firmly pressed against the bed. This can be noted by the observer placing his hand between the heel and the bed. In hemiplegia of organic origin the pressure against the hand increases, but in functional paralysis it is not so great as normal.

2. When a hemiplegic patient attempts to sit up from the recumbent position without using his arms, the paralysed leg is raised higher than the sound one.

3. If the flexed fingers of the paralysed hand are passively extended, the thumb is simultaneously flexed and adducted.

4. Yawning causes a rigid spasm of the paralysed arm with partial extension of the wrist and fingers.

Not uncommonly spontaneous movements of a similar nature may take place ; for example, if the patient is attempting to grip something the wrist may be dorsiflexed.

Convulsive Movements.—These have been described on pp. 232–235.

Rarer types of involuntary movement are *myoclonus* and *torsion spasm.* In myoclonus sudden shock-like contractions occur in the limbs or trunk ; it is sometimes a sequel of encephalitis lethargica. In torsion spasm the trunk is contorted in a freakish manner and the muscles undergo sudden variations of tone (dystonia).

Abnormal Postures (*see also* p. 21).—The posture of the patient, both erect and recumbent, must be observed when possible. Abnormal postures may be observed when the proper control of muscular tone and movement is affected. Lesions of the motor neurones—upper, lower, and extra-pyramidal—and of those tracts such as the posterior columns and cerebellar tracts which convey proprioceptive sensations, may each result in altered posture.

In *hemiplegia* we have an example of an upper neurone lesion causing altered posture. The paralysed arm is adducted, the fingers and wrist flexed, and the forearm pronated. The hip also is adducted, the knee extended, and the foot often inverted and plantar-flexed.

Mention has already been made of the two types of paraplegia—in extension and in flexion—according as the pyramidal tracts are affected alone or with the extra-pyramidal tracts.

Infantile paralysis and other forms of lower neurone lesion cause many different types of posture dependent upon the groups of muscles paralysed. The posture will result at first chiefly from unopposed action of antagonistic groups of muscles, but later the contractures in the paralysed muscles may overcome this and cause a more permanent abnormal attitude of the limb.

Thus a lesion which picks out the extensor muscles of the wrist will result in the familiar ' wrist drop ', seen in certain cases of peripheral neuritis or lesions of the musculospiral nerve.

Lesions of the 5th cervical root, often a result of injury during delivery (obstetrical paralysis), give the characteristic ' waiter's hand ' position, due to internal rotation of the arm by the unantagonized triceps.

The hands often assume peculiar postures in lower neurone lesions involving the anterior-horn cells, anterior nerve-roots, or nerves from the

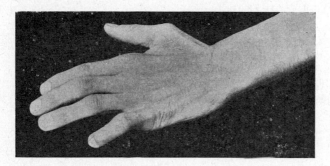

Fig. 186.—Claw-hand, from a case of progressive muscular atrophy. Showing the wasting of the interosseous muscles.

lower cervical and upper dorsal segments. The more important are the claw-hand and the flat-hand.

The *main en griffe* or *claw-hand* results from ulnar paralysis, progressive muscular atrophy, or other lesion causing wasting of the interossei and

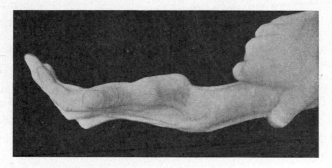

Fig. 187.—Another view of the same hand as in Fig. 186.

lumbricals. The wasting and claw-like appearance of the hand are seen in *Figs.* 186, 187.

The flat hand of median-nerve paralysis is sometimes called the *main de singe* (monkey's hand). The wasting of the muscles of the thenar eminence is mainly responsible for this, and also prevents the power of opposition in the thumbs.

Lesions of the long thoracic nerve result in serratus magnus paralysis, which causes the scapula to stand out—'*winged scapula*' (*Fig.* 188)—when the arms are held outstretched. Slight 'winging' may also result from paralysis of the rhomboids.

The discovery of abnormal postures of this kind should call for careful examination of the part to determine which muscles are paralysed and whether any contractures are present.

Lesions of the extra-pyramidal system such as occur in *paralysis agitans* and *post-encephalitic Parkinsonism* cause an increase of tone in the flexor muscles in particular, and the result is an attitude of flexion (*Fig.* 189). The patient stands with the knees slightly bent, the shoulders drooping, and the chin sunk into the chest. The arms are partially flexed at the elbows and the hands at the

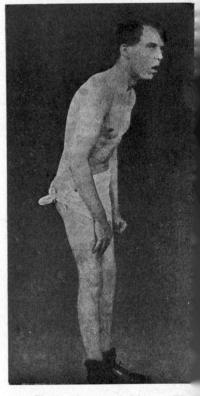

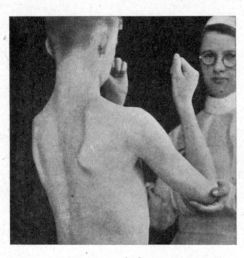

Fig. 188.—Winged scapula from serratus magnus paralysis.

Fig. 189.—Post-encephalitic state. The attitude is one of flexion, especially marked in this case at the hips. (*Prof. Henry Cohen's case.*)

metacarpo-phalangeal joints; but extension occurs at the wrists and interphalangeal joints.

Posterior-column lesions—for example, *tabes dorsalis*—lead to loss of tone in the muscles which sometimes modifies the posture. In tabes the hypotonus often results in abnormal extension at the knee-joints—genu recurvatum (*see Fig.* 182). To preserve his balance the patient also stands with the feet well apart. Cerebellar lesions have a similar effect to posterior column disease but less pronounced.

Even when the patient is *confined to bed*, suggestive postures may be discovered. The retraction of the head and arching of the back (opisthotonos) are valuable signs of meningeal irritation; deviation of the head and eyes to one side is often seen in cerebral hæmorrhage; the contrast between the attitude of flexion and extension in the two types of spastic paraplegia has already been noted.

Finally, all forms of bizarre postures may be assumed in *hysteria*; they have the distinguishing characteristic that they cannot be explained on an anatomical or physiological basis.

Gaits.—The study of the gait is complementary to that of the posture in a neurological case.

The patient should be asked to walk across the floor without shoes or stockings, and with the legs uncovered and *unhampered* by clothes.

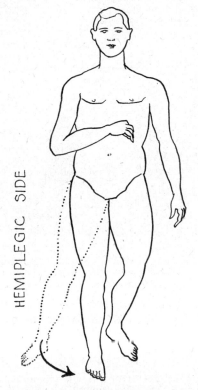

HEMIPLEGIC SIDE

Fig. 190.—Gait in hemiplegia, showing circumduction. (*From Cannon and Hayes'* '*Principles and Practice of Neurology* ', *Heinemann.*)

Spastic gaits are probably the commonest abnormal type. They result from upper motor neurone lesions such as hemiplegia and paraplegia.

In *hemiplegia* the affected limb is stiff and extended with the foot plantar-flexed. To avoid catching the toe against the ground at each step, the limb is sometimes circumducted in the arc of a circle (*Fig.* 190).

The 'scissor' gait of *diplegia* results from contractures in the adductors of the thighs, and is rarely seen save in the cerebral diplegia of children (Little's disease). The legs cross in the act of walking (*Fig.* 191).

Various types of *paraplegia* resulting from spinal cord compression,

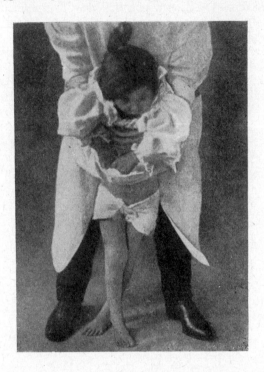

Fig. 191.—Congenital cerebral diplegia. Cross-legged progression. (*From Miller's 'Diseases of Children'.*)

disseminated sclerosis, etc., cause bilateral stiffness of the legs and plantar-flexion of the feet so that the patient walks on the toes.

Lesions involving the posterior columns and cerebellum cause *ataxia*, i.e., an unsteady, uncontrolled gait.

In *tabes* the hypotonia necessitates 'taking in the slack' in the muscles before these can be used effectively. The patient in walking, therefore, picks his feet well off the ground and then slams them down unnecessarily hard.

A somewhat similar gait results from other posterior column lesions, as in subacute combined degeneration and occasionally disseminated sclerosis, though in these two diseases the spasticity resulting from pyramidal tract involvement may mask the ataxia. In Friedreich's ataxia the disorder of gait is chiefly due to involvement of the cerebellar tracts, only to a lesser extent to the posterior column affection.

The ataxia of *cerebellar disease* (tumours, vascular lesions, etc.) is shown by a characteristic reeling or ' drunken man's ' gait with a special tendency to fall to one side, usually to the side of the lesion owing to the loss of muscle tone on that side. Sometimes the affected arm does not swing as the patient walks, and in some cases there is a lack of co-ordination between the trunk and limbs.

The gait in *extra-pyramidal lesions* (paralysis agitans, post-encephalitic states, etc.) is stiff, and the short steps taken by the patient give a quick shuffling appearance, a phenomenon known as *festination*. In classical cases, if pushed gently forwards, the patient appears ' to hurry after his centre of gravity ' (*propulsion*). If pushed backwards he continues in the same direction until he falls or is stopped (*retropulsion*). Lateropulsion is a similar movement sideways, more rarely seen. As in cerebellar disease, the arms do not swing freely, but here both sides are affected, whereas cerebellar signs are generally unilateral. Occasionally in extra-pyramidal disease the syndrome is predominantly unilateral.

Other special types of gait, less frequently observed, are the *waddling gait* of muscular dystrophies caused by weakness of the glutei, the contorted gait of Huntington's chorea, and the *steppage gait* in weakness of the peronei, generally due to peripheral neuritis.

Hysteria may also produce many peculiarities of gait. One special, though uncommon form, generally seen in children, is known as *astasia-abasia*, an inability to stand or walk.

Lastly it is necessary in suspected *myopathies* to watch the way in which the patient rises from the recumbent to the erect posture. In pseudo-hypertrophic muscular dystrophy, this is highly characteristic. The patient rolls over, gets on to his hands and knees, and takes the weight of the body with the hands whilst he extends the knees. He then levers the trunk upright with the hands placed on the thighs (*Fig.* 192). Occasionally paralysis of the extensor muscles of the thighs—e.g., from anterior polio-myelitis—has a similar result.

Motor Power.—When the preliminary observations have been made the examiner proceeds to test the muscular strength of the limbs and trunk. If there is obvious paralysis it is merely necessary to determine the distribution and degree of this. When slight weakness of a limb is the complaint, and also when other neurological symptoms are present without subjective weakness, the examination of motor function must be systematic.

At each important joint the action of the extensors and flexors, abductors and adductors, pronators and supinators, etc., must be tested without any load and then against the resistance of the physician's hand, and compared with the same muscles in the opposite limb. Movements of head and trunk (flexion, extension, and rotation) must be similarly tested. The hand grip can be compared by means of a special instrument, the dynamometer.

The importance of the distribution of muscular weakness has already received attention in discussing the anatomy of the motor system. To recapitulate : In cerebral lesions the paralysis is usually of one or more limbs, or of large groups of muscles such as those controlling the movements of the hands. In spinal disease affecting the tracts, groups of muscles are put out of action corresponding with the level of the lesion. In lower neurone lesions muscular paralysis may also be extensive, as in anterior

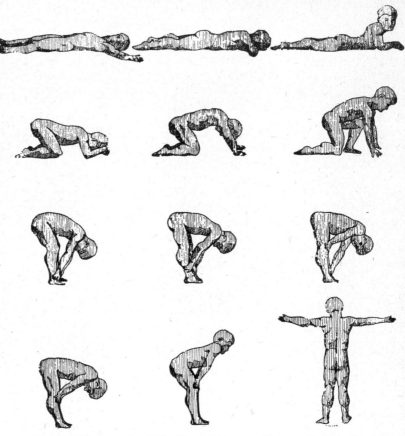

Fig. 192.—Diagrams of a child with pseudo-hypertrophic muscular dystrophy rising by climbing up his legs. (Modified after Lewin.) (From Dr. Roy R. Grinker's ' Neurology ', by courtesy of Charles C. Thomas, Publisher.)

poliomyelitis ; but more commonly the paralysis is localized to smaller groups of muscles according to the segment of the cord, nerve-roots, or nerves affected. The distribution of the paralysis has considerable localizing value, but must be considered in conjunction with sensory changes and those signs which distinguish upper from lower neurone lesions (see table on p. 232).

Electrical Reactions.—These are discussed in Chapter XII.

ILLUSTRATIVE LESIONS OF THE MOTOR NEURONES

Causation.—The common lesions of the motor system, as of other parts of the body, may be grouped pathologically as follows :—

1. *Congenital.*—The child is born with neurological abnormalities or develops them shortly after birth, e.g., cerebral diplegia.

2. *Traumatic.*—There is a history of injury and the onset is sudden in many cases, though traumatic effects are sometimes delayed. Examples include laceration of the brain in head injuries and damage to the spinal cord by fracture of the spine.

3. *Vascular.*—These lesions account for most upper motor neurone types of paralysis. The most familiar examples are cerebral hæmorrhage, thrombosis, or embolism, though similar accidents may occur in the spinal cord. Vascular lesions are suggested by the abruptness of their onset, and by favouring circumstances such as high blood-pressure, arteriosclerosis, valvular disease, and chronic renal disease.

4. *Inflammatory.*—Acute inflammatory lesions produce their effect in a period varying from hours to days. Fever and leucocytosis are usually present. Examples are found in acute anterior poliomyelitis, and to some extent in meningitis and brain abscess in which the motor neurones may be involved.

The chronic inflammatory lesions—syphilis, tuberculosis, leprosy, etc. —produce their effect slowly, and are often difficult to distinguish from degenerative and neoplastic lesions.

5. *Neoplastic.*—Cerebral and spinal tumours may grow slowly, but as they have little room to expand without pressing on delicate tissues the results are extremely serious. As a rule the effects are not purely motor as sensory tracts in the cord are simultaneously involved. Cerebral tumours of the motor cortex may, however, for a long time cause motor symptoms only, e.g., fits and paresis. It is to be remembered that the chronic inflammatory lesions of tuberculosis and syphilis may result in tumour formation which has effects similar to those of neoplasm. Aneurysm more rarely simulates neoplasm.

6. *Degenerative.*—Degenerative lesions affecting the motor tracts are insidious in their effects, in some ways resembling chronic inflammatory diseases. Examples are disseminated sclerosis, amyotrophic lateral sclerosis, and familial spastic paralysis.

Lesions of the Upper Motor Neurone

Hemiplegia (*see also* CEREBRAL HÆMORRHAGE, p. 303).—Vascular lesions are by far the commonest causes of hemiplegia, especially hæmorrhage into the internal capsule. The extent of the paralysis varies with the number of motor fibres affected. In complete hemiplegia the face, arm, and leg are paralysed, but the trunk muscles escape, at least partially.

After an initial period of cerebral shock in some cases, signs of an upper neurone lesion develop on the affected side. The limbs are spastic, the tendon reflexes increased, clonus may be present, the abdominal reflexes are lost, and the plantar response is extensor (Babinski's sign). These release signs and the paralysis are opposite to the side of the lesion, unless this is in the upper cervical regions of the cord or below, when the same side is paralysed. If the patient recovers partially, contractures may occur and the characteristic posture and gait develop. These have been described.

Whatever the position of the lesion these signs of hemiplegia are the same provided *all* the pyramidal tract fibres are affected. From the short account of the anatomy of the motor tract given on p. 227 it follows, how-ever, that a complete hemiplegia more frequently results from a small lesion situated in a region where the fibres are closely crowded together, e.g., the internal capsule, crus, pons, or medulla. In the cortex a small lesion results in a more limited paralysis.

Even where the hemiplegia is complete one limb may be more affected than the other. Thus in internal-capsular hæmorrhage it is common for

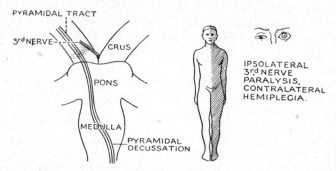

Fig. 193.—Weber's syndrome. A lesion in the crus interrupting the pyramidal tract fibres and simultaneously involving the 3rd nerve. Result: Contralateral paralysis of face, arm, and leg (upper neurone type), with ipsilateral 3rd-nerve palsy (lower neurone type).

slight movement to remain in the leg though the arm is devoid of any. That the fibres of the leg are not so completely destroyed is shown by the quicker recovery of this limb.

Localization of the Lesion.—Certain special features help to localize the lesion causing the hemiplegia. (*See Fig.* 172, p. 228.)

In the cortex, as mentioned, monoplegia, or paralysis of an even smaller group of muscles, is common. Aphasia is a frequent accompaniment if the left side of the brain is affected. Jacksonian fits occur if the lesion is irritative, e.g., tumour or depressed fracture. Of the vascular lesions cerebral thrombosis is the commonest (*see* p. 304).

In the internal capsule the hemiplegia is generally complete, and spread of the lesion (hæmorrhage usually) backwards may result in simultaneous sensory changes and sometimes homonymous hemianopia. (*See Fig.* 175.)

In the crus a form of crossed paralysis may result (Weber's syndrome) in which the 3rd nerve is paralysed on one side and the face, arm, and leg on the other (*Fig.* 193).

Tumours in the interpeduncular space may have a similar effect by pressure on the crus, but polydipsia and polyuria may also be present.

In the pons other types of crossed lesion may occur from involvement of the 6th and 7th nerves at this level. There may be facial paralysis (lower neurone type) on one side and hemiplegia (arm and leg) on the other (*Fig.* 194). If the 6th nerve is also affected the external rectus will be paralysed on the same side as the 7th. Strictly unilateral lesions of the pons are not common, and hemiplegic signs may therefore be present on both sides in variable degrees. The pupils are sometimes pin-point in hæmorrhage. If the fillet is involved, ataxia and loss of deep sensibility may be present on the opposite side.

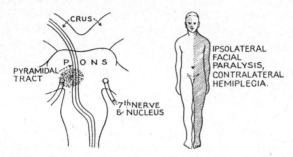

Fig. 194.—Pontine crossed paralysis. A lesion in the pons involving the nucleus of the 7th nerve, causing facial paralysis on the same side, and paralysis of the opposite arm and leg.

Crural and pontine lesions are not common and are generally vascular or neoplastic.

In the medulla crossed paralyses also occur—hemiplegia on one side and paralysis of the 9th, 10th, 11th, or 12th nerves on the other. As in pontine lesions the damage is rarely confined to one side, and frequently extends into the sensory tracts.

In the spinal cord the hemiplegia is on the same side as the lesion (*see* BROWN-SÉQUARD'S SYNDROME, p. 270), but only involves the arm as well as the leg if the cervical region is affected.

Paraplegia.—This word generally means paralysis of both lower limbs, but if the lesion is in the cervical region the arms may also be affected. The signs are similar to those of hemiplegia, but bilateral. The paralysis is generally spastic, though severe lesions of the cord may cause a flaccid paralysis from spinal cord shock (*see also* PARAPLEGIA IN FLEXION AND EXTENSION, pp. 239, 240); the tendon reflexes are increased; the abdominal reflexes lost if the lesion is above this reflex arc; Babinski's sign and clonus are present. Another important sign is loss of sphincter control, not generally present if the pyramidal tract is damaged on one side only.

Pure forms of spastic paraplegia without sensory changes are sometimes seen in disseminated sclerosis, familial spastic paralysis, etc., though even in these diseases other tracts are sometimes affected. Many diseases of the spinal cord are characterized by a combination of spastic paraplegia with sensory changes—for example, compression paraplegia, myelitis, and subacute combined degeneration. They will be described in discussing the sensory system. A short description of disseminated sclerosis may conveniently be given here.

Disseminated Sclerosis (*Fig.* 195).—This is one of the commonest organic nervous diseases. It affects both sexes, usually between the ages of 20 and 40 years, and is generally insidious in its onset. Its progress is marked by remissions in which the symptoms and signs may disappear partially or entirely.

Amongst early symptoms may be mentioned transient pareses, paræsthesiæ (subjective sensory phenomena, *see* p. 264), disturbances of micturition, and ocular symptoms. The ocular manifestations are perhaps most characteristic. Blurring of vision may occur for a few days to a few weeks, indicating a retrobulbar neuritis,

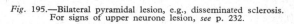

Fig. 195.—Bilateral pyramidal lesion, e.g., disseminated sclerosis. For signs of upper neurone lesion, *see* p. 232.

and may precede cord symptoms by months or years. It is followed in 2–3 months by optic atrophy, especially noticeable in the outer halves of the retinæ. In a developed case, *spastic paraplegia* with the signs just described is perhaps the commonest clinical picture. But as the name of the disease indicates, the lesions are scattered, and before a diagnosis of disseminated sclerosis is justifiable the paraplegia must be accompanied by signs of damage to other parts of the nervous system. The triad of symptoms described by Charcot, *nystagmus*, *staccato speech*, and ' *intention* ' *tremor*, is by no means commonly found, but one of the triad with signs of a spastic paraplegia may suggest disseminated sclerosis, indicating patches of sclerosis in the cerebellum and pyramidal systems. Both nystagmus and staccato speech are defects of postural fixation (tone) due to cerebellar involvement.

Evidence of sclerotic patches in the posterior columns or cerebellar pathways is to be found in *ataxia*, a common symptom, of which the ' intention ' tremor is probably a manifestation. Loss of vibration sensation and of sense of position are more rarely found on objective examination. Damage to other sensory tracts may result in various anæsthesiæ and paræsthesiæ.

Lesions of the Lower Motor Neurone

The lower neurone may be injured or diseased in the cranial nerve nuclei or spinal anterior-horn cells, in the anterior nerve-roots, or in the nerves themselves.

The commonest lesion of the anterior-horn cells is acute anterior poliomyelitis (infantile paralysis). A chronic degeneration of the anterior-horn cells also occurs (progressive muscular atrophy).

The anterior nerve-roots may be damaged by trauma, and more rarely by vascular, inflammatory, and neoplastic lesions. The effects are similar to and frequently indistinguishable from disease of the anterior-horn cells.

Lesions of the peripheral nerves are generally due to trauma or inflammation (peripheral neuritis). The results depend upon the distribution of the nerve and the position in which it is injured. When the nerve is purely motor (e.g., the long thoracic nerve to the serratus magnus) paralysis of the muscles supplied results ; but as the majority of nerves are ' mixed ', i.e., contain both motor and sensory fibres, muscular paralysis is frequently accompanied by sensory changes.

Some examples of lower neurone lesions may now be considered in more detail.

LESIONS OF THE ANTERIOR-HORN CELLS AND OF THE BULBAR NUCLEI

Acute Anterior Poliomyelitis (*Infantile Paralysis*).—This disease is commonest in children and young adults. It is organismal (virus) in origin, and the onset is therefore like other febrile illnesses, with which it is not uncommonly confused until paralytic symptoms appear.

Pain in the back and tenderness of the limbs are suggestive early symptoms. Fever of 102°–104° is often accompanied by signs of meningeal irritation (*see* p. 296), but the diagnosis from meningitis can be made by examination of the cerebrospinal fluid. In 24 to 48 hours a *flaccid paralysis* occurs and establishes the diagnosis. The extent of this is variable. Sometimes only a few muscles are affected ; sometimes the greater part of all the limbs and trunk may be involved. The distribution of the paralysis corresponds with the affected segments of the spinal cord (*see* Table on p. 233) The muscles most commonly singled out are those of the lower limbs, especially the extensors of the thigh, tibialis anticus, peronei, and extensors of the feet and toes.

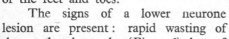

Fig. 196.—Atrophy of the muscles of the left shoulder and upper arm, the result of former infantile paralysis. (*From French's* '*Index of Diagnosis*'.)

The signs of a lower neurone lesion are present : rapid wasting of the paralysed muscles (*Fig.* 196), loss of tendon reflexes, flaccidity, trophic changes in the skin, and alteration in the electrical reactions (R.D.).

Amyotrophic Lateral Sclerosis : Progressive Muscular Atrophy. —These diseases should be regarded as one and the same. They affect the upper and lower neurones in a variable combination, and degeneration of unknown aetiology takes place.

Clinically the commonest form is one in which wasting of the small muscles of the hands (perhaps spreading to the arms) causes weakness and various deformities such as ' claw hand ' and ' flat hand ' (p. 243), without any sensory changes, but accompanied by widespread muscular fibrillation.

The upper neurone involvement shows itself by increased tendon reflexes, especially of the arms, but later of the legs, though the full classical picture with Babinski's sign and lost abdominal reflexes is rarely found.

A somewhat similar condition may result from syphilis, *amyotrophic meningo-myelitis*, but as a rule there is an Argyll Robertson pupillary reaction and mild luetic changes in the cerebrospinal fluid.

Bulbar Paralysis.—Similar chronic degenerative changes to those occurring in the anterior-horn cells may also affect the bulbar nuclei of the cranial nerves, and result in bulbar paralysis of the lower neurone type (*progressive bulbar paralysis*).

The principal symptoms are increasing difficulty in articulation due to paresis of the tongue and lips (hypoglossal nucleus), difficulty in swallowing from paresis of the soft palate and pharynx (10th and 9th nuclei), regurgitation of fluids through the nose, and a nasal voice. The tongue wastes and its movement is more and more limited. The larynx may also be involved. (*See also* CRANIAL NERVES, p. 335.) The process is essentially a chronic one.

More rarely, bulbar paralysis of this type may be an acute process due to acute poliomyelitis, encephalitis, or to vascular lesions. It may also be imitated by affections of the 9th, 10th, 11th, and 12th cranial nerves themselves, especially by diphtheritic neuritis. In myasthenia gravis bulbar symptoms are present, but improve after a rest, only to recur after use of the affected muscles.

Pseudo-bulbar Paralysis.—This term is applied to cases of difficulty in articulation, swallowing, etc., due to *bilateral* involvement of the pyramidal tract fibres to the bulb. It is usually due to bilateral cerebral thrombosis affecting the internal capsular region. Mild bilateral hemiplegic signs are present, together with the bulbar symptoms and generally some emotional instability and progressive dementia.

LESIONS OF THE ANTERIOR NERVE-ROOTS

The anterior nerve-roots contain only motor fibres, which are distributed to the muscles in a segmental fashion so closely resembling that of the anterior-horn cells as to make a diagnosis between a lesion of one or the other impossible unless other signs of spinal-cord disease (e.g., pyramidal-tract signs) are present.

The commonest lesions of the anterior nerve-roots are traumatic, e.g., brachial plexus injuries, and the student's knowledge of anatomy has a direct practical application in such cases. It is not possible here to deal with the many varieties of traumatic lesions of the anterior nerve-roots or the peripheral nerves. One example of a lesion of the anterior nerve-roots may, however, serve as an illustration, namely, the *obstetrical palsy* of Erb-Duchenne type.

Erb-Duchenne Paralysis.—In this condition the 5th cervical anterior nerve-root is torn at birth. The result is a paralysis of the muscles governed by this segment—the deltoid, supinator longus and brevis, brachialis anticus, and biceps. From action of the unopposed muscles the hand and arm are held in the characteristic position shown in *Fig.* 268, p. 364. The arm is adducted and extended at the elbow, and the forearm pronated, giving the ' waiter's hand ' position.

No lesion of an individual nerve could produce such a combination of muscular paralyses, and the cause can be narrowed down to a lesion of the anterior-horn cells or the corresponding nerve-root of the 5th cervical segment. The characteristics of a lower neurone lesion will be present, and the absence of sensory changes will further exclude a peripheral-nerve lesion.

LESIONS OF THE PERIPHERAL NERVES

Traumatic Lesions.—Here again the student must be prepared to work out on anatomical grounds the nerve or nerves affected. The problem is made easier by the *combination of muscular paralysis and anæsthesia* corresponding with the distribution of an individual nerve. The paralysis, again, is of the lower neurone type, and in the area supplied by the sensory fibres of the nerve all types of sensation are lost.

As an example of a peripheral nerve lesion musculospiral paralysis may be taken.

Musculospiral Paralysis.—This is of particular interest to the physician, as not only is the musculospiral the nerve most commonly injured, but it is frequently affected by peripheral neuritis, especially that due to lead poisoning.

The nerve, including its posterior interosseous branch, has a large motor distribution, comprising the triceps, supinator longus, extensor carpi radialis longior and brevior, extensor communis digitorum, etc. When it is injured high up (for example, in ' crutch paralysis ', or ' Saturday night paralysis ' due to pressure on some hard object during alcoholic stupor) these muscles are paralysed in varying degrees. The main result is *wrist-drop*, i.e., an inability to use the extensors of the wrist, and weakness of the extensors of the digits. In cases of lead palsy a peculiar feature is the *escape of the supinator longus* from the general paralysis of muscles supplied by the musculospiral.

The *sensory changes* are limited owing to overlap with other nerves.

Generally the anæsthesia is confined to a small area on the back of the thumb, and the skin between this and the index finger.

Peripheral Neuritis.—The association of muscular weakness with sensory changes, characteristic of a lesion of a single nerve-trunk, is equally characteristic of *multiple neuritis* resulting from more general causes such as infections (diphtheria, influenza, leprosy, etc.) or intoxications (alcohol, arsenic, lead, diabetes, etc.). Many forms of multiple neuritis have distinguishing features, such as the particular nerves affected, or the predominance of sensory over motor changes or vice versa. All have certain symptoms and signs in common. The muscular paralysis accords with the particular muscles innervated by the affected nerves. It is of course lower neurone in type. The neuritis usually involves many nerve-trunks, and the paralysis is often widespread, but is most marked in the distal parts of the limbs, rarely involving the trunk. The sensory changes likewise correspond with the distribution of the nerves, and *all* types of sensation are lost in varying degrees. Paræsthesiæ in the hands and especially feet are common.

As illustrations of the variation of the signs according to the cause of the neuritis, it may be noted that diphtheria affects in particular the oculomotor, 9th, 10th, and other cranial nerves, whilst in other types of neuritis the cranial nerves are rarely affected. The palatal and accommodation paralyses of diphtheria may occur alone or be followed by changes in the limbs. Alcoholic neuritis singles out especially the nerves to the distal parts of the limbs, particularly the legs (foot-drop is common), and subjective sensory changes—especially pain—are common. Lead, on the contrary, picks out the nerves to the extensors of the wrists and forearms, so that wrist-drop is common. Sensory changes are conspicuously absent in lead poisoning. Many similar illustrations will be found by the student in his text-book of medicine.

Associated phenomena such as cardiac manifestations, signs of alcoholism, diabetes or arsenical poisoning are also useful diagnostic aids. Apart from these diffuse forms of toxic neuritis, localized types of unexplained origin, e.g., brachial neuritis and certain forms of sciatica, may occur.

LESIONS OF THE MUSCLES

A few comparatively rare diseases apparently have their pathological seat in the muscles themselves, the motor neurones, both upper and lower, remaining intact. These diseases (myopathies) are often characterized by *muscular weakness*, and their diagnosis is therefore usually made during the examination of the motor system. The more important are the muscular dystrophies, myotonia congenita, myotonia atrophica, and myasthenia gravis.

Muscular Dystrophies.—Muscular atrophy due to primary changes in the muscles, as distinct from neural muscular atrophy, occurs in certain families. This *familial* nature of the dystrophies is all-important in diagnosis. The dystrophies usually appear in childhood, or, in some forms, in adolescence. In many cases, alongside of the wasting of certain groups of muscles, there is apparent hypertrophy of others, really due to overgrowth of fat and connective tissue.

Various types of dystrophy are described, according to the groups of muscles affected, to the age of onset, and to whether pseudo-hypertrophy is present as well as atrophy. The usual types are :—

1. *Pseudo-hypertrophic Muscular Paralysis.*—Boys between the ages of 3 and 10 years are generally affected. The *atrophy* is seen especially in the latissimus dorsi and lower halves of the pectorals, but the biceps, peronei, and hamstrings are also affected. Winging of the scapulæ results from paralysis of the serratus magnus. Lordosis is also common owing to wasting of the flexors of the thighs. By contrast with these wasted muscles, those of the calves and buttocks and the deltoids and spinati are enlarged owing to *pseudo-hypertrophy* (*see Fig.* 181, p. 238). The waddling

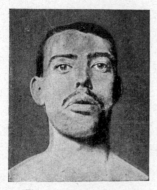

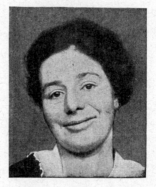

Fig. 197.—Myopathic facies: the loose pout of the lips due to weakness of the orbicularis oris.

Fig. 198.—Myopathic facies: the transverse smile.

(*Figs.* 197 and 198 *by Dr. S. A. K. Wilson; from French's ' Index of Diagnosis '.*)

gait and classical method of rising from the supine to the erect posture are described on p. 247.

2. *Facio-Scapulo-Humeral Type.*—This starts at about the same age as, or somewhat older than, the pseudo-hypertrophic. The distribution of muscles affected is indicated by the name. The facial weakness causes a characteristic myopathic facies with drooping of the lower lip and a ' transverse smile ' (*Figs.* 197, 198). The shoulder-girdle muscles (trapezius, serratus magnus, etc.) and the muscles of the upper arm (biceps, triceps, and pectorals) are involved, causing drooping of the shoulders and winging of the scapulæ (*Fig.* 199).

3. *Juvenile Type.*—This manifests itself later than other varieties, usually in adolescence. The biceps, triceps, supinator longus, and to a lesser extent the quadriceps and glutei, are the paretic muscles.

Myotonia Congenita (*Thomsen's Disease*).—This is a familial disease occurring in children and characterized by *unusually sustained contraction* of any of the voluntary muscles—*myotonia*. On shaking hands the patient

17

is unable to relax his grasp for a few seconds. Similarly on walking, a few seconds are necessary for the proper relaxation of the muscles antagonistic to those actually carrying the limb forward. Once started the patient walks quite well. In spite of this myotonia, there is no rigidity on *passive*

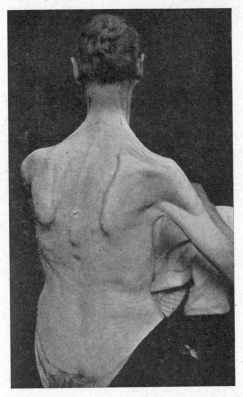

Fig. 199.—Muscular dystrophy. Shoulder-girdle distribution.

movement of the limbs, as in upper neurone lesions. Muscular weakness is only slight in this case.

Myotonia Atrophica (*Dystrophia myotonica*).—In this condition, which occurs usually in the third decade, there is a combination of *muscular atrophy with myotonia*. The muscles particularly affected are those of the neck and face (sternomastoids, masseters, temporals). The face has been described as ' hatchet-like ', and the neck as ' pole-like '. The patient is usually bald and often impotent. The disease is frequently complicated by cataract.

Amyotonia Congenita (*Myatonia Congenita*).—In some cases this disease seems to be related to the muscular dystrophies, as *weakness* of the muscles occurs. The cardinal sign, however, is extreme hypotonus, allowing the limbs to be placed in all manner of grotesque positions. All muscles, save those of the face, may be affected, particularly those of the lower limbs.

Myasthenia Gravis.—In this peculiar disease there is no paralysis or wasting of the muscles, but these *fatigue* very easily. Different groups of muscles are affected. Sometimes the ocular group is singled out and ptosis is then a common feature, the patient complaining that he is unable to keep his eyes open. In other cases of the bulbar type the lips, tongue, facial muscles, etc., show the extraordinary fatigue, and the symptoms of bulbar paralysis (*see* p. 254) may appear, but may improve after rest.

THE SENSORY SYSTEM

ANATOMICAL AND PHYSIOLOGICAL CONSIDERATIONS

As in the case of the motor system the fibres conveying sensation run in relays, but the neurones have a more complex course and are more numerous. Unlike the motor neurones, the sensory fibres are afferent, conveying sensation from the periphery to the brain.

From the peripheral nerves they enter the spinal cord through the posterior nerve-roots and ganglia. In the cord they dissociate to run in different tracts, some ending in the cord itself, some in the gracile and cuneate nuclei of the medulla, some proceeding direct to the thalamus. Most tracts end either directly or through another relay in the thalamus, from which a last relay conveys the sensory impulses to the post-Rolandic area of the cerebral cortex.

The path taken by the different types of sensation is of great importance in clinical neurology.

Path in the Peripheral Nerves.—All types of sensation are conveyed by the peripheral nerves but they arise from special end-organs in the skin, muscles, and tendons. The modes of sensibility include cutaneous sensations, i.e., light touch, cold, warmth, and pain, and deep impressions such as painful and painless pressure, postural sensibility, and vibration sense. There are no special nerves for discrimination and localization, though the end-organs may afford some localizing facilities. The previous distinction of cutaneous sensibility into epicritic and protopathic appears to be without foundation (*Fig.* 200).

Path in the Posterior Nerve-roots.—From the peripheral nerves the various types of sensation enter the cord through the posterior nerve-roots, in which the fibres are arranged in *segmental fashion* similar to the motor fibres in the anterior nerve-roots (*Fig.* 201). Lesions in the posterior roots are not common, but must be considered when segmental anæsthesia is present.

Path in the Spinal Cord.—In the medical wards sensory disturbances are most frequently associated with lesions of the spinal cord. In this part of their course the fibres of sensation are grouped entirely differently from the arrangement in the peripheral nerves (*Figs.* 202, 203).

Touch fibres cross to the opposite side soon after their entry and run in the spino-thalamic tracts (lateral columns). Some also pass up the

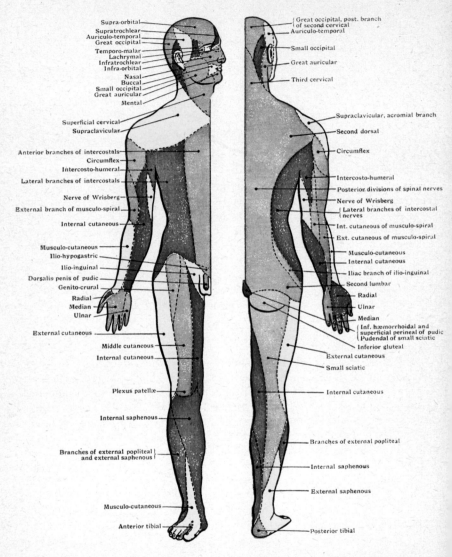

Fig. 200.—The distribution of sensory nerves in the skin. (*By Sir E. Farquhar Buzzard; from French's ' Index of Diagnosis '.*)

posterior columns. These are uncrossed until they reach the fillet. A lesion in the lateral column may thus result in loss of tactile sensation (and pain and temperature—*see below*) on the opposite side below the level of the lesion, together, of course, with motor paralysis on the same side of the type already discussed.

Pain and temperature sensibility is conveyed by fibres which *cross*

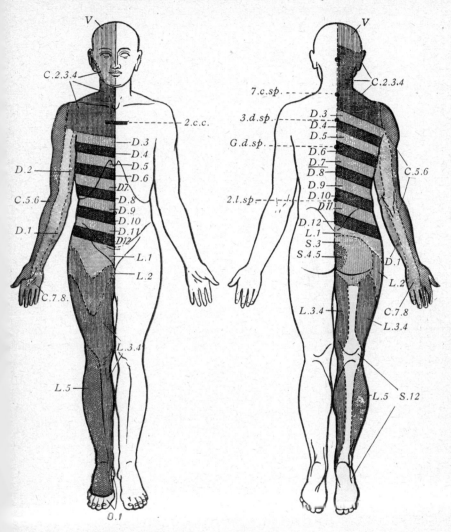

Fig. 201.—The radicular sensory areas of the human body. (*By Sir E. Farquhar Buzzard; from French's ' Index of Diagnosis '.*)

after traversing a few segments of the cord above their point of entrance. In crossing they pass closely in front of the central canal and ascend the opposite spino-thalamic tract to the thalamus. A lesion near the central canal (e.g., syringomyelia or intra-medullary tumour) will involve these fibres and cause a *limited* loss of pain and temperature sense corresponding to the affected segments.

Deep sensibility fibres pass up the posterior columns to the gracile and cuneate nuclei before crossing to the opposite side. Lesions of the posterior columns therefore result in loss of the proprioceptive sensations (muscle,

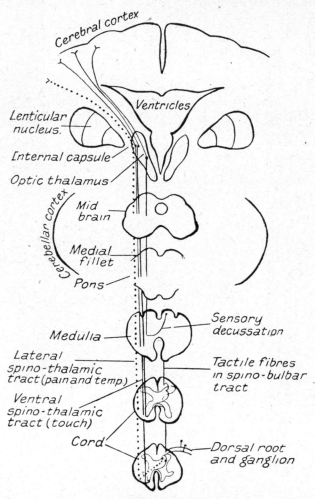

Fig. 202.—Diagram showing course of afferent tracts for cutaneous (exteroceptive) sensations. (*From Roaf's ' Text-book of Physiology ', Edward Arnold & Co.*)

joint, and tendon position ; vibration sense, etc.) on the same side as the lesion. Some loss of touch also occurs.

Path in the Medulla and Brain.—Leaving the spinal cord the sensory paths are continued in the following manner. *Touch* fibres pass through the medulla, pons, and crus in the formatio reticularis, ending in the thalamus. *Pain and temperature* fibres run to the outer side of the medulla separate from the tactile fibres, but in the pons and crus the touch, pain, and temperature paths approximate and pass upwards to the thalamus. *Proprioceptive* sensations differ from pain, temperature, and part of touch, the fibres of which have already crossed in the cord, by continuing uncrossed

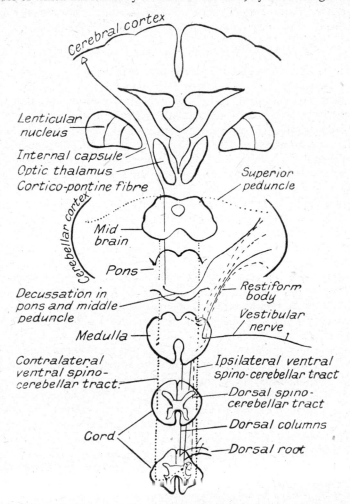

Fig. 203.—Diagram showing course of tracts running to the cerebellum (mainly proprioceptive). (*From Roaf's 'Text-book of Physiology', Edward Arnold & Co.*)

until they reach the fillet, where the superior sensory decussation takes place.

Nearly all sensory fibres end in the thalamus. Some have their final destination there and result in such composite sensations as pleasure, discomfort and pain, hunger, thirst, etc. (*see also* p. 298). Other fibres continue via the internal capsule (*see Fig.* 175) to the sensory cortex behind the fissure of Rolando. The complex forms of sensation appreciated there are described on p. 297 (PARIETAL LOBES).

From these anatomical and physiological data it will be seen that *dissociated anæsthesia*, i.e., loss of some types of sensation, with preservation of others, is most likely to occur in cord lesions, less commonly in midbrain lesions, but very rarely in lesions of the peripheral nerves.

SENSORY SYMPTOMS IN NERVOUS DISEASES

The subjective sensations commonly experienced in disease of the nervous system fall into two groups : (1) *Paræsthesiæ*; (2) *Pain*. Certain phenomena are described under the objective examination, though they may well be appreciated by the patient, i.e., anæsthesia or ataxia.

Paræsthesiæ.—These consist of such sensations as ' pins and needles ', pricking, and numbness. They are common as transient phenomena when the peripheral nerves are stretched or subjected to pressure. A familiar example is the paræsthesia produced by sitting too long with the legs crossed. Equally they may herald serious disease of the nervous system (e.g., disseminated sclerosis, spinal tumour, subacute combined degeneration). The distribution of the paræsthesiæ has localizing value.

In hysteria and neurasthenia complaint may be made of many unusual varieties of sensory disturbance—creeping sensations in the skin, bursting sensations, etc.

Pain.—Pain impulses, interpreted as pain in the consciousness, are carried by the nervous system whatever their origin may be, but the description of pain as a symptom of visceral disease is considered under the various systems. Special types of pain associated with lesions of the nervous system need mention here.

Neuralgia.—Pain along the course of a nerve or its branches is termed neuralgia. Apart from trigeminal neuralgia, which is considered separately (p. 328), neuralgia may occur in the distribution of the peripheral nerves —intercostal, brachial, and sciatic neuralgia. The pain experienced may not be associated with any gross lesion of the nerve, though in some cases slight changes—e.g., a mild neuritis, or adhesions between the nerve and its sheath—are present. *Sciatica*, neuralgia in the course of the sciatic nerve, is often of this type. The pain is made worse by stretching the nerve. If the sciatica is due to an actual neuritis, of course objective signs (anæsthesia, hyperæsthesia, muscular weakness) will also be present. Neuralgia may also be a symptom of pressure or irritation ; for example, pelvic growths not uncommonly produce bilateral sciatica.

If the irritation is of nerve-roots rather than individual nerves, the pain will have the segmental distribution of a root lesion (*see below*).

Causalgia.—This is an unusual type of burning pain, often occurring after limb injuries in cases where the nerve damage is comparatively slight.

Root Pains.—These are often of a neuralgic type, but are characteristically *increased by coughing and sneezing*. They follow the distribution of the particular root or roots affected, and may at first be unaccompanied by objective evidence of root irritation. It is therefore of great importance to ascertain the exact distribution of pains in the trunk. Examples may be seen in the *girdle pains of tabes* and the half-girdle pains of *herpes zoster*, an affection of the posterior-root ganglia associated with a vesicular rash in the same area as the pain. Root pains may also be distributed to the limbs.

Tumours arising from the meninges of the cord frequently produce pain of a root type, at first confined to one side, later spreading to the other. The ' lightning pains ' of tabes are an example of a root pain in the limbs.

Visceral Pains.—Excluding pains due to visceral disease, pains of a visceral type may occur in the well-known *visceral crises* of tabes. The commonest of these is the gastric crisis, in which epigastric pain and vomiting may erroneously suggest a diagnosis of gastric ulcer.

Headache and *Thalamic Pain* are considered elsewhere (pp. 293, 298).

PHYSICAL SIGNS: EXAMINATION OF THE SENSORY SYSTEM

Probably no more tedious task falls to the physician's lot than testing sensation, and so often the results are disappointing and conflicting, depending as they do upon the patient's intelligence, attention, and co-operation, any of which may be faulty. Yet in all neurological cases a thorough investigation of the perceptions of sensations is valuable, and in many the diagnosis depends chiefly upon this.

The examination must test *tactile sensation and discrimination, deep sensibility, perception of pain and temperature, joint and vibration sense, and stereognosis.* It may be necessary to test for *ataxia.*

When the exact localization of the lesion is of direct therapeutic importance, as in spinal-cord tumours, the *areas of disturbed sensibility should be carefully charted* (simple line drawings of the body are readily obtainable). This is the more important as it enables the observer to appreciate changes in the distribution of anæsthesiæ, etc., which may take place from time to time.

Tactile Sensation.—This is best tested by gently touching the skin with a wisp of cotton-wool; the patient's eyes should be covered. If an area of *anæsthesia* is found, it should be carefully compared with the corresponding area on the opposite limb or part of the body. The anæsthesia may be graded as slight (*hypo-æsthesia*) when sensation is merely dulled, or complete when it is entirely absent. If the touch is more acutely felt than normal, *hyperæsthesia* is said to be present. If it is felt as a perverted sensation, e.g., tingling or pain, the term *paræsthesia* or *dysæsthesia* describes it.

Tactile Discrimination.—This is tested by determining at what distance apart two points of a compass can be distinguished as separate entities (usually about 2–3 cm.).

Deep Sensibility (*Pressure Pain*).—This may be tested by firm pressure with a blunt object such as a pencil, or by pinching the muscles, tendons, etc.

Testicular pain on squeezing is another form of pressure pain, often absent in tabes.

This type of sensation is often present when cutaneous sensibility is lost.

Pain.—Cutaneous pain may be tested by pricking the skin with a pin or needle, taking care not to press heavily lest pressure pain be induced. The interval between the prick and the patient's response should be noted, and the patient's expression observed as to whether it corresponds with his statement of his sensations. The term *analgesia* signifies absence of the sense of pain, and in dissociated anæsthesia the part may be analgesic without being anæsthetic.

Temperature.—Two test-tubes of water, cold and warm, may be conveniently used. They should be interchanged frequently so that the patient cannot guess which is being used.

Sensations of Joint Movement and Posture.—The joint must be moved passively, making sure that the muscles to it are completely relaxed. In the case of the great toe, for example, the patient should be conscious when it is passively extended or flexed *without moving it himself*. When the limb (especially the upper) is put in a certain position it should be possible for the patient to put the opposite limb in a similar position.

Vibration Sense.—This is tested by placing a tuning fork of low pitch over the superficial bones, e.g., tibia, phalanges, etc. The patient is normally conscious of a vibratory tremor.

Stereognosis.—The patient should be asked to identify some familiar object by touch alone, e.g., a key or coin. The recognition of variations in weight is called *barognosis* or the *kinetic sense*, and is tested by asking him to compare the weight of different objects (e.g., coins).

Ataxia.—The proper co-ordination of movement depends amongst other factors upon the integrity of the sensory paths in the posterior columns and cerebellar tracts, and it is not out of place to consider here the various ways of testing for ataxia.

In the *arms* the proper co-ordination of movement may be tested by asking the patient to touch the tip of the nose with the index finger of each hand in turn (*Fig.* 204). He should be able to do this accurately both slowly and rapidly. Ataxia of the arms is not infrequently seen in disseminated sclerosis and cerebellar lesions, less commonly in syringomyelia, cervical tabes, etc.

In the *legs* ataxia is best observed by watching the patient's attempt to walk along a chalked line on the floor (*see* GAITS, p. 245). In bed the ' heel-to-knee ' test (*Fig.* 205) may be made. The patient is instructed to touch each knee in turn with the opposite heel, as accurately as possible. The degree of ataxia in the affected limb may be roughly gauged by the clumsiness of the attempt. Ataxia in the legs is well seen in tabes and other lesions (Friedreich's ataxia, subacute combined degeneration, etc.) where the posterior columns are diseased. It also results from cerebellar lesions.

It is important to note that in the posterior-column (sensory) type of ataxia, the inco-ordination can be partially corrected by ocular impressions.

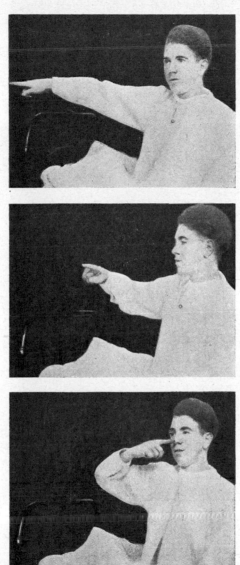

Fig. 204.—Method of testing for ataxia in the arms. This method also demonstrates the presence of any ' intentional ' tremor.

The ataxia is therefore made worse by closing the eyes. In cerebellar ataxia, on the contrary, the degree of ataxia is little influenced by ocular impressions. These facts are made of use in *Romberg's sign*. The patient first stands with the eyes open and brings the heels as closely together as possible without losing his balance. The eyes are then closed, and normally the patient sways but slightly. In posterior column lesions, such as tabes, he often sways to the extent of falling if unsupported. In sensory ataxia (posterior-column lesions) an error of projection is often present, e.g., when the patient attempts to touch the nose with the finger he fails to do so. This differs from the jerky movements of the arm in intention tremor (p. 241) which is essentially a manifestation of cerebellar ataxia.

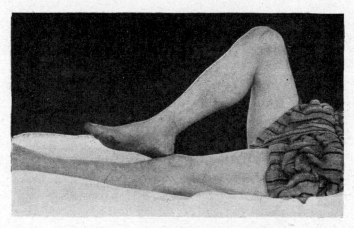

Fig. 205.—Testing for ataxia in a recumbent patient. The ' heel-to-knee ' test.

Other features of cerebellar ataxia (dysmetria and dysdiadochokinesia) are considered on p. 299.

It must be remembered that the sensory impulses upon which co-ordinated movement depends may be interrupted in the brain itself—for example, in the thalamus or post-central gyrus. Cerebral lesions which injure these parts may therefore result in ataxia. Examples are seen in thalamic tumours or vascular lesions, internal-capsular hæmorrhage, post-Rolandic cortical tumours, etc.

ILLUSTRATIVE LESIONS OF THE SENSORY NEURONES

A few diseases affect chiefly the sensory neurones, but many involve concurrently the motor neurones. As lesions of the motor neurones have already received attention, it will be convenient to use as illustrations some diseases in which sensory and motor neurone lesions are combined, but in which the sensory changes are more notable.

Lesions of the sensory neurones have a similar causation to those of the motor system (*see* p. 249).

Localization.—The localization of a lesion of the sensory neurones depends partly on the distribution of the disturbance of sensation and partly on its type. This has been partially discussed in the sections on anatomy and physiology, and may be recapitulated here.

From an *anatomical* point of view lesions of the peripheral *nerves* result in anæsthesia corresponding to the distribution of the sensory fibres ; segmental anæsthesia results from *root* lesions. Complete transverse lesions of the *spinal cord* cause anæsthesia in the limbs and trunk below the level of the lesion. Unilateral lesions result in the dissociation of anæsthesia found in the Brown-Séquard phenomenon (*see* p. 270). Lesions of the *brain-stem* may also result in dissociation, some types of sensation being lost on the same side of the body, some on the contralateral side. Lesions

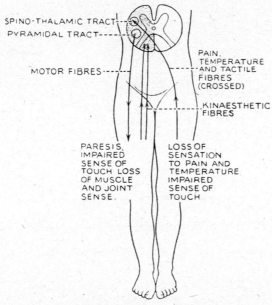

Fig. 206.—Brown-Séquard syndrome. Hemisection of the cord. As touch has a double pathway, it may be impaired on each side as shown in diagram, or may be preserved on both sides.

of the *thalamus, internal capsule,* or *cortex* result in hemi-anæsthesia affecting the face, arm, and leg on the opposite side of the body.

As regards the *type* of anæsthesia, *all varieties* of sensation may be lost in peripheral-nerve lesions and complete transverse lesions of the spinal cord. *Dissociated anæsthesia,* e.g., abolition of pain and temperature sense with preservation of touch sensibility, may result from lesions in the grey matter of the cord near the central canal. Such a lesion may occur in syringomyelia and intramedullary tumours which interrupt the pain and temperature fibres. Dissociated anæsthesia also results from brain-stem lesions (particularly the medulla), as in syringomyelia of these parts, or thrombosis of the posterior inferior cerebellar artery. A rather different type of dissociation takes place in the Brown-Séquard syndrome (*Fig.* 206).

The *loss of proprioceptive sensations* (joint movement, vibration sense, etc.) with little or no loss of tactile, thermal, or pain sensibility, is characteristic of lesions of the posterior columns (tabes, subacute combined degeneration, etc.) or of their continuation fibres to the medulla.

When anæsthesia is *central* in origin (thalamus, internal capsule, and cortex) it is rarely so complete as in peripheral lesions, and it affects the distal parts of the limbs more than the proximal.   It is further characteristic of thalamic lesions that the response to sensory stimulation is exaggerated and frequently perverted (touch may produce an unpleasant sensation almost amounting to pain).   Spontaneous pain may also occur.   In lesions of the sensory cortex the higher types of sensation are impaired (astereognosis, barognosis, etc.) (*see also* p. 297).

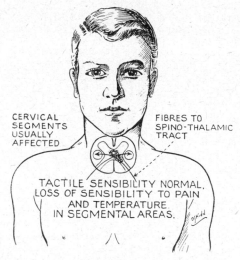

CERVICAL SEGMENTS USUALLY AFFECTED

FIBRES TO SPINO-THALAMIC TRACT

TACTILE SENSIBILITY NORMAL, LOSS OF SENSIBILITY TO PAIN AND TEMPERATURE IN SEGMENTAL AREAS.

Fig. 207.—Syringomyelia. Cavitation near central canal of cord. The sensory changes are irregularly distributed in the cervical, pectoral, and shoulder-girdle regions, according to the particular segments affected by the syrinx.

Brown-Séquard's Syndrome (*Fig.* 206).—Although not common, this phenomenon is an excellent illustration of one type of dissociated anæsthesia.   The lesion consists of a hemisection of the cord and is usually *traumatic* (e.g., stab wound), though tumours and other conditions occasionally produce the same effect.

On the side of the lesion the sensations from tendons, muscles, and joints, vibration sense, and tactile discrimination are lost.   *On the opposite side* pain and temperature sense are abolished and to a lesser extent touch. In addition, motor and vasomotor signs are added : on the side of the lesion there is paralysis of the upper neurone type, and signs of vasomotor paresis.   A limited lower neurone paralysis may also be present, corresponding with the segments of the cord affected.

Syringomyelia (*Fig.* 207).—Allusion has already been made to this disease.   Pathologically it is an overgrowth of neuroglial tissue, usually with central cavitation, probably congenital, situated in the grey matter of the spinal cord near the central canal. It thus interrupts the pain and temperature fibres crossing here, but only affects part of the touch fibres, those in the posterior columns remaining intact. *Pain and temperature sense are therefore lost whilst common touch and postural sensibility are preserved.* Injuries due to the non-appreciation of pain and heat may first call attention to the disease. Charcot's joints may occur in the upper limbs in cases of long standing.

Motor signs are also generally present. If the lesion extends into the anterior-horn cells there will be a lower neurone type of paralysis corresponding with the spinal segments affected. As these are usually the lower cervical and upper dorsal segments the *paralysis affects the small muscles of the hand*, as in progressive muscular atrophy.

Involvement of the lateral columns often gives *pyramidal tract signs on one or both sides*, but the degree of paralysis is rarely great. More rarely the posterior columns are damaged, with corresponding loss of deep sensibility, etc. (tabetic type). A rare type of syringo-

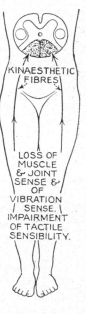

Fig. 208.—Tabes. Lesion of the posterior columns. The lumbar and sacral segments are generally affected.

myelia affects the brain stem—*syringobulbia*. Here the bulbar nuclei are affected, and dissociated anæsthesia may be present.

Tabes Dorsalis (*Locomotor Ataxia*) (*Fig.* 208).— This disease is an example of a degenerative lesion resulting from syphilis. It affects the sensory neurones (principally) and is largely confined to the posterior nerve-roots and the posterior columns of the spinal cord. The disease also implicates the cranial nerves in most cases and thus provides valuable confirmatory clinical signs. Both the symptoms and physical signs are mainly sensory.

Amongst early *symptoms* must be mentioned *pains*. These may be of the 'lightning' variety—hot sharp pains generally in the limbs striking them at right angles, or 'girdle pains' due to the root changes. Other common subjective sensations are a feeling of *walking on air* or cotton-wool (due to light anæsthesia of the soles of the feet), and the band-like sensation often experienced round the chest (cuirass sensation) which corresponds with an area of analgesia. Interference with the vesical and rectal reflexes (tabes affects especially the lumbar and sacral roots and segments of the cord) may result in *difficulty in beginning micturition*, often with retention. More rarely defects in the bowel action result. Usually much later the patient may complain of *unsteadiness* in walking, or a tendency to fall when he stands with the eyes closed (p. 268). These symptoms are due to the ataxia which develops from loss of proprioceptive sensations. The *visceral crises* (gastric, laryngeal, renal, cardiac, etc.) are analogous to the lightning pains, consisting of sharp pain simulating that due to visceral disease, sometimes accompanied by other visceral symptoms. They often occur early in the disease, sometimes leading to an erroneous diagnosis. The commonest is the gastric crisis in which abdominal pain, vomiting, and skin hyperæsthesia are usually found, imitating an acute abdominal catastrophe.

The *physical signs* result partly from the damage to the posterior nerve-roots and posterior columns and partly from cranial-nerve involvement. Loss of tendon reflexes due to interruption of the sensory limb of the reflex arc is exemplified by the *absent knee- and ankle-jerks* (reflex centres in the lumbosacral region). Ankle-jerks are generally lost much earlier than the knee-jerks. Areas of anæsthesia and even more commonly *analgesia* occur on the trunk and limbs. Analgesia may also be found on the nose and lips, though common touch is preserved. *Deep sensibility* is impaired, and pain is no longer produced by testicular pressure, or squeezing the calf muscles, or a delay may be appreciated in the perception of pain, e.g., on squeezing the tendo Achilles. The ulnar nerve when rolled under the fingers at the elbow is also frequently analgesic. *Ataxia* is not usually an early sign, but before it results in the characteristic gait (*see* p. 246) it can be demonstrated by *Romberg's sign* (p. 268). Cranial-nerve signs are often early manifestations of tabes. The more important are the *Argyll Robertson pupil*, *optic atrophy*, and *ptosis*, the last being partly responsible for the ' tabetic facies ' (*see Fig.* 243, p. 322).

Lastly, in tabes, trophic disorders may occur in the limbs, causing *perforating ulcers* and *arthropathies* (Charcot joints, *see* p. 53). The exact mechanism by which these are produced is not fully understood, but the loss of sensations from the parts is undoubtedly an important factor.

Compression of the Spinal Cord (*see also* Cauda Equina Lesions).— Compression of the cord illustrates a combination of motor and sensory phenomena varying in type and degree according to the nature of the compressive lesion. There are a number of common causes which may be responsible, e.g., fractured spine, tuberculous caries, extramedullary tumours, arachnoiditis, malignant disease, and so forth. As in many diseases the symptoms vary with the rapidity with which the compression occurs. In sudden catastrophies such as fracture of the spine, immediate paralysis and loss of sensation below the level of the lesion results. When the compression is more slowly produced as by tumour there are often pains in the limbs or round the trunk due to root irritation. These are increased by sneezing, coughing, and movements of the spine and often precede other signs. Later the general symptoms consist of progressive paraplegia with characteristic upper motor neurone signs together with sensory loss and sphincter paralysis. Localization of the lesion is helped by the segmental distribution of the paralysis and sensation and by alteration of the reflexes which can be assigned to special segments of the cord (*Fig.* 209).

Useful evidence of compression is also obtained by examination of the *cerebrospinal fluid*. The protein is greatly increased without any cellular increase (compression or Froin's syndrome). Occasionally the increase of protein is so great that spontaneous coagulation occurs and the fluid may assume a yellow colour, *xanthochromia*. The fluid removed from above the level of the obstruction, e.g., by cisternal puncture, remains normal (*see also* p. 418). Compression of the jugular veins in such a case does not cause the usual rise in cerebrospinal fluid pressure as measured with a manometer attached to a lumbar puncture needle.

Certain types of intramedullary tumour of the cord do not produce

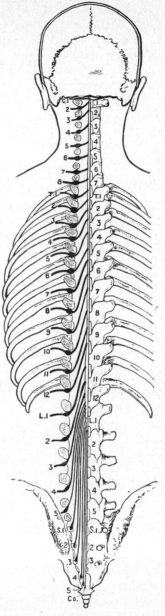

Fig. 209.—Diagrammatic representation of the origin of the spinal nerves, showing the position of their roots and ganglia respectively in relation to the vertical column. The nerves are shown as thick black lines on the left side. (*From Cunningham's ' Text-book of Anatomy ', Oxford Medical Publications.*)

these compression symptoms but tend to imitate other lesions of the spinal cord such as syringomyelia.

Myelitis (*Myelo-malacia ; Softening of the Spinal Cord*).—The term myelitis is used broadly to indicate sudden lesions of the spinal cord due to inflammatory or vascular causes. The pathological changes in most cases suggest that thrombosis in the arteries plays the greatest part in the disease. Many cases are syphilitic. Some of these are chronic in course resulting from a slowly progressive syphilitic meningo-myelitis.

In most instances the cord is affected as a whole—*transverse myelitis*— though only part may suffer (e.g., Brown-Séquard syndrome). Transverse myelitis interrupts all the sensory pathways, and there will be *loss of all types of sensation* below the lesion. Further, the organic reflexes are interfered with, and *retention or incontinence results*. The *motor symptoms* vary.

18

Owing to the severity of the lesion there is generally a *flaccid paralysis* at first, *followed by the usual spastic paraplegia.* Even from the onset, however, the signs of pyramidal tract disease are present (Babinski's sign and absent abdominal reflexes). Trophic changes are prominent, and *bed-sores* occur early and progress alarmingly.

Subacute Combined Degeneration (*Fig.* 210).—The degeneration of the spinal cord which occurs in certain cases of pernicious anæmia (more rarely without anæmia or in other blood diseases) is another example of combined motor and sensory lesions of the cord. In this case the onset of symptoms and signs, and their progress, is gradual.

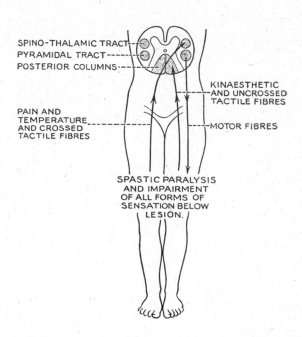

Fig. 210.—Subacute combined degeneration. Lesion of lateral and posterior columns. The different groups of fibres shown exist on *each* side of the body, but to simplify the diagram have been divided between the two sides. All afferent fibres should properly be shown entering the spinal cord through the posterior horns.

Symptoms in the form of *paræsthesiæ* usually occur first (numbness or tingling in the hands), followed later by unsteadiness of gait, ultimately resulting in gross *ataxia* due to degeneration of the posterior columns. *Vibration sense* is also lost. Simultaneously the pyramidal tracts are affected, with a consequent *spastic paraplegia* and other signs of upper motor neurone disease. In many cases the *peripheral nerves* are also involved and the case may resemble one of multiple peripheral neuritis rather than a cord lesion. This is sometimes described as the flaccid type, as contrasted with the spastic type when the lateral columns are extensively involved. In severe cases, and in the terminal stages, the increased tendon reflexes may become diminished or lost and the paralysis flaccid. Disturbances of micturition and defæcation, and trophic changes in the skin, may occur as in other spinal cord diseases.

Friedreich's Ataxia.—This disease also illustrates the effects of a simultaneous involvement of motor and sensory tracts. The disease is familial, and usually becomes manifest in childhood.

The cerebellar tracts are affected, causing *ataxia* both of the arms and legs which is not made worse by closing the eyes. The ataxia is the more pronounced as commonly the posterior columns are also affected to a slighter extent. Affection of the pyramidal tracts gives *signs of an upper motor neurone lesion*, especially Babinski's sign and spasticity. The tendon reflexes are, however, *lost* as in tabes, owing to an interruption of the sensory limb of the reflex arc. The diagnosis is confirmed by the presence of *nystagmus, head tremor, scanning speech*, and of *deformities*, especially pes cavus and scoliosis.

Other types of familial ataxia are described bearing a close resemblance to Friedreich's disease.

Cauda Equina Lesions.—These result in combined motor and sensory symptoms varying considerably in distribution according to the particular nerve-roots affected.

Their characteristic features are a *saddle-shaped area of anæsthesia* over the genitalia, perineum, and buttocks, with *disturbances of micturition and defæcation*—especially retention of urine—and motor paralysis of the lower neurone type affecting all or several groups of muscles in the lower limbs. Both the anæsthesia and muscular paralysis have a root distribution.

REFLEXES

Reflex action is an immediate motor or secretory response to an afferent sensory impulse. For clinical purposes such reflex action is spoken of as a ' reflex ', of which several types are differentiated :—

1. Deep or tendon reflexes.
2. Superficial or skin reflexes.
3. Organic or visceral reflexes.
4. Tonic reflexes.

In health these should be present, and, in the case of deep, superficial, and tonic reflexes, equal on the two sides of the body. It must be recognized, however, that past disease, or some present disability not necessarily of neurological significance, may modify them. Thus the knee-jerks may be lost as a result of diphtheria many years previously, or the abdominal reflexes absent owing to laxity of the abdominal wall after repeated pregnancies.

The clinical importance of reflexes depends partly on their *localizing* value, and partly on the information they give as to the *integrity of the neurones*, sensory and motor, which form the reflex arc. If the tendon reflexes of the arm are altered, this will place the lesion higher than if those of the legs only are modified. Again, exaggeration of the deep reflexes is an important sign of an upper motor neurone lesion, whilst their loss is commonly found in lesions of the lower motor neurone or afferent sensory path.

DEEP OR TENDON REFLEXES

These reflexes are elicited by striking a tendon and so stretching it. This forms the sensory impulse which passes up afferent nerve-fibres to the spinal cord.* Commissural fibres convey the impulse to the anterior-horn cells, which discharge a motor impulse to the muscles supplied from that segment.

Diminution or absence will result if the reflex arc is interrupted by injury or disease. It may be interrupted in the motor limb (e.g., anterior poliomyelitis, peripheral neuritis); in the sensory limb (e.g., tabes, posterior-root tumours, etc.) or in the spinal cord itself (tumours, syringomyelia, etc.). Tendon reflexes are also abolished by spinal cord shock, e.g., severance of the cord. Lesions of the muscles themselves (dystrophies, involvement in scar tissue, etc.) will of course prevent the muscular contraction which is the visible evidence of the reflex. Certain more general causes lead to *bilateral* loss of tendon reflexes, e.g., pneumonia, coma, and greatly increased intracranial pressure, but *the loss has not the same clinical significance as unilateral loss.* Lastly it must be borne in mind that in some persons the deep reflexes are sluggish and occasionally absent without pathological cause. Abolition of a reflex by a segmental lesion of the cord is particularly valuable in localization (*see* LEVEL OF REFLEXES, p. 285).

Exaggeration of the deep reflexes is just as commonly found in functional as in organic nervous disorders, and has not the same clinical importance as absent reflexes. Nevertheless if it is accompanied by other evidence of an *upper neurone lesion*, it is an important confirmatory sign, especially when unilateral and of high degree. The exact reason for this increase in the tendon reflexes is not fully understood, but it appears that the upper neurone normally restrains the lower, and this restraint is removed by lesions of the pyramidal tract. Amongst functional disorders of the nervous system causing exaggerated tendon reflexes, the commonest is neurasthenia, but other states of hyperexcitability of the nervous system (e.g., strychnine poisoning, tetanus, etc.) have a similar effect.

Alternative reflexes are occasionally seen in circumstances in which a reflex would usually be abolished. For example, in lesions of the 5th

---

* Some doubt exists in the case of the knee-jerk as to whether this mechanism holds good, as the time taken for the motor response is too short for the whole arc to be traversed.

and 6th cervical segments the radial-jerk (p. 280) may respond abnormally by flexion of the fingers without the characteristic supination of the forearm.

The more important deep reflexes, and the methods by which they are elicited, follow.

Knee-jerk.—If the patient is able to sit, he should cross one leg over the other and allow the upper leg to hang loosely. A sharp tap on the patellar ligament then produces a contraction of the quadriceps extensor of the knee, which *can be felt* if the observer's hand is placed over the lower part of the front of the thigh. The leg is momentarily shot forward if the contraction is sufficiently marked, owing to the extension of the knee-joint.

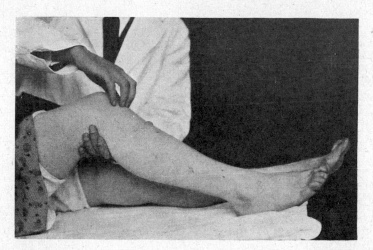

Fig. 211.—Knee-jerk. Method of eliciting knee-jerk in a recumbent patient.

If the patient is recumbent, his leg should be supported behind the knee with one hand and the patellar tendon tapped with the fingers of the other (*Fig.* 211).

When the knee-jerks are apparently absent they may be reinforced by *Jendrassik's method*. The patient is asked to lock his hands and try to pull them apart whilst the physician strikes the patellar tendon (*Fig* 212). This is one method of producing a slight general increase of tone. Other muscular efforts or strong emotions have a similar effect.

Apart from diminution or exaggeration of the knee-jerks, certain special responses may be observed occasionally. In chorea they may be *sustained*, that is, after the contraction of the quadriceps has occurred, the leg seems to hover momentarily before falling to the resting position. Somewhat similar is the *pendular* knee-jerk of acute cerebellar disease, present on the same side as the lesion. In myasthenia gravis the knee-jerks and other reflexes *tire rapidly* in common with voluntary muscular action.

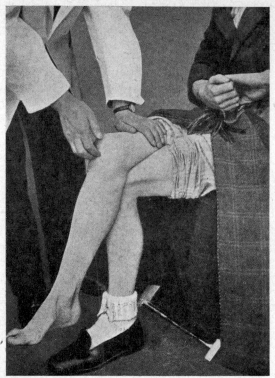

Fig. 212.—Knee-jerk. Method of eliciting knee-jerk in an ambulatory patient. Reinforcement by Jendrassik's method. The patient is 'reinforcing' the knee-jerks by pulling his clasped hands apart, whilst the observer strikes the patellar ligament.

Suprapatellar-jerk.—The leg is extended at the knee-joint. The observer places one finger in close contact with the thigh just above the

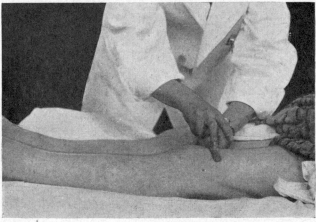

Fig. 213.—Elicitation of suprapatellar-jerk.

patella and strikes it (*Fig.* 213). The result is a quick upward movement of the patella. This reflex is generally obtained when the knee-jerks are exaggerated from pyramidal tract disease, but less commonly in functional states.

Ankle-jerk.—The patient should kneel with one or both knees on a chair. The tendo Achillis is then struck with the hand or a percussion hammer (*Fig.* 214), causing the foot to be briskly plantar-flexed.

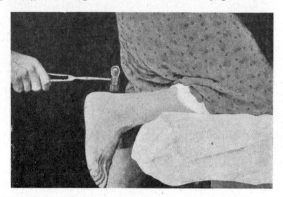

Fig. 214.—Ankle-jerk. A tap on the tendo Achillis causes contraction of the gastrocnemius.

Triceps-jerk.—The arm is supported at the wrist and flexed to a right angle. The triceps tendon is struck just proximal to the point of the elbow (*Fig.* 215), and the resulting contraction of the triceps causes extension at the elbow.

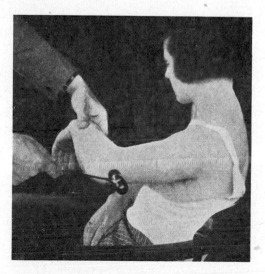

Fig. 215.—Triceps-jerk. Percussion of the triceps tendon causes contraction of the muscle with extension at the elbow.

Biceps-jerk.—The elbow is flexed to a right angle and the forearm slightly pronated. One finger is placed over the biceps tendon and struck with another or with a percussion hammer (*Fig.* 216). The result is a contraction of the biceps causing flexion and slight supination of the forearm.

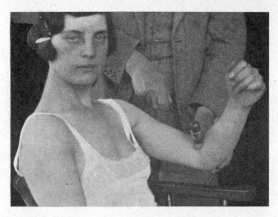

Fig. 216.—Biceps-jerk. A tap on the biceps tendon causes contraction of the biceps and flexion of the forearm.

Radial-jerk.—This is a periosteal, not a tendon, reflex, but falls into the group of deep reflexes. The elbow is flexed to a right angle and the forearm placed midway between pronation and supination. The styloid process is tapped with a percussion hammer (*Fig.* 217). The result is

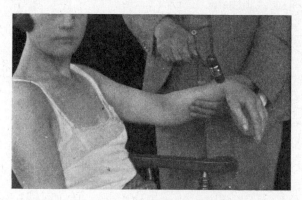

Fig. 217.—Radial-jerk. A sharp tap on the styloid process of the radius causes flexion at the elbow and partial supination of the forearm.

a contraction of the brachioradialis causing flexion at the elbow and partial supination of the forearm.

The *ulnar jerk* is similarly performed, the tap being made on the styloid process of the ulna, the result being adduction of the hand and pronation of the forearm.

Jaw-jerk.—The jaw is allowed to relax and the mouth to hang open loosely. A wooden spatula is placed over the lower teeth on each side in turn and percussed with the finger (*Fig.* 218). The result is a contraction of the corresponding masseter, with partial closure of the mouth.

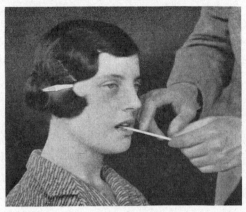

Fig. 218.—Jaw-jerk. The wooden spatula is placed on the lower teeth of each side of the jaw in turn. A tap on the spatula causes contraction of the corresponding masseter.

Clonus.—Closely allied to the tendon reflexes is clonus, a series of involuntary contractions of certain muscles initiated by stretching their tendons. Clonus is usually found when the tendon reflexes are grossly

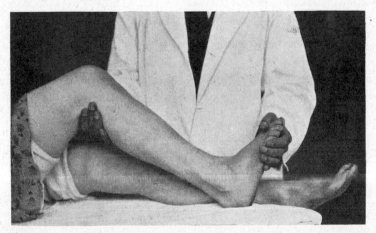

Fig. 219.—Ankle-clonus. The foot is sharply dorsiflexed. If clonus is present the calf muscles give a series of jerky contractions.

exaggerated, and is therefore commoner in organic (upper neurone) than functional nervous disorders. It is of more significance when it is increased by continuing and increasing the stimulus (stretching the tendon) than if it is abolished. The former type is called 'true' or 'inexhaustible' clonus, the latter 'spurious' or 'exhaustible'. In many cases, however, the spurious clonus may become true as the malady progresses. Clonus occurs in two main types in clinical practice—ankle-clonus and patellar-clonus.

Ankle-clonus.—Ankle-clonus is elicited by sharply pressing up the foot into the dorsiflexed position (*Fig.* 219). This results in contractions of the calf muscle leading to plantar flexion of the foot, and in upper motor neurone disease the contractions usually continue so long as pressure is made. True clonus generally occurs with the foot in plantar flexion and is increased by dorsiflexion of the foot. The spurious forms occur with

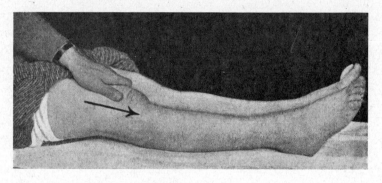

Fig. 220.—Patellar-clonus. The patella is pressed firmly and sharply downwards in the direction of the arrow. If clonus is present a series of jerky contractions of the quadriceps take place, continuing whilst pressure is exerted.

the foot in any position and tend to diminish and become irregular as the foot is pressed up.

Patellar-clonus.—With the leg extended at the knee, the patella is forced downwards by the observer's fingers (*Fig.* 220). Contractions of the quadriceps pull the patella upwards and continue so long as pressure is exerted.

SUPERFICIAL (CUTANEOUS) REFLEXES

These include the plantar responses, abdominal reflexes, cremasteric reflex, cilio-spinal reflex, and corneal reflex. All consist of a contraction of certain muscles when the skin over a particular area is stimulated by stroking, pinching, etc. They are *lost or diminished, or altered*, in upper motor neurone lesions. Exaggeration of them is of less importance.

Plantar Reflex.—If the sole of the foot is stroked gently but firmly with the thumb-nail or a match-stick, the great toe becomes plantar-flexed and there is sometimes a contraction of the tensor fasciæ femoris. The stimulus should be applied to the outer half of the sole. This is the normal *flexor response* which occurs in adults (*Fig.* 221). It may be absent without organic disease, especially if the feet are cold or damp.

In infants before the pyramidal tracts are myelinated the response is different. It consists of slow dorsiflexion of the great toe and occasionally spreading of the small toes in a fan-like manner. In adults such a response is *always pathological*, and is known as the *extensor plantar response* or

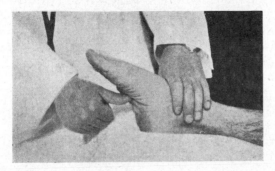

Fig. 221.—Plantar reflex. Normal flexor response.

Babinski's sign (Fig. 222). If the hand is placed behind the thigh a simultaneous contraction of the hamstrings can be felt.

The extensor response can also be elicited by squeezing the calf muscles (Gordon's sign) or by stroking firmly down the inner aspect of the tibia (Oppenheim's sign), but these signs are rarely positive when Babinski's

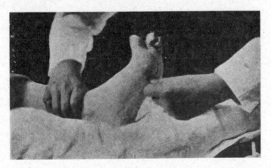

Fig. 222.—Plantar reflex. Extensor response. Babinski's sign.

sign is negative and are thus not of great value. They are, moreover, merely methods of applying a stimulus over a wider field, from which the same response may be evoked.

Babinski's sign indicates that the pyramidal tracts are out of commission. This may be a temporary affair, as in some types of coma (e.g., barbiturate and aspirin poisoning) and after epileptic fits, but as a permanent phenomenon it is found almost constantly in all lesions of the upper motor neurone (e.g., in cerebral hæmorrhage, disseminated sclerosis, subacute combined degeneration, etc.) and it has great significance in distinguishing an organic from a functional lesion, in which latter it *never* occurs. Occasionally in paraplegia in extension a crossed response is obtained, namely, a Babinski sign on the stimulated side, and a plantar flexion of the opposite foot.

Abdominal Reflexes.—To elicitate these reflexes the handle of a pen or some similar object is drawn firmly but lightly across the abdominal wall, on each side in turn (*Fig.* 223). In a healthy young adult the natural response is a contraction of the underlying abdominal muscles and a deviation of the linea alba to the same side. The response is generally brisker in the upper part of the abdomen (*epigastric reflex*).

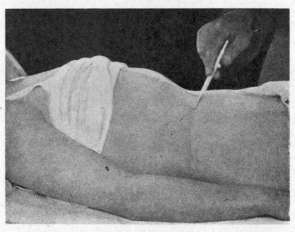

Fig. 223.—Abdominal reflex. The skin of the abdomen is lightly stroked with a pencil. Brisk contraction of the underlying abdominal muscles normally occurs.

In infants the abdominal reflexes are not present, and in adults obesity or laxity of the abdominal wall may abolish them. Acute abdominal lesions may also abolish these reflexes, but from the neurologist's point of view the most important cause of *absence* or *diminution* is a lesion of the pyramidal system. It is of greater significance, too, if the reflex is lost on one side only (e.g., in hemiplegia).

One of the commonest nervous lesions in which the abdominal reflexes are lost is *disseminated sclerosis*.

Cremasteric Reflex.—This reflex consists in a retraction of the testicle by the cremaster muscle when the inner side of the thigh is stimulated by stroking the skin or pressure over Hunter's canal. It is often difficult to elicit in older men, though easy in children. Loss occurs in upper motor neurone lesions, but is rarely of importance unless unilateral. It is not to be confused with the *dartos reflex* in which the scrotum contracts under the influence of cold.

Cilio-spinal Reflex.—If the skin of the neck is pinched, the pupil normally dilates. The sympathetic trunk and pathway in the spinal cord must be intact for this reflex to occur, and its abolition is therefore suggestive of a lesion of these.

Corneal Reflex.—Blowing on one cornea normally produces blinking in both eyes. This reflex may be abolished in coma of any type. If it is abolished on one side only, a lesion of the efferent limb (7th nerve) is likely, but if on both sides the afferent sensory limb (5th nerve) is probably interrupted. This reflex is important in the early diagnosis of 5th-nerve lesions, testing as it does for anæsthesia of the cornea.

Pharyngeal Reflex.—Irritation of the pharynx with a spatula produces contraction of the pharyngeal muscles. This may be absent in hysteria.

Segmental Levels of some of the Commoner Reflexes* :—

Deep Reflexes		Superficial Reflexes	
Knee-jerk	L. 2, 3, 4	Plantar reflex	S. 1, 2
Ankle-jerk	S. 1, 2	Abdominal reflexes	D. 7-11
Triceps-jerk	C. 6, 7, 8	Cremasteric reflex	L. 1
Biceps-jerk	C. 5, 6		
Radial-jerk	C. 7, 8		
Ulnar-jerk	C. 8, D. 1		
Jaw-jerk	Pons		

ORGANIC OR VISCERAL REFLEXES

There are many visceral reflexes, such as those for uterine contractions, the oculo-cardiac reflex, and the cutaneo-gastric reflex, which are of little immediate value in the examination of a neurological case.

The reflexes for *micturition* and *defæcation* are, however, of prime importance.

Micturition.—This is a reflex act which can be voluntarily controlled to a considerable extent by higher centres in the brain. It is normally initiated by a voluntary effort, but once started becomes a reflex act which is difficult to interrupt. The reflex path is partly through plexuses in the bladder wall and partly in the pelvic plexuses. The innervation of these plexuses is from the sympathetic (from L. 3, 4, and 5 segments) and parasympathetic systems (S. 2 and 3, nervi erigentes).

The stimulus for this reflex is distension of the bladder with urine. This stimulus passes to the spinal cord by way of the nervi erigentes and rami communicantes. Controlling centres are situated in the spinal cord at various levels, so that although the reflex arc is left intact, spinal cord and cerebral lesions still result in defects in micturition. In disseminated sclerosis, for example, precipitancy of micturition results from loss of the influence of these controlling centres. The patient cannot control the urgent desire to pass urine.

Retention and *incontinence* of urine may occur from interference with consciousness (e.g., cerebral hæmorrhage) without affection of the local reflex mechanism in the spinal cord. When retention has occurred and

---

* Slight variations of these levels are given by different authors.

the distension is sufficiently great, incontinence may result from partial overflow.

In spinal cord lesions with complete paraplegia, similar *retention with overflow* may occur, but it is sometimes followed by *automatic micturition* in which part of the bladder content is discharged at certain fairly fixed intervals.

In all cases in which incontinence occurs it is essential to examine the abdomen for evidence of bladder distension.

In most cases the patient gradually recovers from the bladder effects of lesions of the brain and spinal cord, the bladder becoming capable of expelling larger quantities of urine and the residuum becoming daily smaller.

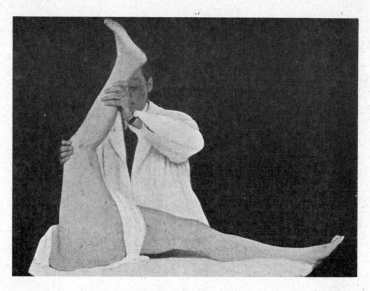

Fig. 224.—Kernig's sign. Negative response. The leg can be well extended.

In cauda equina disease, however, the reflex arc is itself interrupted and the incontinence is therefore prolonged or permanent.

Defæcation.—The bowel action may be embarrassed, causing constipation (analogous with retention of urine) or incontinence of fæces, especially after purgation (analogous with incontinence of urine).

Mass Reflex.—The mass reflex occurs in severe spinal-cord lesions. After a period of flaccid paralysis with retention of urine and constipation, there occurs with paraplegia in flexion a periodic involuntary evacuation of the bladder and rectum. On the application of a stimulus (pin-prick or stroking the sole of the foot) to any point below the level of the lesion, especially in the midline of the body, the legs are vigorously drawn up, Babinski's sign occurs, the skin sweats below the lesion, and the bladder is evacuated. This phenomenon is known as the mass reflex.

TONIC REFLEXES*

Certain reflexes bear a close relationship to those found in decerebrate animals. Some are evidence of disease, some occur in health.

Brudzinski's Neck Sign.—This is a tonic reflex which occurs in meningitis. It consists in flexion of the legs when the neck is passively flexed on the chest.

Kernig's Sign.—Although not a 'tonic' reflex, Kernig's sign, in common with Brudzinski's sign, occurs chiefly in *meningitis* and is conveniently described here.

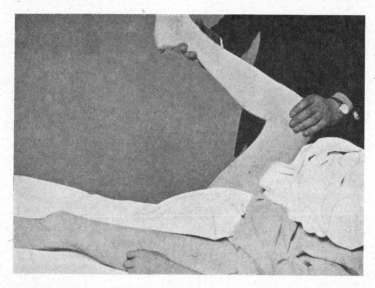

Fig. 225.—Kernig's sign. Positive response. The leg cannot be extended to more than a right angle when the thigh is well flexed on the abdomen. From a case of meningococcal meningitis.

The patient should be recumbent. The thigh is flexed as far as possible on the abdomen, and an attempt is then made to extend the knee-joint. Normally the leg can be well extended (*Fig.* 224). When, however, Kernig's sign is positive, the attempt is resisted by *contraction of the flexors* of the knee and causes *pain*, due to stretching of the sacral nerve-roots and meninges (*Fig.* 225).

---

* *See also* Associated Movements, p. 241.

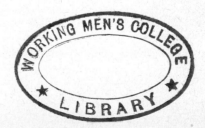

CHAPTER IX

THE NERVOUS SYSTEM (continued)

THE BRAIN

SPEECH DEFECTS

SPEECH is one of the highest functions of the human mind. It is not surprising, therefore, that it is disordered in many gross diseases of the brain which affect other mental functions. For speech to be carried out normally not only must the higher centres of the brain be intact, but the motor mechanism which controls the muscles of articulation must be perfect. Disorders of speech can thus be divided at once into two groups : (1) Those affecting the higher centres in the brain—*aphasia*, a disturbance of speech as an intellectual function ; (2) Those interfering with the motor execution of speech—*dysarthria* or *anarthria* (see TWELFTH CRANIAL NERVE, p. 335, and BULBAR PARALYSIS, p. 254).

Aphasia.—The study of aphasia is highly complicated, and the many elaborate concepts which have been evolved to clarify the problem have frequently only served to make it more confusing. The older view that two principal types of aphasia, motor and sensory, exist, still has much to commend it from the point of view of simplicity, providing the student does not draw too sharp a distinction in his mind between the two, but allows for mixtures of both types, which almost invariably occur in every clinical case. The conception of sensory and motor aphasia arises from a consideration of the way in which language is built up in the child mind. Sight and hearing take the first part. The repetition of the same sound evokes in the child's mind a particular mental impression. Similarly a visual impression repeated in association with a word causes that word to be identified with the object seen. The two types of sensory impression, auditory and visual, are usually received at the same time. We point to a book and say ' book ' to the child, and, with repetition, the word ' book ' eventually produces the mental image of that article. Conversely the sight of a book recalls to the mind the sound of the word.

Other sensations besides hearing and sight take part in the formation of speech, notably the appreciation of the form and size of objects (stereognosis) and the sense of smell.

In time the child learns to speak, that is, to call into action those parts of the brain which control the mechanism for understanding and emitting words. The use of a word conjures up in the mind an auditory, visual, or other sensory image. With mental development, not only in the child but in the adult, this process of speech becomes more intricate, but the later acquired faculties of speech, for example, foreign languages, do not take such deep root as those upon which the foundations were laid. Further, speech has an emotional as well as an intellectual character and the former is more primitive and less disturbed by lesions of the speech centre.

The symptom aphasia implies above all a *loss of speech comprehension*. It is possible, and indeed not uncommon, for an aphasic person to speak words which he does not understand. On the other hand, speech may be impossible owing to paralysis of the articulatory mechanism (anarthria) without aphasia being present.

Sensory Aphasia.—In sensory aphasia impressions upon which speech is based become meaningless. The patient may hear words which convey nothing to him (*word-deafness*), or may see written words which have lost all meaning (*word-blindness*). These types of aphasia may be recognized by asking the patient to perform some simple command. A *spoken command* —" put out your tongue "—will not be executed if the patient does not grasp the meaning of the words. The same *command in writing* will test whether he appreciates the meaning of written words. In sensory types of aphasia the patient often misnames objects shown to him (*nominal aphasia*).

In testing for different types of aphasia the possibility of paralysis of the muscles of articulation or of the right hand when the patient is asked to write must not be overlooked.

Motor Aphasia.—Motor aphasia may be surmised if the sensory appreciation of words appears normal and the articulatory apparatus is unharmed, yet the patient is unable to speak words *which have a meaning* both to him and the listener.

This type of aphasia may be obvious if the patient is quite unable to speak at all or if he utters unintelligible sounds. Often the earliest change is the loss of names, so that the patient circumvents the use of the name by a phrase, as one does with a limited knowledge of a foreign language. It may be specifically tested by asking him to name common objects after first ascertaining that no gross sensory aphasia is present. In motor aphasia the faculty of writing is usually lost (*agraphia*), but in testing for its loss the possibility of paresis of the right arm or hand must first be excluded.

Although this account of aphasia has been simplified and the scheme of examination reduced to a minimum, it is necessary to add that as speech is one of the highest intellectual functions, it is usually disturbed as a whole, and great patience and more elaborate questioning are essential to unravel the complicated problems that are presented by so many clinical cases of aphasia. The interested reader is advised to consult a standard text-book of neurology.

Localizing Value of Aphasia.—If the patient is right-handed the presence of aphasia establishes the lesion in the left side of the brain. Motor aphasia is usually caused by lesions in front of the fissure of Rolando, whilst lesions behind it may cause sensory aphasia. The whole area which may be involved in aphasia is considerable, and extends from the posterior ends of the 2nd and 3rd frontal gyri to the upper temporal area and the lower part of the parietal region. The zone includes the island of Reil. (*Fig.* 226.)

The vascular lesions, especially embolism and thrombosis, which cause aphasia, can usually be localized with greater certainty by the extent

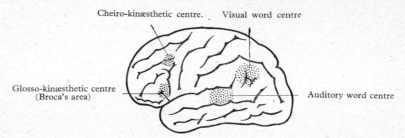

Cheiro-kinæsthetic centre.   Visual word centre

Glosso-kinæsthetic centre (Broca's area)

Auditory word centre

Fig. 226.—Diagrammatic representation of the left cerebral hemisphere, showing the chief centres concerned with speech. (*From French's ' Index of Diagnosis '.*)

of concomitant paralysis, but aphasia may sometimes have a topographical diagnostic value in cerebral tumours.

Alterations in Type of Speech.—Speech is often altered in character without being lost. Some types of abnormal speech may be recognized spontaneously, but others are made apparent when the patient attempts to repeat certain difficult phrases. In lesions of the basal ganglia speech is unusually *slow* ; in disseminated sclerosis it has an interrupted character described as *staccato* or *scanning*. The speech of general paralysis of the insane (G.P.I.) is *slurring and tremulous*, most obviously so when the patient tries to say difficult words such as ' artillery ' or ' constitutional '. A slurring speech is also found in Friedreich's ataxia. An explosive element is often characteristic of the speech in cerebellar lesions. In bulbar paralysis, whether of nuclear or supranuclear origin, all stages between difficult speech and complete absence may be present, and the patient frequently mumbles indistinguishable sounds although fully aware of what he wishes to say.

CEREBRATION AND CONSCIOUSNESS

The brain is an organ concerned in the higher functions of cerebration and consciousness apart from its work in connexion with motor power, sensory reception, and the maintenance of the vital phenomena of respiration, cardiac action, etc. The functions of cerebration and consciousness are often the first to be disordered in brain disease, and in the examination not only of neurological but of all cases, it is necessary to form some estimation of the intellectual activity of the individual and to observe any deviation from the normal.

The examination of these higher functions of the brain is chiefly based upon intelligent and systematic questioning and upon observation of the patient's behaviour, habits, and mode of life. Physical examination plays a smaller part in the diagnosis of cerebral disease than accurate history-taking, though associated lesions of the motor or sensory cortex and of the cranial nerves frequently form an integral part of the clinical picture, which must be considered as a whole.

Cerebration.—The general *intelligence* of different individuals varies enormously, but the patient's relatives are often able to assist in determining whether his mental activity has changed of late. Inquiry should be made about his *memory*, and simple tests made to confirm the patient's statements.

Mental disease should be suspected when hallucinations, delusions, or gross abnormalities of conduct are present.

Hallucinations are false sensory impressions. The patient, for example, hears sounds or sees sights which do not exist.

Delusions imply false beliefs. The patient may believe himself to be another person, or to be unusually wealthy, or to be the object of persecution by others.

Abnormalities of conduct are perhaps most difficult to define, unless the individual is well known to the practitioner. Here, again, the patient's relatives are usually the first to recognize those early changes in temperament (irritability, moroseness), in morality, and in business acumen, which may be of such importance in incipient mental disease.

During the interrogation, note will be made of undue garrulity or effusiveness, of negativism and peculiar mannerisms, and of abnormal repetition of words or phrases, which may be important in mental disease. Phobias and undue anxiety are often found in neurasthenia.

This book has no concern with the diagnosis of mental disease *per se*, but the few points mentioned need consideration in those cases, especially neurological ones, in which psychical changes are an essential part of the disease—e.g., G.P.I. and some cerebral tumours.

Disturbances of Consciousness.—Mental function naturally depends upon full consciousness. This may be lost partially, *stupor*, or completely, *coma*, apart from the physiological cyclical loss of consciousness which we know as sleep. The partial unconsciousness which is accompanied by restlessness of the body and mind is called *delirium*. All phases of this state are seen, from tossing and turning in bed with periodic chattering, to the wilder types in which the patient throws himself about and struggles violently, frequently shouting at the top of his voice. These changes in consciousness are often found in severe cerebral lesions such as trauma, vascular insults, and tumours, but may be caused by fever, poisoning, and toxæmias, which exert an indirect effect upon the brain.

Coma.—Coma is defined as a state of unconsciousness from which the patient cannot be aroused. The depth of unconsciousness may, however, vary considerably, and in semi-comatose states it is sometimes possible to wake the patient by strong external stimulation. In every patient who is deeply comatose *the breathing is stertorous*, and *the deep reflexes are abolished*. Incontinence of urine and fæces usually occurs, though the urine may be retained.

Although a complete account of the causes of coma cannot be given here, the principles upon which a diagnosis is made in a comatose patient may be discussed briefly.

The patient must first be examined for signs of *injury*, especially to the skull. Concussion, fracture of the skull, and hæmorrhage from the middle meningeal artery are common causes of coma. Next the patient should be examined for signs of *paralysis*. In an unconscious person this may be done by lifting each limb in turn and comparing the two sides. The paralysed limb falls limply and heavily to the bed, the opposite normal limb preserves sufficient tone to allow it to sink more gently. The tendon reflexes may be abolished on the affected side and the superficial reflexes altered (*see* REFLEXES, p. 275). It is necessary to repeat here that Babinski's sign may be found in many cases of coma without gross damage to the pyramidal system (*see* p. 283). Paralysis associated with coma is frequently the result of cerebral vascular lesions ; less commonly it is found in cerebral tumour, meningitis, and other intracranial lesions. Examination of the *optic disks* may show evidence of pre-existent disease in the form of papillœdema, optic neuritis, or retinitis. The condition of the *pupils* should also be noted. Pin-point pupils are characteristic of morphine poisoning and pontine hæmorrhage. Irregularity is often found in cerebral lesions affecting the third nerve or sympathetic. In coma due to cerebral hæmorrhage the pupils dilate (especially on the side of the lesion) as death becomes imminent.

The possibility of *metabolic toxæmias* should next be considered. With this in mind the *urine should be tested*. The presence of *albuminuria* calls for further examination for signs of uræmia. This condition is often marked by fits between which the patient lies comatose. Numerous epileptic fits may also result in coma, a condition known as status epilepticus. *Glycosuria*, especially when combined with ketonuria, would lead to a diagnosis of diabetic coma. Hyperglycæmia would be found by blood-sugar analysis. In a known diabetic, coma without glycosuria might suggest insulin poisoning. The blood-sugar would be low and no ketonuria would be present. Further, the onset of coma is more rapid, the patient flushed and restless. Fits may occur. The presence of sugar in the urine does not exclude hypoglycæmia as the urine may have been excreted into the bladder before the fall in blood sugar.

Lastly, clues to *poisoning* must be diligently sought when other causes for the coma are not apparent. Poisons found in the patient's possession or within his access, the pricks of hypodermic needles, and the odour of the breath may all yield valuable data. The breath should be smelt in all cases. Alcoholism, ketosis, and certain poisons may be suspected in this way.

Frequently the examination must proceed on these lines without any history as to the mode of development of the coma, but when the patient's relatives or friends can be interviewed they should be questioned about his past history, especially as to any previous disease and alcoholic or drug-taking habits. The manner in which the coma developed, whether gradual or sudden, should be ascertained, and whether the patient has had any similar attacks before. Inquiry should be made for any associated symptoms, such as headache, fits, vomiting, or paresis, at the onset of the condition.

SYMPTOMS AND SIGNS OF INCREASED INTRACRANIAL PRESSURE

Whatever the cause of a rise of intracranial pressure, certain common symptoms result. The most important of these are headache, vomiting, papillœdema, disturbances of cerebration, fits, and bradycardia.

Headache.—This is such a common complaint in everyday life and so often due to trivial causes that it is often only its persistence over a considerable period of time which arouses suspicion of an intracranial lesion. Headache due to increased intracranial pressure has no definite distinguishing character, though it is often increased by stooping, coughing, or sneezing, which aggravate the intracranial tension. The headache is usually worse in the morning. Its position is but rarely any guide to the site of the lesion, though exceptions occur, especially in the case of gummata and tumours involving the skull bones.

When the headache does not appear to be of cerebral origin, the physical signs of disease in other systems must be sought if the symptom is to be explained. The more important details of examination are as follows. Look for :—

1. *Reflex causes*, especially errors of refraction, focal sepsis (teeth, tonsils, sinuses, etc.).

2. *Toxæmias*, e.g., constipation, metabolic diseases, and low-grade fevers (e.g., undulant fever and tuberculosis).

3. *Evidence of system disease* in : (*a*) Cardio-vascular system ; (*b*) Genito-urinary system ; (*c*) Hæmopoietic system ; (*d*) Digestive system.

4. *Psychic causes.* Worry and mental over-activity are fruitful causes of headache, apart from the pure neuroses of neurasthenia and hysteria, in which headache is one of the most frequent complaints. In headache of psychogenic origin the symptom is often described in extravagant terms, though the patient's state may not suggest severe pain.

5. *Migraine.* Inquire for other symptoms of migraine if this type of headache is present. The migrainous headache is classically *unilateral* (though the side may vary in different attacks), occurring in attacks which usually begin in the morning and increase in severity during the day. They are accompanied by *nausea* and *vomiting* in a few hours, and the patient may have the characteristic *visual disturbances* consisting of scotomata, ' fortification figures ', or coloured lights in zig-zag formation. These precede the headache and last some minutes.

The non-cerebral causes of headache have been briefly considered here as they frequently enter into the differential diagnosis. Moreover, it is probable that many headaches such as those of anæmia or high blood-pressure are caused by alteration in intracranial tension, either an increase or a decrease. According to Head some types of visceral disease produce referred pains in the head, which are also described by the patient as headache.

In some cases the cause of the headache can be elucidated easily if the student has some such scheme as the one described, but when the headache is not associated with other symptoms or signs the diagnosis may be extremely difficult.

Vomiting.—Typical cerebral vomiting is not preceded by nausea, and is sometimes projectile in character. This is often seen in meningitis. In children especially, the gastric contents may be ejected quite forcibly through the mouth. Vomiting due to increased intracranial pressure is, however, *not commonly of this cerebral type*. It may resemble other forms of sickness preceded by nausea.

Papillœdema (*Choked Disk*).—This is the sign of greatest importance in the diagnosis of increased intracranial pressure. The patient may complain of impaired vision, which is confirmed by the discovery of scotomata, especially for colours. In many cases no *subjective* visual changes are present, emphasizing the necessity of examining the retinæ in all neurological cases. The objective sign consists in swelling of the optic-nerve-head to an extent of several dioptres. (*See also* SECOND CRANIAL NERVE, p. 313.)

Mental Changes.—Mental confusion and apathy are common in most cases of increased intracranial pressure (*see* CEREBRATION AND DISTURBANCES OF CONSCIOUSNESS, p. 291) and stupor or coma follow in severe unrelieved cases.

Fits (*see also* p. 233).—It is important to remember that generalized convulsions resembling idiopathic epilepsy are a commoner manifestation of increased intracranial pressure than localized fits. Fits occurring first in middle life should emphasize the necessity of excluding organic cerebral disease.

Bradycardia.—The general rise of intracranial pressure in time causes slowing of the heart-rate owing to its effect on the vagal centres in the medulla. This sign is of most value when the normal heart-rate for the individual is known. The blood-pressure often rises as a compensatory measure in proportion as the pulse-rate decreases.

CEREBRAL LOCALIZATION

It is interesting in vascular lesions, but a vital necessity in tumours and some inflammatory diseases of the brain, to localize the lesion as accurately as possible. Upon this will depend the success of any operative treatment, and the accuracy of the prognosis. The earlier the anatomical diagnosis can be made the more likely is the treatment to be successful, not only because the encroachment of even a simple tumour upon the brain substances is attended by grave results, which increase the longer the tumour remains, but also because the *slight localizing signs of the early stages often disappear* when the intracranial pressure rises further. Moreover, the disturbances of consciousness which have been mentioned (impairment of intellect and increasing stupor) soon render the patient unable to help in the diagnosis of the condition by his accurate history.

This preamble emphasizes the necessity for paying due attention to the slightest focal signs in the early stages of intracranial disease. These signs depend upon abolition or alteration in function of the various parts of the brain and the cranial nerves which proceed from it. Some areas—for example, the motor area—have well-defined functions, the loss or alteration of which will almost certainly occur when a lesion affects them. Others—for instance, the frontal lobes—may be the seat of gross changes without symptoms or signs of real localizing value. In this connexion it is well to note that supra-tentorial tumours are relatively silent, whilst below the tentorium lesions generally produce early focal signs.

Those *focal signs are of greatest value which appear earliest*, for they are more likely to be due to the original lesion. The same signs appearing later may merely result from secondary changes in the neighbourhood of the lesion, e.g., meningitis or thrombosis.

Local signs are of even greater value in the diagnosis of cerebral lesions than general ones, for whereas such signs as headache, vomiting, and optic neuritis may be caused by renal disease, blood diseases, and other conditions, local signs such as paresis or disturbances of sensibility indicate a local lesion. Sometimes a combination of signs is known to be associated with a particular type of tumour. For example, a medulloblastoma is the commonest cerebral tumour of childhood, and causes a combination of headache, vomiting, and papilloedema, oculomotor pareses, mild ataxy, and later signs of meningeal irritation and coma. Such a combination indicates not only the position of the tumour in the vermis and surrounding structures, but the pathological nature of the tumour. Local signs may now be discussed in more detail, and grouped according to the various parts of the brain.

The Meninges.—The meninges form a continuous membrane over the whole brain and extend down to cover the spinal cord. The pia and arachnoid are in close contact in most places, and between them circulates the cerebrospinal fluid, which is more plentiful in the ' cisterns ', where the pia and arachnoid separate from one another to accommodate it. The pia-arachnoid follows the convolutions of the brain closely and carries the blood-vessels in its substance.

These facts explain the necessity for considering the meninges, both cerebral and spinal, as a whole, and of remembering that some of the symptoms and signs in meningeal disease may be due to spread of the disease process into the brain itself and to the cranial nerves which are partly or completely ensheathed by the meninges.

Whatever the cause of meningeal irritation, the symptoms and signs are similar. They will be modified by the part of the membranes which are most affected, e.g., cerebral or spinal; by the actual pathology, e.g., inflammation, hæmorrhage, etc.; and by the rapidity with which the membranes are affected. They may be conveniently grouped as follows :—

1. *Symptoms and Signs of Increased Intracranial Pressure (see* p. 293).— Headache, vomiting, and sometimes optic neuritis may result from the increased tension on the meninges by the accumulating cerebrospinal fluid between the pia and arachnoid, and also by the pressure which this exerts on the brain. These signs occur early. The *headache* is frequently referred to the nape of the neck and may be very severe. *Vomiting* may be of the cerebral type. *Optic neuritis* is not common, and true papillœdema is unusual.

2. *Essential Signs of Meningeal Irritation.*—The characteristic phenomenon of *neck rigidity* occurs early, and later changes to definite *head*

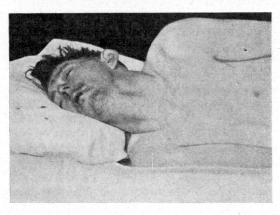

Fig. 227.—Head retraction. Case of cerebrospinal meningitis. Note also the herpes.

retraction (Fig. 227). To test neck rigidity the observer attempts passively to flex the head on the chest and with his other hand notes the tautness of the neck muscles. When the spinal meninges are much affected *opisthotonos* occurs : the body is arched backwards and held rigidly, so that in extreme cases it may rest on the occiput and heels only. This sign is but one example of the *generalized muscular rigidity* which occurs in meningeal irritation. Other methods of testing this are described under Kernig's and Brudzinski's signs (*see* p. 287).

3. *Signs of Brain Involvement.*—Especially in cases of cerebral meningitis some spread of the disease process may take place to the brain itself. The resulting signs depend upon the extent and degree of this. As examples may be mentioned motor phenomena such as fits and paresis, mental disturbances, and so forth.

4. *Signs of Cranial-nerve Involvement.*—Ocular pareses resulting in inequality of the pupils and squint are common. Lesions of the 7th and 8th nerves are also not infrequent. These lesions are common in acute

meningeal disease, especially meningitis in all forms, but are also observed in chronic forms of basal meningitis.

The Pre-frontal Lobes.—These lobes are believed to be the seat of intellectual activity. By their connexions with the motor zone in the pre-Rolandic area they are also concerned in the origination of muscular movement. The symptoms which result from disease in these lobes are therefore chiefly *disturbances of the highest forms of cerebration*—thought, memory, reasoning, and so forth—often leading to dementia. The patient is sometimes abnormally jocular. *Apraxia* may also occur, i.e., the inability to perform a particular movement although the patient is aware of what he wishes to do and has no paralysis preventing him from doing it. The character of the lesion will modify the symptoms produced. In the case of G.P.I. the mental symptoms predominate ; in tumour the general signs of increased intracranial pressure may long precede any focal signs. The tumour may eventually extend into the pre-Rolandic and other areas and so give clues to its situation.

The Frontal Lobes (Motor Area).—*See* MOTOR SYSTEM, p. 227.

The Parietal Lobes.—These are concerned in the reception of all types of sensory impulses which are elaborated into the final cortical conceptions of sensation. Some of these are grouped under the term stereognosis (p. 266). In *astereognosis* the patient is unable to recognize the form and shape of familiar objects. Astereognosis is only pathognomonic of parietal lobe lesions when the paths of sensation in other parts of the brain (thalamus, fillet, etc.) and spinal cord are intact (*see also* SENSATION, p. 259). In every case, therefore, it is necessary to test the integrity of the simpler forms of sensibility (touch, muscle, and joint sense).

Other complicated forms of sensation are appreciated in the cortex, notably the sense of position of the limbs in space and the range of movement when the joints are passively moved by the observer. The finer distinctions between grades of temperature and the faculty of point discrimination are also lost in cortical lesions involving the parietal area. Apraxia may occur.

Tumour is the commonest lesion, and it may extend forward into the pre-Rolandic area, causing motor symptoms ; or backwards into the occipital region, causing hemianopia.

The Temporo-sphenoidal Lobes.—The temporal lobe is the final receptor for hearing from the opposite side of the body, though the cochlear divisions of the 8th nerves are connected with both sides of the brain. Owing to these bilateral connexions lesions of the temporal lobe do not cause deafness, but auditory aphasia may result. Convulsions are not uncommon.

In the case of tumour, extension may take place to the pre-Rolandic area, causing motor symptoms ; to the post-Rolandic region, with sensory symptoms ; or to the optic radiation, causing quadrantic hemianopia. Pressure of the tumour downwards on to the tentorium may cause homolateral cerebellar symptoms.

If the *uncinate gyrus* of the temporo-sphenoidal lobe is involved curious perversions of smell may occur, which occasionally form the aura of epileptiform attacks. Jackson's ' dreamy states ' may also occur, in which the patient complains of a sense of unreality difficult to define.

The Occipital Lobes.—In these lobes are situated centres for the final reception and interpretation of visual impressions. Lesions of them usually result in hemianopia of the homonymous type or occasionally of the quadrantic type (*see* p. 317 and *Fig.* 230, p. 312). Word-blindness and inability to read may also result if the angular gyrus is affected.

The Thalamus.—This large basal ganglion is the final cell-station for all types of sensation before these are passed along new relays of fibres to the cerebral cortex. The visual fibres also pass through the pulvinar of the thalamus on their way to the occipital cortex. The sensations received in the thalamus are *crude* perceptions of pain and temperature (but not touch), gross joint movements, or merely a sense of comfort or distress or a general ' sense of awareness '.

The results of a thalamic lesion are :—

Hemianæsthesia, excessive sensibility to painful stimuli, spontaneous pains, and misinterpretation of other stimuli (e.g., light touch or tickling may give an unpleasant sensation), ataxia, hemianopia (if the pulvinar is involved), and choreiform movements from concurrent involvement of the corpus striatum. These signs are present on the side opposite to the lesion.

Lesions of the thalamus are commonly vascular or neoplastic. If vascular they are rarely confined to the thalamus, but involve the internal capsule, so that hemiparesis is also present.

The Cerebellum.—This part of the brain lies closely packed below the tentorium in intimate contact with the pons and medulla and the cranial nerves which take origin in the neighbourhood. It is not surprising, therefore, that lesions of the cerebellum are frequently accompanied by signs of involvement of these neighbouring structures.

The cerebellum has elaborate connexions with other parts of the nervous system, notably with the vestibular nerve, the cerebral cortex and pons, and the spinal cord. These connexions make the explanation of cerebellar symptoms complex, but, in general, muscular co-ordination depends upon the connexions of the cerebellum with the higher parts of brain, whilst tone and equilibrium are more particularly associated with its connexions with the lower parts. Modern work tends to assign disturbances of equilibrium to the flocculo-nodular lobe, whilst hypotonia and disorders of movement appear to be related to the neo-cerebellum.

The main *clinical* features of cerebellar lesions can be summarized as follows :—

1. *Loss of Muscle Tone (Hypotonia).*—The limbs are unduly flaccid and can be moved through unusually large ranges of movement. The hypotonia is generally accompanied by slight weakness, because perfect muscular action is impossible with atonic muscles. The disturbance of postural fixation or tone accounts for most of the physical signs which

are elicited. Not only are the muscles in action affected, but also those passively maintaining the background of correct posture.

2. *Muscular Inco-ordination.*—This is seen in the ataxic (drunken) gait so often present. The patient suffers from *vertigo* with a tendency to fall to the affected side. Ataxia in the arms may be demonstrated by asking the patient to pronate and supinate the forearms rapidly and comparing the two sides. On the affected side this cannot be properly accomplished (*dysdiadochokinesia*). Intention tremor is another example. When the patient attempts to touch the nose with the finger, the arm and hand become increasingly shaky until the nose is reached. The precision of movement which depends upon the appreciation of the force and rate of muscular contraction is also lost. This is known as *dysmetria.*

3. *Ocular Disturbances.*—The commonest is *nystagmus* (oscillations of the eyeball—*see* p. 325), usually lateral, but sometimes rotary. In lateral nystagmus the quicker component is generally away from the lesion, the slower towards it. Nystagmus is again a defect of postural fixation and can be regarded as an intention tremor of the oculomotor muscles. Occasionally *skew deviation* is observed, one eye being turned upwards and outwards, the other downwards and inwards.

4. *Altered Postures.*—The position of the head is sometimes altered. It is retracted, with the face turned upwards towards the lesion. When the middle lobe is affected a position may be assumed similar to that of meningeal disease—the head retracted, the back arched, and the legs extended. The natural tendency of the patient to lean towards the side of the lesion may be over-corrected, producing an abnormal attitude.

These signs of cerebellar disease are present chiefly *on the side of the lesion.* Signs may be present on the opposite side due to involvement of surrounding structures. This is particularly so in tumour. Pressure on the pons causes signs of pyramidal-tract involvement on the other side, with oculomotor paresis on the same side. The 6th nerve, owing to its propinquity, frequently suffers in cerebellar tumours, with consequent paralysis of the external rectus (*see also* CRANIAL NERVES, p. 322).

5. *Speech Defects.*—These generally take the form of ' staccato ' speech, in which each syllable is pronounced as though it was a word. Here the muscles of articulation are affected by the defect of postural fixation.

In tumours of the cerebellum the general signs of increased intra-cranial pressure are more marked than in supratentorial lesions.

The Cerebello-pontine Angle.—Lesions in this region present a peculiar combination of symptoms and physical signs which is almost pathognomonic, and is usually due to tumours, especially those growing from the acoustic nerve. The signs produced are :—

1. *Cerebellar signs* similar to those just described.

2. *Signs of pressure on the pons and medulla,* which are often pushed over by the growth. This displacement causes upper motor neurone signs on the opposite side of the body, rarely amounting to a definite paralysis owing to the gradual nature of the compression.

3. *Signs of cranial nerve involvement.* The most important of these is deafness, which is to be expected owing to the usual origin of the tumour from the 8th nerve. Tinnitus is also present in some cases. The 6th nerve is the next most commonly affected, and external rectus paresis results. If the 5th nerve is damaged some sensory loss generally occurs over the face, and pain of a neuralgic type may be present. Loss of the corneal reflex is an early sign. Slight facial weakness may be caused by pressure on the 7th nerve. In the diagnosis of tumours of the cerebello-pontine angle from those of the cerebellum itself, stress should be laid on the early involvement of the cranial nerves.

The Neighbourhood of the Pituitary Fossa.—Lesions in this region may involve the pituitary body or surrounding structures. The hypothalamus is thought to exercise an important controlling influence over the pituitary, and it is not possible at present completely to separate the effects of a pituitary from a hypothalamic lesion. Indeed a lesion primarily of one may affect the other. In the case of tumour the optic chiasma is usually pressed upon, causing various hemianopias, the commonest being the bitemporal variety. Tumours of the pituitary itself result in the endocrine dyscrasias (acromegaly, gigantism, Fröhlichs' syndrome) which have been mentioned in Chapter II. Lesions in this region, e.g., specific meningitis, may also produce diabetes insipidus, a condition characterized by polydipsia (excessive thirst) and polyuria.

The Cerebral Vessels.—Blockage of these vessels by embolism or thrombosis results in varying clinical pictures depending on the distribution of the vessel, which is not always constant. The more important results may be summarized as follows :—

Internal Carotid.—Contralateral hemiplegia and loss of spatial and discriminative senses. In a left-sided lesion, motor and sensory aphasia. Blindness on the same side when the lesion occurs before the ophthalmic artery is given off.

Anterior Cerebral Artery.—Various forms of hemiplegia in combination with other symptoms such as mental deterioration, dysphasia. Special tendency to weakness and sensory changes of a cortical type in the lower limb.

Middle Cerebral Artery.—Hemiplegia and hemi-anæsthesia (cortical type) on the opposite side, particularly in the face, tongue, and upper limb. Aphasia of various types common : sometimes occurs alone.

Posterior Cerebral Artery.—Crossed homonymous hemianopia with escape of macula.

Basilar Artery.—Quadriplegia with bilateral anæsthesia—generally fatal. Various forms of crossed paralysis.

Superior Cerebellar Artery.—Ipsilateral cerebellar signs with choreiform movements. Various anæsthesias on the contralateral side.

Posterior Inferior Cerebellar Artery.—Sudden onset of intense vertigo, with vomiting and forced movements. The patient is forced into the prone position with that side of the face, corresponding with the side of the lesion, in contact with the pillow. Nystagmus and hypotonia occur, and when the acute phase is passed, a typical unilateral cerebellar syndrome is present. Involvement of the lateral medulla may give various types of crossed sensory loss. For example, pain and anæsthesia may occur in the distribution of the fifth nerve on the affected side, and numbness of the whole of the opposite side of the body. Other cranial nerve nuclei may be involved, including the 6th, 7th, 8th, 9th, and 10th, giving corresponding signs.

THE DIAGNOSIS OF INTRACRANIAL DISEASE

It is not sufficient in the diagnosis of intracranial disease to consider only the symptoms and signs which have been discussed in this chapter. To form a complete clinical picture the state of the whole nervous system must be envisaged, particularly the integrity of the cranial nerves, the motor and sensory systems in the spinal cord and nerves, and the sympathetic nervous system. Only in this way is it possible to avoid explaining symptoms and signs falsely, as due to lesions of the brain, when they are in fact due to affections of other parts of the nervous system. Equally the converse holds good.

The symptoms and signs have been described in such a way as to emphasize the prime importance of anatomical diagnosis. In a delicately fashioned organ such as the brain, enclosed moreover in a rigid case, the skull, almost every lesion is a serious one, and even a simple tumour is ' malignant ' in its results.

When the topographical diagnosis has been made as accurately as possible, the examiner turns to the pathological diagnosis. From this point of view lesions of the brain may be grouped as follows :—

1. Traumatic.—The history is of most importance here, but although the symptoms and signs are usually apparent at once (concussion, depressed fracture, etc.), it must be recognized that some effects are delayed for a considerable time. For example, meningeal hæmorrhage may not occur for twenty-four to forty-eight hours after the accident, and skull injuries may produce epileptic fits or headache for months or years after.

2. Vascular.—Trauma may, of course, produce vascular lesions, but the commonest are the spontaneous forms—embolism, thrombosis, and hæmorrhage. The characteristic of all vascular lesions is the *suddenness of onset without trauma*. The effects of embolism are instantaneous, those of hæmorrhage may take minutes to hours to develop, and those of thrombosis are even more gradual, but rarely take longer than twenty-four hours to reach their maximum. Vascular accidents (hæmorrhage and thrombosis) are not unusual secondary changes in new growths and inflammatory masses, and their dramatic suddenness may obscure the underlying chronic lesion. The internal capsule is the commonest site for vascular lesions.

3. Inflammatory.—The onset of inflammatory lesions is fairly rapid, but a few days are generally required before the symptoms and signs become obvious. *Fever* is present in some cases, though not by any means in all. Leucocytosis may be present. Some of the more chronic inflammatory lesions (e.g., tuberculosis and syphilis) may imitate the results of neoplasm closely : indeed, in many cases these chronic infections result in tumour formation which differs in its effects very little from neoplasm.

4. **Neoplasm.**—New growth, as in other parts of the body, may grow slowly or rapidly, and the general rule holds good that the effects are proportionate to the rapidity of development. The cerebral tumour differs in two most important respects from other tumours. It is growing in contact with very delicate tissues which are easily destroyed, and it is growing inside a cavity, the cranium, which allows little room for expansion. The results of even small tumours are correspondingly disastrous. The possibility of tumour arises especially when focal cerebral signs appear gradually, or if signs of increased intracranial tension are present.

5. **Degenerations.**—Certain cerebral diseases are classed as degenerative, though further understanding of their pathology may eventually lead to re-classification. In general paralysis of the insane, for example, degenerative changes are found in the brain and meninges, but these are now known to be the results of the insidious effects of the *Spirochæta pallida* and its toxins. In other mental diseases, and in such diseases as amyotrophic lateral sclerosis and paralysis agitans, the degenerative processes have no known cause. Degenerative lesions are relatively uncommon, and the diagnosis depends on exclusion of other causes of the condition. In mental diseases it is of prime importance for the physician to exclude a physical basis.

ILLUSTRATIVE DISEASES OF THE BRAIN AND MENINGES

Cerebral Injuries.—Trauma to the skull is serious on account of damage to the brain. This may be clearly recognizable in lacerations or rupture of meningeal or cerebral vessels which may cause objective signs during life, or distinguishing post-mortem findings. Often these grosser changes are associated with fracture of the skull. In the case of concussion, however, serious clinical manifestations may be present with minor pathological changes.

Concussion.—All grades of this condition are seen, varying from a state in which the patient is merely dazed and " sees stars " to one of coma of varying depth and duration. In the stage of recovery automatism is common and sometimes mental confusion and delirium. Headache, dizziness, and irritability may persist for weeks.

Fracture of the Skull.—The force required to fracture the adult skull is generally considerable, and symptoms of concussion are usually pronounced. If the fracture is *depressed*, pressure on or laceration of the brain will occur, with resulting symptoms varying with the locality (*see* CEREBRAL LOCALIZATION, p. 294). A depressed fracture over the motor area may, for example, produce Jacksonian fits or localized paresis. Fracture of the *base of the skull* is often associated with paresis of the cranial nerves. Bleeding, and escape of cerebrospinal fluid through the mouth, nose, and ears, are also found. When a fracture of the skull is followed by œdema or hæmorrhage into the brain, *cerebral compression*, a common event, results. The loss of consciousness is deeper—true coma, which may last for some hours or days. The pupils may be contracted at first, later dilated. Some of the signs of increased intracranial pressure may be present, especially brady-cardia and respiratory arrhythmias (Cheyne-Stokes breathing).

It should be noted that a fracture of the skull may exist without any of the symptoms mentioned, and radiological examination is necessary in every case.

Chronic Subdural Hæmorrhage.—Sometimes a comparatively minor injury to the skull may result in a gradual leakage from the cortical veins, and a hæmatoma is formed causing pressure symptoms and therefore sometimes confused with cerebral tumour unless the history of trauma is elicited. The symptoms may manifest themselves in a few days, weeks, or months after the injury and concussion may not have occurred. Head-ache, vomiting, drowsiness, mental confusion, and bradycardia are common, but subject to remarkable fluctuation, seldom seen in tumour to the same extent. Papillœdema of moderate degree may develop. Variable changes in tendon and superficial reflexes result and drowsiness changes to stupor or later, coma and death, if unrelieved.

Subarachnoid Hæmorrhage.—The usual cause is the leakage or rupture of a congenital aneurysm on the circle of Willis. Sometimes in older persons a degenerate artery bursts, or trauma may be responsible. The clinical manifestations vary. Meningeal symptoms—slowly or suddenly produced—include head retraction, Kernig's sign, pyrexia, and other signs which may lead to a wrong diagnosis of meningitis. The truth is established on lumbar puncture when pure blood or heavily stained fluid is withdrawn. After settling, the supernatant fluid remains straw-coloured, thus distinguishing the blood from that due to imperfect lumbar puncture.

In other cases the picture is that of a severe cerebral hæmorrhage, though the localizing symptoms are not so obviously on one side.

Cerebral Hæmorrhage.—Cerebral hæmorrhage or apoplexy is one of the commonest vascular lesions of the brain. It most frequently results from rupture of the lenticulo-striate artery, ' the artery of cerebral hæmor-rhage ', a branch of the middle cerebral artery which supplies blood to the neighbourhood of the internal capsule. Cerebral hæmorrhage is there-fore usually associated with disturbances of motor power—paralysis (*see* MOTOR SYSTEM, pp. 232 and 249). The symptoms and signs to be expected in the rarer types of cerebral hæmorrhage may be gathered from the details already given about cerebral localization.

The patient usually suffers from high blood-pressure and arterio-sclerosis and is of the apoplectic type (*see* p. 20). Sometimes there are *premonitory* symptoms, such as headache and vertigo, transient aphasia, paræsthesiæ, or paresis, but these are often absent. The *onset* is abrupt with vertigo, which in a few minutes, during which the brain tissue is ploughed up, causes the patient to fall. Shortly he is *unconscious*, with the stertor, sweating, and abolition of reflexes found in coma (*see also* COMA, p. 291). Signs of *increased intracranial pressure* are present during this stage owing to accumulation of extravasated blood, œdema of the brain, and impairment of the circulation of the cerebrospinal fluid. The patient often vomits, the pulse becomes slower, and respiration may be slower and modified to the Cheyne-Stokes type. The temperature falls at first, but rises after twenty-four hours if the patient lives, owing to the toxic effects of the absorbed blood. The cerebrospinal fluid in most cases contains blood within a few hours of the hæmorrhage.

The local signs in an internal-capsular lesion are usually those of a *hemiplegia* on the side of the body opposite the lesion. Face, arm, and leg are generally affected, the trunk to a lesser extent owing to its bilateral cortical innervation (*see Fig.* 172, p. 228). Aphasia may be present if the lesion involves subcortical fibres on the left side. Conjugate deviation often occurs, i.e., the head and eyes are persistently turned in one direction (*see* p. 323).

The paralysis is at first flaccid, due to cerebral shock, but if the patient recovers it becomes spastic with other signs of an upper motor neurone lesion (*see* p. 232). During the flaccid stage the paralysed limbs drop lifelessly when they are raised from the bed, and the cheek on the affected side puffs out with each expiration. The paralysed leg looks broader than its fellow owing to the flaccidity.

When a comatose patient has signs of a recent hemiplegia the diagnosis is usually confined to vascular lesions. Hæmorrhage must then be distinguished from thrombosis and embolism, both of which produce similar effects, and the possibility of hæmorrhage into a tumour must not be overlooked.

Cerebral Thrombosis.—Thrombosis often causes a localized paralysis, e.g., one arm, because the cortical vessels are involved, but if the clotting extends to the parent middle cerebral, hemiplegia may occur as in cerebral hæmorrhage. The appearance of the paralysis is slower, over a period of hours and sometimes with fluctuations over a few days. Consciousness may not be lost when smaller vessels are affected, but unconsciousness may result later, though it is rarely so profound as in cerebral hæmorrhage. Cerebral thrombosis may occur in young persons as well as old, and often starts during sleep.

Cerebral Embolism.—This becomes the probable diagnosis when a complete hemiplegia occurs instantaneously without any loss of consciousness, especially in a young person. A confirmatory sign of great importance is the discovery of any lesion from which emboli are likely to be dislodged, e.g., valvular endocarditis and auricular fibrillation.

Hypertensive Encephalopathy.—Whenever cerebral symptoms suggestive of gross vascular lesions are encountered, the possibility of an acute hypertensive crisis has to be considered. A sudden rise of blood-pressure to 250 mm. or more may result in symptoms very similar to those of cerebral tumour or the cerebral vascular lesions just outlined. Headache, vomiting, papilloedema, fits, hemiparesis, hemianopia, or other local signs, may lead to an erroneous diagnosis unless the possibility of essential hypertension is carefully considered. Doubt may still exist until the patient recovers with the recession of physical signs which would persist in other organic lesions.

Lead encephalopathy may produce similar signs.

Meningitis.—The symptoms of meningeal irritation have already been described (p. 296). The most important disease producing them is meningitis, an inflammation of the meninges. Less commonly subarachnoid hæmorrhage is responsible. Meningitis may be caused by the specific meningococcus in cerebrospinal and posterior basic meningitis, by the tubercle bacillus, by the pneumococcus, and by other non-specific organisms. Whichever organism is responsible, the results are similar, though special clinical signs may help in distinguishing one type from another. Tuberculous meningitis is often suggested by a long prodromal period and by the discovery of other tuberculous lesions. Cerebrospinal meningitis is rapid in onset, often found in epidemics, and sometimes accompanied by a petechial or roseolar rash, which has given it the name ' spotted fever '. Pneumococcal meningitis would be a likely diagnosis if signs of pneumonia were found, or in cases of pneumococcal otitis media. It may also be a primary infection.

Other types of meningitis are rarer. Infections introduced by trauma to the skull, or from sinus or middle-ear disease, less frequently enter the diagnostic field. *Serous meningitis* is of unknown cause, possibly toxic. It has similar clinical signs, but lymphocytosis occurs in the cerebrospinal fluid without change in the sugar or chlorides. The term *meningismus* is given to a condition of meningeal irritability due to toxæmia without any actual inflammation of the meninges. It occurs especially in pneumonia. The headache is said to cease when delirium begins, whereas in meningitis it continues.

The diagnosis, not only of the type of meningitis, but of the disease itself, is not complete without examination of the cerebrospinal fluid. The fluid is usually under pressure, turbid or even purulent in coccal forms of meningitis, though crystal-clear in the tuberculous form. Microscopically the cell-count is increased and the causal organism is usually found. The protein is increased and the sugar and chlorides diminished.

Meningitis is an inflammatory disease and *fever* is a symptom. It is variable in degree, and the pulse-rate may be proportionately increased at first, but later tends to become slower owing to the increase in intracranial pressure.

Encephalitis.—Inflammation of the brain itself has been mentioned as occurring to some extent in meningitis. It may also result from traumatic and inflammatory lesions of the skull. Following certain virus

20

diseases such as measles, small-pox, and vaccinia, cerebral or spinal symptoms may occur in association with renewed fever. This has been called *infective encephalo-myelitis*. So-called *polio-encephalitis* is of uncertain origin and probably not related to infantile paralysis. Its manifestations include spastic hemiplegia and cranial nerve palsies. The localized form of encephalitis resulting in cerebral abscess will be considered later.

Undoubtedly the most important inflammatory disease of the brain is encephalitis lethargica.

Encephalitis Lethargica.—This disease is an infection of the brain with a virus, as yet unknown. Its infective origin is supported by its occurrence in epidemics and by fever as an initial symptom. Almost any part of the brain may be involved, and the symptoms and signs are accordingly protean.

In its early stages the disease has little to distinguish it from febrile infections such influenza, characterized by general malaise, diffuse pains, and fever. The most important early diagnostic features are *alteration in sleep rhythm* and transient *cranial-nerve paresis*. Sleep is usually excessive ; the patient is drowsy in the daytime, though at night he may complain of insomnia. This symptom may persist for weeks or months. The depth of drowsiness is rarely so great as in the stupor of increased intracranial pressure and the patient can generally be aroused from it. Ocular disturbances, such as diplopia, ptosis, squint, and pupillary changes, are the most frequent manifestations of cranial-nerve involvement, though other nerves may be affected. In severe cases delirium and coma commonly lead to a fatal conclusion.

In taking the history of a patient suspected to have post-encephalitic symptoms, it is necessary, if the information is not supplied voluntarily, to inquire specially whether the patient had any influenzal symptoms or double vision at the onset of his illness.

Motor symptoms of an upper neurone type are rare, but involuntary movements, both choreiform and myoclonic, may be a notable feature of the acute stage.

During the convalescent phase, or sometimes months or a year or two after, the patient develops in many cases the most characteristic sequelæ. These resemble closely the features of paralysis agitans, the *mask-like, expressionless facies* (Figs. 228, 229), and the *rigidity* and *attitude of flexion*, but *tremor* is not so common, though sometimes a fine flutter of the closed eyelids is noted (*see* PARALYSIS AGITANS, p. 310). To these the name post-encephalitic Parkinsonism is generally given. These symptoms and signs indicate that the disease attacks the basal ganglia and extra-pyramidal system. Apart from Parkinsonism, mental and moral deterioration are common after-effects, especially in children. Occasionally *oculo-gyric* crises are seen in which the eyes roll upwards and the head becomes retracted for some minutes.

Examination of the *cerebrospinal fluid* is important in suspected encephalitis lethargica, if only to exclude other cerebral and meningeal

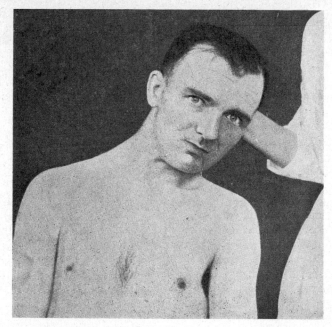

Fig. 228.—Post-encephalic state. The Parkinsonian mask and dribbling of saliva are characteristic. The torticollis is unusual. (*Prof. Henry Cohen's case.*)

lesions. The fluid is clear, may be under increased pressure, and may show a slight protein increase. The sugar, however, is not diminished as in meningitis, and there is little, if any, cellular increase.

Cerebral Tumour.—The diagnosis of cerebral tumour is an excellent example of the general mode of neurological diagnosis, in which the lesion must first be localized and its nature then ascertained. The *localization* has already been considered (*see* p. 294), but a short résumé under the headings of the symptoms and signs is not out of place.

Disorders of intellectual function, including changes in memory, reasoning, and moral faculties, should direct attention to the frontal lobes, especially when other more positive localizing features are absent.

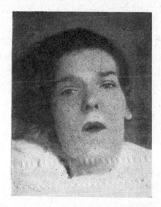

Fig. 229.—Parkinsonian facies in encephalitis lethargica.

Motor phenomena such as Jacksonian fits and paresis point to lesions in the pre-Rolandic area and the neighbouring subcortical regions. Paralysis with involvement of the cranial nerves suggests lesions in the mid-brain—crura, pons, or medulla. They are more fully described under the motor system, p. 250.

Cortical sensory disturbances, i.e., astereognosis, loss of point discrimination, and of the perception of small variations in temperature, suggest a lesion of the parietal lobe.

Aphasia may suggest parietal lobe involvement if of the auditory type, a lesion of or near the angular gyrus when visual, or an affection of Broca's area (in front of the lower part of the pre-Rolandic area) when essentially motor. Aphasia is a sign which must be used with caution for localizing purposes, owing to the difficulty in analysing different types.

Perversions of smell, when local nasal causes have been excluded, may throw suspicion on the uncinate gyrus.

Hemianopia, especially homonymous and quadrantic types, is found in lesions of the optic radiation and occipital cortex.

Cranial-nerve palsies are of great localizing value, and are particularly found when the tumour is situated at the base of the brain.

Disturbances of equilibrium and muscle tone are the most important symptoms suggestive of cerebellar tumours.

It must not be forgotten that tumours are rarely localized to one area, and may spread to others, causing new signs to appear. The possibility of tumour may first arise when any localizing signs are present, especially when these appear gradually over a period of some months. If signs of increased intracranial pressure (*see* p. 293) occur concurrently, the diagnosis becomes more certain. The reverse, however, is commonly the case, namely, the signs of increased intracranial pressure occur early and the localizing signs only later. In such cases the careful exclusion of other diseases causing the triad of headache, vomiting, and optic neuritis may establish a diagnosis of tumour, but its position may remain uncertain. Of the general signs, it is to be noted that papilloedema and vomiting are often more pronounced in subtentorial than supratentorial tumours.

In the diagnosis of the *nature of a tumour* the patient's age takes a prominent part. Carcinoma, which is always secondary, is naturally found in older people. A primary focus should be sought. Most other tumours are commoner in younger persons. Cerebellar tumours are often tuberculous, especially in children, and the lungs and lymphatic glands should be examined for evidence of tuberculosis. In no case must the Wassermann reaction be omitted, and if it is deemed advisable to perform a lumbar puncture (an operation which must not be undertaken lightly owing to the risk of death by medullary compression), the cerebrospinal fluid must be examined for evidence of syphilis. Gummata do not often reach sufficient size to produce the general signs of cerebral tumour, but local signs due to irritation of the motor cortex or paralysis of the cranial nerves are common. Endotheliomata contrast with gummata. The former press upon, the latter replace, the brain substance. The general signs are, therefore, as a rule more pronounced in endotheliomata. Auscultation over the parietal region of the skull may discover murmurs which have great diagnostic value in vascular tumours, e.g., angioma of the meninges.

Cerebral Abscess.—A cerebral abscess is a common type of tumour. It most frequently arises from suppuration in the middle ear or nasal sinuses, which must always be examined in suspected cerebral tumour. Rarer causes such as disease of the skull bones, metastasis from bronchiectasis or pulmonary abscess, or from a general pyæmia, must also be borne in mind, and the necessary examination made to find the primary focus of infection.

The symptoms are often vague, in itself an indication of the apathy, mental deterioration, and drowsiness which are usually present. Headache may be a feature, and also other signs of increased intracranial pressure, but they are rarely so convincing as in tumour. The patient's general condition is usually poor, with pallor, wasting, and in some cases pyrexia. Localizing signs are often slight or absent, but may include evidence of pyramidal tract damage on one side, aphasia, and various types of hemianopia. These signs appear more particularly when the abscess is in its common site, the temporo-sphenoidal lobe. In some cases meningeal signs may also occur, in which case, examination of the cerebrospinal fluid may be helpful in diagnosis (*see* p. 418).

Thrombosis of the Lateral Sinus.—This is another complication of otitis media, and in some of its features (headache, mental confusion) resembles cerebral abscess, with which it is often associated. Engorgement and tenderness of the veins in the mastoid region and of the internal jugular vein are the important signs. Rigors, sweats, and high temperature are generally present.

General Paralysis of the Insane.—This disease is an illustration of a chronic infection of the brain and its meninges which results in degenerative changes. The infection is a late syphilitic one, and ten to twenty years commonly elapse between the primary infection and the resulting nervous lesion. The localization of the disease is essentially in the frontal lobes and the meninges. It therefore disturbs the higher intellectual functions of the pre-frontal lobes and the motor functions of the pre-Rolandic area.

The onset is insidious. *Mental changes* are usually noticed by the patient's relatives and friends. He becomes neglectful and careless in his work, his memory fails, his judgement in family and financial matters is impaired, and his moral outlook deteriorates. Later more gross symptoms appear, especially delusions of the grandiose type. The patient imagines himself a great personage or the possessor of untold wealth and acts accordingly, with disastrous results to himself and his family.

Gradually, objective signs appear. The *speech* becomes slurred, and syllables are missed out in speaking and writing. Instead of British the man may say ' Brrish ', in place of artillery, ' artllry '. *Tremors* of the lips, tongue, and hands may be obvious, but if not should be looked for in all cases. The *motor* signs are at first slight. General bodily weakness is present, but slowly the patient becomes bedridden, with signs of upper motor neurone paralysis of the limbs. The *Argyll Robertson pupil* (*see* p. 323), and in some cases optic atrophy, are present as in other forms of cerebrospinal syphilis. The *cerebrospinal fluid* may be under increased pressure and shows an increase in protein and a high cell-count consisting chiefly of lymphocytes. The colloid gold curve (*see* p. 420) is of the paretic or luetic type, and the Wassermann reaction is positive.

Paralysis Agitans.—This disease is a good example of a degenerative process probably affecting the basal ganglia (corpus striatum). It appears insidiously in elderly persons, and it is characterized by two principal physical signs, which depend on disordered function in the extra-pyramidal system. These are : (1) Muscular rigidity ; (2) Tremors.

The *muscular rigidity* causes stiffness in using the limbs, resulting in a characteristic shuffling gait. The patient appears to hurry in the direction he is going (*festination*), or if gently pushed backwards may continue in this direction (*retropulsion*), gathering speed and tending to fall unless stopped. The *attitude* is one of flexion, the head depressed on the chest, the shoulders bowed, the knees and elbows slightly bent. The rigidity of the facial muscles gives a characteristic immobility to the face which is known as the *Parkinsonian facies* (*see Figs.* 228, 229). The expression is fixed and staring ; the patient smiles little or not at all ; the mouth is often slightly open and saliva dribbles away.

The *tremor* is not always present, but in many cases is the first sign observed. It is described as ' pill-rolling ' owing to the characteristic movement of the thumb and index finger. Later the tremor extends to the whole hand, to the leg on the same side, and finally to other parts of the body. Both rigidity and tremor may for a long time be unilateral. It may be momentarily controlled by an effort of will, or by muscular movement, only to return when these cease.

Reference has already been made to the resemblance of post-encephalitic Parkinsonism to the degenerative form of paralysis agitans.

Arteriosclerotic Parkinsonism.—Here the basis of the striated lesion is vascular so that hypertension and arteriosclerosis are generally found. Clinically the condition has a more rapid course than paralysis agitans and mental deterioration is common. Tremor on the other hand is uncommon.

The sequel of Parkinsonism from lethargic encephalitis, cerebral arteriosclerosis, degenerative lesions of the basal ganglia, and more rarely causes such as manganese poisoning, illustrates the frequency with which a neurological syndrome results from many differing pathological causes which must be ascertained before diagnosis is complete.

THE CRANIAL NERVES

A systematic examination of the cranial nerves is essential in every neurological case. Not only may primary lesions of the nerves, their nuclei, or their cerebral controlling centres be found, but the secondary involvement of these by diseases of the brain or its meninges frequently gives most important localizing data.

If there are signs of irritation or paralysis of a cranial nerve it is necessary to consider whether the lesion is situated in the upper or lower motor neurone, just as in the case of paralysis of the limbs, though it may be stated at once that the lower neurone lesions are by far the commoner. When the lesion has been localized, its pathology must be determined. The common pathological processes responsible for cranial-nerve paralysis are similar to those mentioned in the case of diseases of the motor neurones (see p. 249)—namely :—

1. *Trauma*, e.g., fracture of the base of the skull.

2. *Vascular lesions* (hæmorrhage, thrombosis, and embolism). These may affect the supranuclear centres or the nuclei themselves. Extravasation of blood around the base of the brain may affect the nerve-trunks.

3. *Inflammatory lesions*, e.g., meningitis and encephalitis, and neuritis of the nerve itself, especially diphtheritic neuritis, etc.

4. *Neoplasm*, e.g., tumours in the region of the nerve nucleus or in the course of the nerve.

5. *Degenerative lesions*. Not common, but an example is seen in optic atrophy.

The First or Olfactory Nerve.—This nerve is not of great clinical importance. Its anatomical position renders it liable to be damaged by tumours projecting from the lower surface of the frontal lobes on to the olfactory bulb, or by fractures involving the anterior fossa. The result will be loss of the sense of smell, *anosmia*. The patient often confuses this with loss of the sense of taste, as flavours depend upon the sense of smell, not on the sense of taste. In bilateral olfactory lesions, only the primary sensations of taste (sweet, bitter, sour, and salt) remain.

The perception of smell appears to be situated in the uncinate and hippocampal gyri, lesions of which may be associated with perversions of smell. Similar perversion may occur as an aura in epilepsy, and in insane persons.

EXAMINATION.—The 1st nerve must be *tested by substances which do not stimulate the sensory endings of the 5th nerve.* Ammonia and acetic acid, therefore, must not be used. Peppermint, turpentine, and oil of cloves are suitable, and should be applied to each nostril in turn.

The Second or Optic Nerve.—This is the most important of the cranial nerves. Not only does it serve the most highly organized special sense, that of sight, but it spreads out into the retina, the examination of which so often reveals signs of disease in other parts of the body.

A few important *anatomical facts* must be recalled. The impressions of light from the whole of each retina are taken in the optic nerve to the optic chiasma. Here the fibres from the left half of each retina pass into the left optic tract, those from the right half to the right optic tract. Most of the fibres of each optic tract pass on to the external geniculate body ; some to the pulvinar of the optic thalamus and to the superior quadrigeminal body. From these lower visual centres the fibres make their way, via the optic radiation on each side, to the occipital cortex. Through the medial part of each optic tract communication is established between this optical system and the oculomotor nuclei. The pupillary reflexes are also controlled through special fibres in the optic nerve which leave the optic tract to reach the superior quadrigeminal bodies, which in their turn communicate with the third nerve nucleus.

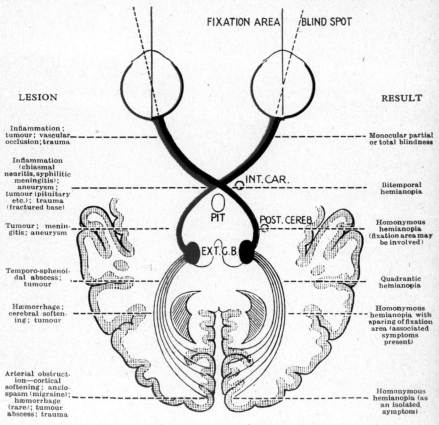

Fig. 230.—Course of visual fibres. On the left side are shown the common lesions in the various parts of the course of the fibres, on the right the results of the lesion. INT. CAR., Internal carotid artery; PIT., Pituitary body; POST. CEREB., Posterior cerebral artery; EXT. G. B., External geniculate bodies. (*Diagram constructed by Mr. A. McKie Reid.*)

The various parts of these optical paths may now be considered in relationship to their surrounding structure. The nerve itself may be involved as it enters the orbit, or by lesions in the anterior fossa of the skull or of the contained frontal lobes. The chiasma lies in close contact with the pituitary body and the internal carotid arteries, and may be damaged by lesions of these structures such as pituitary tumour or carotid aneurysm; also by meningeal changes such as arachnoiditis following skull injury. Each optic tract, as it diverges from its fellow in front of the interpeduncular space, winds round the corresponding crus in close association with the posterior cerebral artery which supplies it. The tract may be affected by disease either of the artery or of the crus. Finally, each optic radiation passes in close proximity to the internal capsule and lenticular nucleus, and after plunging far into the temporo-sphenoidal lobe sweeps round the posterior horn of the lateral ventricle to the region of the calcarine fissure of the occipital lobe in the posterior fossa of the skull.

The effects of lesions in the different parts of these visual pathways will be seen in *Fig.* 230.

EXAMINATION OF THE OPTIC NERVE AND ITS CONNEXIONS.—The patient must first be asked whether he has noted any visual changes. His visual acuity may then be tested, and an ophthalmoscopic examination of the retina and optic disks made. Finally the visual fields may be tested.

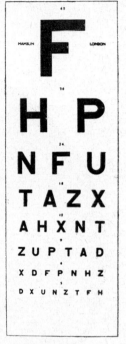

Fig. 231.—Snellen's test types. (*By courtesy of Messrs. Hamblin.*)

Visual Acuity.—Acuity of vision is tested by means of special charts (Snellen types) with lines of print of varying size (*Fig.* 231). Each eye is tested separately. Central visual acuity is conventionally recorded as a fraction. For example, if the patient standing at six metres distance can read only the largest type, which he should be able to read at sixty metres, his visual acuity is said to be 6/60. Similarly, if he can read no further down the type than that line which should be read at eighteen metres, his visual acuity is stated to be 6/18, and ability to read the penultimate line (line 7 in diagram) is expressed as 6/6, i.e., normal vision.

Opthalmoscopic Examination.—The retinæ and optic disks (*Fig.* 232) can be examined with an electric ophthalmoscope even by the inexperienced, and it cannot be over-emphasized that the student should use every opportunity of becoming familiar with the physiological variations in the fundus, and the commoner types of pathological changes. These include changes in the optic disk or nerve-head such as pallor, swelling (papillœdema and optic neuritis), hæmorrhages, cupping, and atrophy; and various forms of retinitis, either primary or associated with constitutional disease such as blood dyscrasias, renal disease, and diabetes. The retinal changes are described briefly in connexion with the diseases in which they occur.

Papillœdema (choked disk) : This means swelling of the nerve-head, i.e., where the optic nerve emerges through the lamina cribrosa of the sclera to spread out into the retina. The swelling is usually caused mechanically by increased intracranial pressure which results in internal hydrocephalus, though not all cases are explained in this way. The commonest cause of the increased pressure is *cerebral tumour*. Less common causes are meningitis and cerebral abscess and hæmatoma, whilst gumma of the brain or meninges and cerebral hæmorrhage are rarely responsible.

Pathogenesis of papillœdema (*Fig.* 233): The subarachnoid space of the optic nerve-sheath is in direct communication with the cerebral

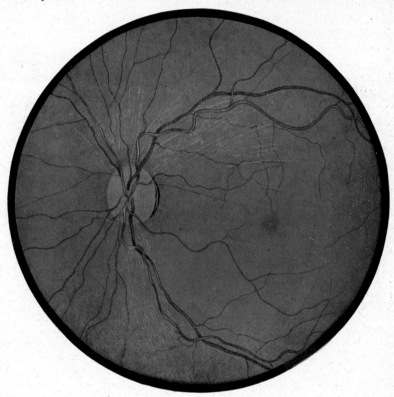

Fig. 232.—NORMAL DISK.—Note clearly defined disk of pinkish colour; at the temporal margin is a black choroidal crescent. The vessels are rather more tortuous than usual, but sharply defined, and the veins are larger and darker than the arteries. The general fundus (remainder of the retina) is uniformly red. (*By kind permission of the Oxford University Press. Drawing by Messrs. Hamblin.*)

subarachnoid space. The retinal artery, vein, and lymphatics run in the nerve, and cross the subarachnoid space of the nerve-sheath about half-an-inch behind the eyeball. Increased pressure in the cerebral subarachnoid space is transmitted into the nerve-sheath. The relatively thin walls of the vein and lymphatics, with the low pressure of their fluid contents, permit them to be compressed more than the artery. The inflow of blood to the retina is practically unchecked, whilst the outflow of venous blood and lymph is obstructed. This results in increased transudation of lymph and œdema of the nerve-head or papilla.

The swelling may be measured by noting the difference between the highest plus lens required to bring a vessel *on* the disk into sharp focus and the highest plus lens required to bring the same vessel into focus after it has left the disk and is lying on the level part of the adjacent retina. The swelling is measured in dioptres (3 dioptres = 1 mm. of swelling).

Other features to be noted are the engorgement of the veins and blurring of the disk margin.

Optic neuritis or papillitis (*Fig.* 234): In this condition the veins are very full and hæmorrhages often occur on the disk or in the neighbouring retina. The disk is not so raised as in papillœdema, rarely more than to the extent of two dioptres, though the swelling extends farther into the surrounding tissues. Optic neuritis may result from syphilis, disseminated sclerosis, renal disease, methyl alcohol poisoning, etc.

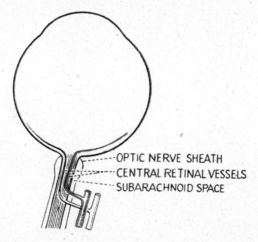

Fig. 233.—Pathogenesis of papillœdema. (*Diagram by Mr. A. McKie Reid.*)

The term *retrobulbar neuritis* describes an inflammation of the optic nerve which produces symptoms rather than physical signs, because it affects the optic nerve behind the disk. The patient's sight is affected, generally as a central scotoma which may lead to complete blindness. At first no changes are found on examination of the disk, though optic atrophy may eventually result. The condition is frequently unilateral, and results from disseminated sclerosis and occasionally also from infections of the accessory nasal sinuses.

Optic atrophy (*Fig.* 235): Optic atrophy may be *consecutive* to papillœdema or optic neuritis. A few cases follow retrobulbar neuritis. Other cases are *primary*, as in tabes, G.P.I., and when the optic nerve is damaged by tumour or trauma, or in poisoning with lead, methyl alcohol, tryparsamide, etc. True *secondary* optic atrophy results from degeneration of the ganglion cells of the retina, as in retinitis pigmentosa, etc.

If the atrophy is consecutive, examination shows the disk to be pale, its edge irregular, and the lamina cribrosa blocked with organized exudate, remnants of the previous œdema of the nerve-head. In primary types the disc is pale and sharply defined like a full moon in a retinal sky. The lamina cribrosa is well-marked and the absence of small vessels on the disk is notable.

Fields of Vision.—Whenever the visual field is found to be abnormal by rough tests, accurate charts should be prepared by perimetry. As a rough test it is often sufficient to make the patient gaze straight ahead

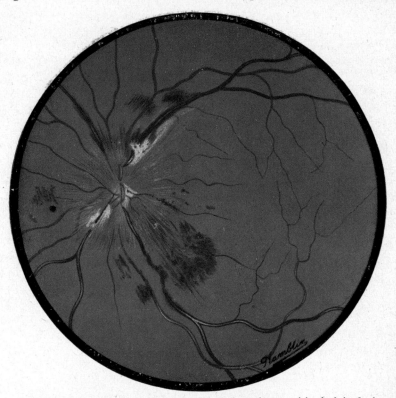

Fig. 234.—OPTIC NEURITIS.—The disk is raised above the general level of the fundus and its edge is obscured by the radial striations of the œdematous nerve-fibre layer. The veins are relatively engorged, and white and hæmorrhagic exudates are seen in the surrounding retina. (*By kind permission of the Oxford University Press. Drawing by Messrs. Hamblin.*)

at a fixed object, and then to move a small white object (e.g., a pin with a white head) from the periphery to the centre of the visual field in two diameters at right angles to one another. When a perimeter is used, a record must be made of the visual field for each colour separately (white, red, green, and blue). The colour fields are the first to be restricted in most cases. Lastly, it is essential not to overlook central scotomata, i.e., patches of impairment in the central area of the field of vision.

Blindness in the whole of the visual field occurs from lesions of the retina or optic nerve, less commonly from occipital lobe lesions. Blindness in one-half of each visual field is known as *hemianopia*. If it affects the same—that is, right or left—half of each field it is called right or left *homonymous hemianopia* (*Fig.* 236). This occurs, for example, in lesions of the optic tract and also of the optic radiation. If the right side of one field and the left side of the other are affected, the condition is known as *crossed* or *heteronymous hemianopia*. There are two types of this, bitemporal hemianopia (*Fig.* 237) when the outer half of each visual field is affected,

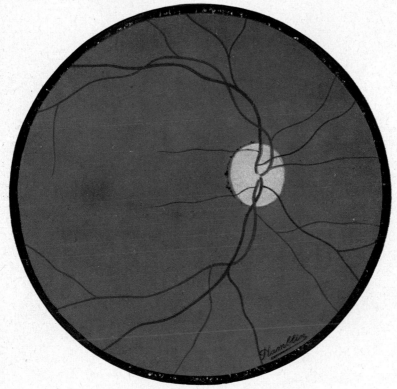

Fig. 235.—PRIMARY OPTIC ATROPHY.—The disk is pale and stands out vividly against the red fundus; the margin is sharply defined. The vessels are attenuated (By kind permission of the Oxford University Press. Drawing by Messrs. Hamblin.)

and binasal hemianopia when the inner halves are involved. Bitemporal hemianopia not infrequently results from tumours of, or adjacent to, the pituitary body. Nasal hemianopia is usually unilateral, and may result from lesions in the same region.

Quadrantic defects ('quadrantic hemianopia') (*Fig.* 238) occur from lesions involving the optic radiations or, less commonly, the occipital lobe. The restriction of the visual field is less than one half, usually about one quarter. It is to be observed that most forms of hemianopia are irregular, and in their early stages both homonymous and crossed hemianopia may appear quadrantic. This is particularly so when the temporal loop of the optic radiation is affected.

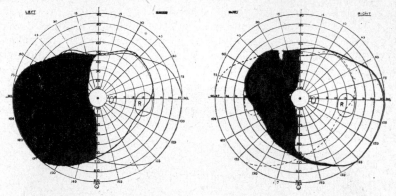

Fig. 236.—LEFT HOMONYMOUS HEMIANOPIA.—Tumour right parietal lobe; male, aged 50. Visual acuity; right and left eyes 6/6. Fixation area spared. Perimetry with white object 5 mm. in diameter—daylight. (Constructed by Mr. A. McKie Reid.)

Oculomotor and Pupillary Innervation (the Third, Fourth, Sixth, and Sympathetic Nerves).—

ANATOMICAL CONSIDERATIONS.—The muscles which move the eyeball and those which are responsible for the pupillary reactions are all innervated

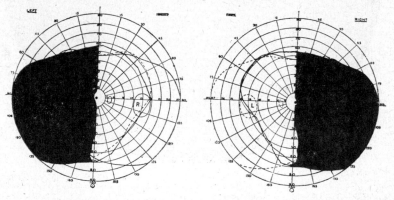

Fig. 237.—BITEMPORAL HEMIANOPIA.—Pituitary tumour, six years' history. Visual acuity: right eye 6/9, left eye 6/24. Sparing of fixation area. Perimetry with 5-mm. white object—daylight. (Constructed by Mr. A. McKie Reid.)

by the 3rd, 4th, 6th, and sympathetic nerves, and these nerves are tested together.

The 3rd nerve emerges at the upper border of the pons, passes through the cavernous sinus and sphenoidal fissure, and supplies all the external ocular muscles except the superior oblique and rectus externus. It also sends fibres to the levator palpebræ superioris, and, through the ciliary ganglion, controls the muscles of accommodation (the sphincter of the pupil and ciliary muscle).

The 4th nerve and its fellow decussate in the superior medullary velum, and each winds round the crus and enters the orbit through the sphenoidal fissure to supply the superior oblique.

Both the 3rd and 4th nerves have their nuclei in the floor of the aqueduct of Sylvius.

The 6th nerve appears between the pons and medulla, and also passes through the cavernous sinus and sphenoidal fissure to enter the orbit.

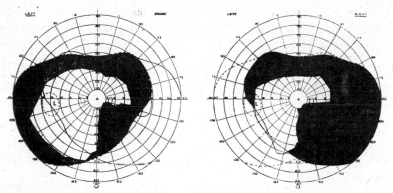

Fig. 238. QUADRANTIC HEMIANOPIA.—Subcortical hæmorrhage left parietal lobe; male, aged 58. Accompanied by weakness of right arm and leg and blurring of speech. Visual acuity: right eye 6/12, left eye 6/9. Perimetry four months after onset with 2-mm. white object—daylight. (*Constructed by Mr. A. McKie Reid.*)

It supplies the external rectus. Its nucleus is in the floor of the fourth ventricle.

The *sympathetic* fibres concerned with the oculomotor mechanism arise in medullary centres, and run in the spinal cord to the 1st, 2nd, or 3rd dorsal segments, from which the sympathetic trunk runs upwards, some of its fibres passing to the Gasserian ganglion, thence by ciliary branches of the 5th nerve to the pupil. The sympathetic fibres innervate the dilator muscle of the pupil, the involuntary fibres in the levator palpebræ superioris, and the small muscle of Müller which bridges the sphenomaxillary fissure.

The oculomotor muscles work in unison so as to secure conjugate movements of the eyes in a vertical or lateral plane, during which the visual axes remain parallel and in convergence. This simultaneous action of the oculomotor muscles is obtained by special centres in the brain-stem, in close association with the nuclei of the 3rd, 4th, and 6th nerves. These centres probably control the reflex movements of the eyes, whilst similar conjugate movements of voluntary origin are under control of the higher cortical centres.

EXAMINATION.—To test the *ocular movements* the patient's head must be fixed and he must be asked to move the eyes in turn to the right, to the left, upwards, and downwards as far as possible in each direction. Any limitation of movement is noted (*see Fig.* 243).

The patient should be asked if he sees double (*diplopia*), and note should be taken of squint (*strabismus*), drooping of the eyelid (*ptosis*), or oscillation of the eyeballs (*nystagmus*).

The condition of the *pupils* should be observed, whether they are equal in size and regular, whether abnormally dilated or contracted, and whether they react normally to light and accommodation.

In testing the reaction to light the patient should focus on a distant point and the lighting should not be too bright. Each eye is covered in turn with the hand and the pupil contracts when the hand is taken away. An alternative method is to shine an electric torch into each eye in turn.

In testing the reaction to accommodation the patient is told to look at the far wall of the room. The observer's finger is then suddenly held vertically about six inches in front of the patient's nose and the patient is told to look at it. The pupils should contract equally as he accommodates for the finger, and dilate as the finger is moved away.

A *consensual* reflex may be obtained by shining a light into one eye and noting the contraction of the pupil in the other. The value of this reflex is in the recognition of retrobulbar neuritis, one of the earliest signs of disseminated sclerosis. If the afferent path of the reflex arc for pupillary reactions is interrupted by retrobulbar neuritis, the direct response to light will be lost. But the efferent limbs of the reflex arc (from the 3rd nerve nuclei) are intact, so when a light is shone into one eye the other pupil will contract, though it may show no response to direct light.

COMMON LESIONS.—These are usually lower motor neurone lesions, i.e., affecting the nuclei or nerves. Upper motor neurone lesions, e.g., cerebral hæmorrhage or thrombosis affecting the cortical or mid-brain centres, are rarer and often transient.

Third Nerve Paralysis.—If this is complete, the eye is immobile except in the direction it is moved by the rectus externus (*Figs.* 239–241). It cannot be moved upwards, downwards, or inwards. There is usually external strabismus with downward deviation owing to the unopposed action of the 6th and 4th nerves. Diplopia results in most cases, the type varying with the muscles principally involved, but it may be masked by ptosis. There is ptosis (*Fig.* 242), owing to paresis of the levator palpebræ superioris, and there is compensatory wrinkling of the forehead on the same side. This wrinkling, due to over-action of the frontalis muscle, may raise the eyelid and mask the narrowing of the palpebral fissure, especially if the ptosis is slight. If the fingers are pressed firmly on the eyebrow against the bone, however, so as to prevent the eyelid from being raised by the frontalis, the ptosis at once becomes apparent. The pupil is fixed and dilated owing to unopposed action of the sympathetic on the dilator pupillæ. In 3rd and 6th nerve paralyses *secondary deviation* may also be observed, i.e., the non-paralysed muscles force the eye farther

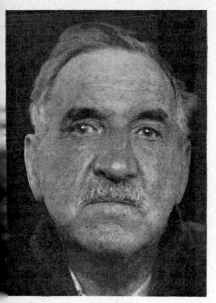

Fig. 239.

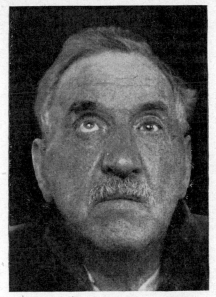

Fig. 240.

Figs. 239-241.—LEFT THIRD NERVE PARALYSIS.—
Fig. 239.—Patient looking straight ahead: note narrow palpebral fissure and dilated pupil.
Fig. 240.—Patient looking upwards; the left eye does not move upwards owing to paralysis of the left superior rectus.
Fig. 241.—Patient attempting to look to the right; the left eye does not move owing to paralysis of the right internal rectus.

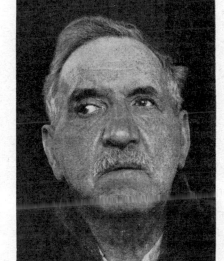

Fig. 241.

21

to the canthus than normal and this in its turn results in *erroneous projection*, so that the patient points farther to one side than the object really is.

Sometimes only portions of the nucleus of the 3rd nerve are affected,

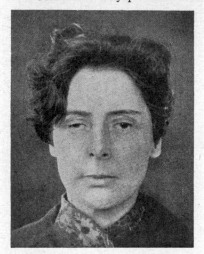

Fig. 242.—Tabetic facies, showing ptosis. The unequal ptosis gives the face a suggestive appearance.

and the result is paresis of individual ocular muscles such as the superior or inferior rectus, or the inferior oblique. This happens especially with central lesions involving the 3rd nucleus, whilst peripheral lesions of the nerve give complete paralysis.

Fourth Nerve Paralysis.—Superior oblique paralysis is difficult to determine objectively, but on looking downwards the patient complains of diplopia, particularly when the eye is adducted, i.e., turned towards the nose.

Sixth Nerve Paralysis. — The patient is unable to move the eyeball outwards (*Fig.* 243). Contraction of the internal rectus eventually leads to internal strabismus with corresponding diplopia.

If the 6th nucleus is paralysed abduction is limited, i.e., the patient is unable to look toward the side of the lesion with the affected eye, but the unaffected eye moves normally.

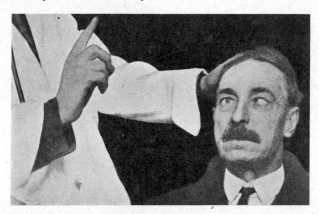

Fig. 243.—Testing the ocular movements. On looking to the extreme right, the right eye remains fixed owing to paralysis of the right external rectus (6th nerve), but the left eye moves normally.

The descriptions which have been given of an oculomotor paralysis apply only to lower motor neurone lesions. If the lesion is *supranuclear* individual ocular muscles are not affected, therefore squint and diplopia do not occur. Instead, muscles controlling a particular movement are paralysed. In most cases this results in *conjugate deviation*, in which the eyes are persistently turned towards the side of the lesion, as the centres enabling the patient to gaze to the side opposite from the lesion are paralysed.

Cervical Sympathetic Paralysis (Fig. 244).—The pupil is contracted owing to unopposed action of the 3rd nerve ; the eye recedes into the orbit, as the muscle of Müller which normally pushes it forwards is paralysed. Slight ptosis occurs from paresis of the involuntary muscle fibres in the upper eyelid, and sweating may be absent on the affected side of the head and neck. This combination of myosis, enophthalmos, ptosis, and anhidrosis is known as Horner's syndrome.

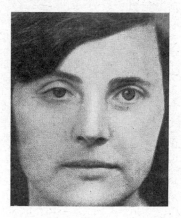

Fig. 244.—Sympathetic nerve paralysis. The right sympathetic nerve was resected at operation (Mr. J. B. Oldham). The corresponding eye shows ptosis, causing narrowing of the palpebral fissure, and myosis from unopposed action of the 3rd nerve.

Pupillary Abnormalities.—Make sure first that no mydriatics have been used recently.

The pupils may be abnormally dilated (*mydriasis*) in conditions of sympathetic over-activity, e.g., hyperthyroidism and anxiety, or from the adhesions of iritis. They are contracted (*myosis*) in cerebro-spinal syphilis, especially tabes, in morphine takers, and sometimes in arteriosclerosis.

Inequality in the size of the pupils is common in lesions of the 3rd nerve or sympathetic affecting one side only, and in diseases such as syphilis or iritis which may produce more advanced changes on one side. The sympathetic may be involved by lesions of the spinal cord such as syringomyelia and hæmatomyelia.

Irregularity may result from the synechiæ of iritis, but syphilis and encephalitis are sometimes responsible.

The *Argyll Robertson* pupil is of great importance as a sign of cerebro-spinal syphilis. It is seen most conclusively in tabes, but also occurs in G.P.I. and meningo-vascular syphilis. It consists in a lack of response to light with presentation of the response to accommodation. In its most complete form it is associated with myosis (contracted pupil), irregularity of the pupil, and atrophy of the iris. The pupil also fails to react to mydriatics These various components cannot be anatomically explained by a lesion of a single area of the brain, such as is suggested for the site of the A.R. pupillary response, namely, the grey matter around the aqueduct in the mid-brain. None the less a combination of these components helps to distinguish the A.R. response of syphilis from the less complete forms sometimes found in other diseases such as chronic encephalitis and other mid-brain lesions, in which the pupil fails to respond to light, but is often large and free from irregularity.

The myotonic pupil is a rare condition which may erroneously suggest tabes, especially as the knee-jerks are sometimes absent. The pupils are, however, regular and of normal size. The reaction to light is lost and that to accommodation sluggish. The condition is generally found in young women and is unexplained, but it is not associated with clinical or spinal-fluid signs of syphilis.

Diplopia.—Double vision has been referred to under paralysis of the oculomotor nerves. The patient may complain spontaneously or only after questioning that he sees double. The diplopia may be present in all positions of the eye, but increases when an attempt is made to move the eye in that direction towards which the paralysed muscle would normally move it.

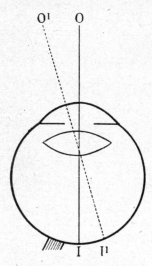

Fig. 245.—Diplopia and false projection (*see* text). O, Fixation spot; O′, Fixation spot or object falsely projected to nasal side of space; I, Image at macula; I′, Image on temporal side of macula. (*Diagram by Mr. A. McKie Reid.*)

The symptom results from strabismus because the images from the two eyes do not fall on corresponding parts of the retina and two images are seen instead of the one which is the normal result of binocular vision (*Fig.* 245). The visual axis is a line drawn from the point of fixation through the nodal point of the eye so as to cut the retina in the macula lutea. If an image falls on the retina to the temporal side of the macula it is projected to the nasal side of space (in front of the observer), and vice versa. In paralysis of the internal rectus it may be impossible to direct the eye so that the image of the fixation point falls on the macula. The image falls on the retina to the temporal side of the macula and the object is falsely projected to the nasal side of the fixation spot. True fixation and projection take place in the unaffected eye, and hence crossed diplopia occurs. When the squint is of long standing the patient may learn to disregard the false image, and diplopia no longer occurs.

The position of the images as seen by the patient is often useful in determining the nature of the ocular paresis. The false image is the one seen by the paralysed eye, the true one by the normal eye.

Candle test : In a dark room a red glass is placed in front of the right eye and a green glass in front of the left, and a lighted candle held in front of the patient. The image of the candle as seen by one eye is red and by the other green. The patient's head is kept stationary and the candle is moved about at a distance of 4 ft. in front of him. The following data are ascertained :—

1. Are there one or two images?
2. If two, is the red flame to the right or left of the green (i.e., is it a homonymous or a crossed diplopia)?

3. Which image is the true image and which is the false? The patient is asked to point to the *red* candle. If he points at the *true* flame, the image as seen by the eye wearing the red glass is the true image, and vice versa.

4. He is then asked to state, when the candle is moved into different positions, the relative positions of the two images. These are charted as in *Fig.* 246.

Interpretation of chart (see also legend beneath figure):—

1. Homonymous diplopia is due to abductor paralysis and crossed diplopia to adductor paralysis.

2. When an eye is adducted, that is, turned towards the nose, the superior oblique acts purely as a depressor and the inferior oblique as an elevator.

3. A false image moves towards a position into which the paralysed muscle would move the eye—that is, the false image makes that movement which the eye has lost.

Every possible combination of paralysis cannot be given and explained, nor has any account been taken of complicating factors, such as : (*a*) Secondary contracture of antagonistic muscles ; (*b*) Fixation of the object with the paralysed eye when this eye has the better visual acuity ; (*c*) Heterophoria or muscle-imbalance which may be unmasked by the paralysis.

Moreover, the candle test is purely subjective, and, in a patient of low intelligence or where the intelligence is obscured by intracranial disease, an accurate diagram may be difficult or impossible ; but a knowledge of the action of the muscles and a grasp of the principles underlying the test will help to elucidate most cases of ocular palsy.

Strabismus (Squint).—This sign has been mentioned as occurring in oculomotor pareses. Many cases of squint are non-paralytic and are called concomitant. The main difference between paralytic and concomitant squint may be summarized as follows :—

Paralytic Strabismus	*Concomitant Strabismus*
1. Known cause and sudden onset	1. Gradual onset in early childhood
2. Diplopia present	2. No diplopia
3. Limitation in ocular movements	3. No limitation of movement
4. Deviation of visual axis varies as the gaze is turned in different directions	4. Deviation of visual axis does not vary
5. No amblyopia (blindness)	5. Eye may be amblyopic
6. False projection	6. No false projection
7. Vertigo may occur	7. No vertigo

Nystagmus.—This consists in oscillations of the eyeball in a lateral, vertical, or rotatory manner. It may be a physiological phenomenon, as after rapid rotation of the body, or the introduction of cold or hot water into the ear, or watching the scenery from a railway carriage. Some cases are congenital. When not explained by such causes it is *always a sign of organic disease*, but slight nystagmoid jerks have not this significance, and may occur in toxæmias and exhaustive states.

The patient should be asked to look to the extreme right and left in turn, then upwards, and finally downwards. In lateral nystagmus the

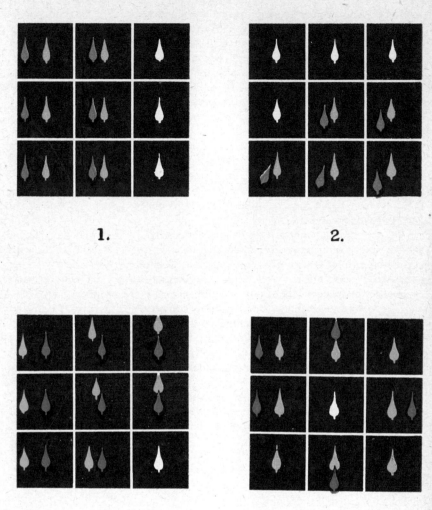

1.   2.   3.   4.

PATIENT'S RIGHT

Fig. 246.—CANDLE TEST FOR DIPLOPIA.—The *red* flame represents the image seen by the *right* eye. The *green* flame represents the image seen by the *left* eye. The white represents the fused images—that is, absence of diplopia.

1. *Right External Rectus Paralysis.*—Homonymous diplopia; false image referable to right eye; diplopia increased on attempted abduction.

2. *Right Superior Oblique Paralysis.*—Diplopia on infraduction or depression; false image referable to right eye; false projection increased on adduction.

3. *Left Internal and Superior Recti Paralysis.*—Crossed diplopia on looking to right; vertical diplopia on looking to left; false image referable to left eye.

4. *Complete External Ophthalmoplegia of Right Eye.*—False projection in every attempted movement; false image referable throughout to right eye.

oscillations may be equally rapid in both directions (pendular nystagmus), or rapid in one direction (cerebral component) and slower (vestibular component) in the other (rhythmic nystagmus). The latter is the commoner type.

Before nystagmus is given a neurological significance, certain ocular causes must be excluded. The more important of these are congenital and early infantile nystagmus occurring in cases of congenitally malformed eyes, albinism ; opacities of the media such as leukoma of the cornea and congenital cataract ; and the occupational nystagmus of coal-miners.

As a physical sign in nervous disease nystagmus indicates a lesion of the cerebellum, vestibular apparatus, or the pathways in the pons and medulla between these. The commonest diseases in which it is found are *disseminated sclerosis*, tumours and other *lesions of the cerebellum*, lesions of the vestibular nerve, tumours and syringomyelia affecting the pons or medulla, and Friedreich's ataxia.

The Fifth or Trigeminal Nerve.—

ANATOMICAL CONSIDERATIONS.—This nerve has motor and sensory roots. Both have their nuclei in the pons. The sensory nucleus also makes connexions with the medulla and spinal cord through the substantia gelatinosa. The motor and sensory roots emerge from different parts of the brain, but come closer together as they approach the Gasserian ganglion on the petrous portion of the temporal bone. Into this ganglion the sensory root enters, but the motor portion lies beneath the ganglion and later joins the inferior maxillary division of the 5th nerve.

From the Gasserian ganglion the three divisions of the 5th nerve emerge : (1) Ophthalmic ; (2) Superior maxillary ; (3) Inferior maxillary. These divisions are responsible for reception of sensation from the greater part of the face, forehead, parietal and temporal regions, nasal and buccal mucosæ, and conjunctiva.

The inferior maxillary division makes connexions through the lingual and facial nerves with the chorda tympani, which is responsible for the sensation of taste in the anterior two-thirds of the tongue. The motor fibres of the same division innervate the muscles of mastication, of which the most important are the temporals, masseters, and pterygoids.

EXAMINATION.—The sensory, motor, and gustatory functions of the nerve must be tested.

Sensation.—Sensation may be tested as elsewhere in the body by the use of cotton-wool and a pin over each area of the face supplied by the three divisions of the 5th nerve. A light wisp of cotton-wool touching the cornea normally produces closure of the eye, but if there is anæsthesia of the cornea the reflex will be abolished. The same result may be obtained by blowing lightly on the conjunctiva. If the 5th nerve has been paralysed for some time serious effects may appear, especially ulceration of the cornea and dryness of the nasal and buccal mucous membrane, with anosmia and difficulty in chewing.

Motor Power.—The position of the teeth should be noted to see if there is any deviation of the jaw. The patient may then be asked to bite on a soft piece of wood with each side of the jaw in turn. The depth of indentation of the teeth gives some idea of the comparative strength of the temporals and masseters. The side-to-side movements (pterygoids) may be tested by asking the patient to move the jaws in a ruminating manner against the resistance of the observer's fingers. If the lesion is in the upper neurone the paresis is rarely marked owing to bilateral cortical innervation. The *jaw-jerk* will be increased in upper neurone lesions and decreased or abolished in those of the lower neurone. Wasting of the muscles of mastication will also be present in lower neurone lesions of considerable standing, giving the face and temple on the affected side a hollowed-out appearance.

Taste.—The sensation of taste is tested in suspected lesions not only of the 5th, but of the 7th and 9th nerves. The anterior two-thirds of the tongue may show loss of taste sensation in 5th or 7th nerve lesions, and the posterior third when the glossopharyngeal nerve is affected.

Substances which are sweet, salt, sour, and bitter (sugar, salt, vinegar, and quinine) should be used in turn by placing a little on one half of the anterior two-thirds of the tongue. The patient should not speak, but write down what he tastes. A weak galvanic current is recognized as a metallic taste, and is particularly useful in testing the posterior third (glossopharyngeal nerve).

LESIONS.—These do not differ from those described on p. 310 for all the cranial nerves. Special mention may be made, however, of pontine lesions (vascular and neoplastic) which involve the 5th nucleus whilst producing pyramidal tract and other characteristic signs. Outside the pons the nerve may be involved by tumours at the base of the brain, especially in the cerebello-pontine angle, and more rarely the Gasserian ganglion or individual branches may be affected by tumours, neuritis, etc.

Trigeminal Neuralgia.—This affection of the 5th nerve needs special consideration in view of its frequency. Any or all of the three sensory branches may be involved, and the patient complains of severe lancinating pain over the distribution of the affected divisions or their smaller branches. The second and third divisions are usually primarily affected, but the first may follow. Localized tenderness is usually present over the same area. Trigeminal neuralgia comes in attacks, at first short, but later of long duration. Long periods of freedom are common. Sometimes no cause is found for it ; sometimes contributory factors such as carious teeth, sinus infection, and overwork are present.

The Seventh or Facial Nerve.—

ANATOMICAL CONSIDERATIONS.—The facial nerve arises from its nucleus in the pons, where its fibres course around the nucleus of the 6th nerve. The nerve emerges in the cerebello-pontine angle in company with the 8th nerve. Both enter the internal auditory meatus, but later the 7th nerve leaves the 8th and runs in the aqueduct of Fallopius to its point of exit at the stylomastoid foramen. Thereafter the nerve is distributed to the facial muscles, all of which it supplies except the levator palpebræ superioris (3rd nerve). In its course through the aqueduct the facial nerve gives off two branches which have localizing value : (1) the nerve to the stapedius ; (2) the chorda tympani.

In cases of facial paralysis it is often possible, if these anatomical data are borne in mind, to determine fairly accurately the part of its course in which the nerve has been damaged. Simultaneous involvement of the 6th nerve is suggestive of a pontine lesion ; concurrent affection of the 7th and 8th nerves is common in lesions at the cerebello-pontine angle ; excessive response to sounds in one ear indicates that the lesion has also affected the nerve to the stapedius in the aqueduct, and loss of taste over the anterior two-thirds of the tongue implies that the 7th nerve has been damaged in the aqueduct before the origin of the chorda tympani. In

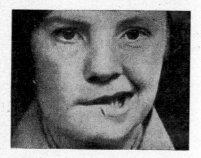

Fig. 247.—Facial paralysis (lower neurone type). The patient is attempting to show the teeth. The right side is paralysed and the angle of the mouth does not move.

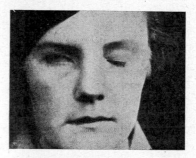

Fig. 248.—Facial paralysis (lower neurone type). The patient is attempting to close the eyes, only with partial success on the paralysed side.

the commonest type of facial lesion, Bell's palsy, these collateral signs are not commonly present, as the nerve is affected either at or after it has left the stylomastoid foramen, or sometimes in its course through the temporal bone. In some cases herpes of the geniculate ganglion may be responsible.

EXAMINATION.—The examination of the facial nerve is primarily designed to test the movements of the facial muscles. The patient should be asked in turn to show the teeth (Fig. 247), puff out the cheeks, wrinkle the forehead by looking upwards, and close the eyes (Fig. 248).

Taste on each half of the anterior two-thirds of the tongue should be tested as described on p. 328. Finally, note should be taken of any abnormal acuity of hearing on the affected side.

LESIONS.—

Facial Paralysis.—This results quite commonly from both upper and lower neurone lesions, though the latter are more frequent.

Upper neurone paralysis : This only affects the muscles of the lower part of the face, as the occipito-frontalis and orbicularis palpebrarum muscles are bilaterally innervated from the cortex. The angle of the mouth droops, the paralysed cheek is puffed out loosely with each expiration. On the other hand, the forehead can be wrinkled normally, and the eye closed (cf. lower neurone lesions).

The abnormal signs are on the opposite side to the lesion in supranuclear affections and on the same side in nuclear or infranuclear.

Lower neurone paralysis (Bell's palsy): If the paralysis is complete the whole side of the face is smooth and free from wrinkles. The lower eyelid droops and the angle of the mouth sags. Saliva may dribble away from the mouth and tears flow over the lower lid. In attempting to look upwards or frown, the wrinkling on the normal side contrasts with the

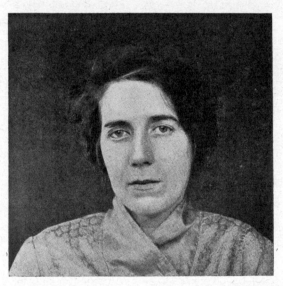

Fig. 249.—Bilateral facial paralysis. In repose the face would pass as normal, though the skin has lost its normal wrinkles. (*Prof. Henry Cohen's case.*) (Cf. *Fig.* 250.)

smoothness of the affected side. The patient is unable to close the eye, and also rolls it upwards in the attempt, due to the mechanical effect of the fibres of the levator palpebræ superioris, supplied from the third nerve, which are partially inserted into the eyeball (*Figs.* 249, 250). The mouth cannot be moved so as to expose the teeth, and when the cheeks are puffed out the paralysed side balloons more than normal.

The electrical reactions are those of a lower neurone lesion (*see* p. 389) and help to distinguish doubtful cases from those due to supranuclear lesions.

If the paralysis does not improve quickly, conjunctival infections may result from inability to close the eye. Later, contractures may draw up the corner of the mouth and make it difficult on superficial observation to determine which is the paralysed side.

Eighth or Auditory Nerve.—
ANATOMICAL CONSIDERATIONS.—This nerve is peculiar in consisting of two nerves which subserve different functions, the cochlear that of hearing, the vestibular that of equilibrium.

The *cochlear nerve* carries auditory impressions from the ganglion spirale to the auditory nuclei in the medulla and thence by way of the fillet, posterior corpora quadrigemina, and optic thalamus to the brain (*see* CEREBRAL LOCALIZATION, p. 294).

The *vestibular nerve* carries impulses from the semicircular canals which are concerned chiefly in the appreciation of change in posture, and

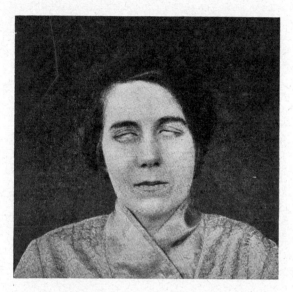

Fig. 250.—The same case. The patient is attempting to close the eyes.

impulses from the otoliths upon which depend the maintenance of a particular posture in a perfect state of equilibrium. The nerve terminates in nuclei within the medulla, which communicate with the cerebellum and mid-brain, and by way of the vestibulo-spinal tract with the spinal cord. The vestibular nuclei thus bring into harmony all parts of the central nervous system concerned in maintenance of muscle tone and balance.

Between the internal auditory meatus and the medulla, the cochlear and vestibular nerves run as a common trunk, the auditory nerve, which passes in close contact with the 7th and 5th nerves through the cerebello-pontine angle, where it is not uncommonly injured.

EXAMINATION.—Examination of the auditory nerve necessitates testing separately the functions of the cochlear and vestibular nerves. In lesions of the 8th nerve in its peripheral course both nerves are affected, but the functions of each division may be separately impaired by intramedullary or other central lesions and by lesions affecting separately the ganglion spirale or ganglion of Scarpa.

The following *symptoms* and *signs* may attract attention to disease of the auditory nerve : deafness, tinnitus (cochlear), and vertigo (vestibular).

Deafness.—This may be noticed by the patient or only discovered by test. It is important first to exclude local causes such as perforation of the drum or wax in the external meatus before proceeding to examine further the nature of the deafness.

Each ear is then tested in turn for its auditory acuity by finding the maximum distance at which a watch can be heard, whilst the other external meatus is closed by means of the finger or a plug of wool. The two ears may then be compared and the results expressed as a fraction as in Snellen's eye charts. If deafness is present in both ears a standard must be taken from a normal person for the particular watch used.

When the presence of deafness has been established the examiner next determines whether it is *nerve deafness* or *middle-ear deafness*. The patient with otitis usually hears better in noisy surroundings. Two special tests are also employed, as follows :—

Rinne's test : A tuning fork is placed on the mastoid process and the patient asked to say immediately he ceases to hear it vibrate. It is then quickly transferred to the external auditory meatus, where it should still be audible if the tympanic membrane and ossicles are conducting normally ; such a result is expressed as Rinne + ve ; but if owing to middle-ear disease the vibrations cannot be heard at the external meatus, the result is Rinne — ve ; expressed differently, conduction of sound by way of the middle ear is more delicate than through bone. If nerve deafness (bone conduction) is present, the tuning fork will not be heard well through the mastoid process, but, if heard at all, will be louder at the meatus.

Weber's test : The tuning fork is placed over the vertex of the skull. Normally it is heard equally well in both ears. In middle-ear disease it is heard better in the affected ear (Weber + ve), as the fused ossicles make conduction through the skull bones complete. In nerve deafness the tuning fork will not be heard on the affected side (Weber — ve).

Tinnitus.—This symptom is variously described by the patient as ringing, buzzing, hissing, singing, or other form of noise in the ear. It may precede deafness as a symptom of 8th nerve disease. It is also common in diseases which indirectly disturb the auditory apparatus, e.g., high blood-pressure, and anæmia, and after exhibition of drugs such as salicylates and quinine. It does not occur in deafness of central origin.

Vertigo.—This is a sensation of giddiness or loss of sense of position in relationship to surrounding objects. Sometimes the patient feels himself rotating (subjective vertigo) ; in other cases surrounding objects appear to rotate (objective vertigo).

Vertigo depends upon abnormal movements in the endolymph and stimulation of the endings of the vestibular nerves. It is therefore often modified by posture, which alters the position of the semicircular canals. It is a common symptom, occurring not only in 8th nerve disease, but in many general conditions such as arteriosclerosis, high blood-pressure, intestinal disturbances, poisoning with alcohol and tobacco, increased intracranial pressure, and so forth. These conditions modify labyrinthine function.

Ménière's Syndrome.—In its most intense form this is usually found in labyrinthine disease. It consists of vertigo, sometimes so extreme that the patient is thrown to the ground, accompanied by nausea and vomiting as reflex vagal effects. The aural origin is suggested by concurrent tinnitus and the deafness which follows, usually in one ear.

Labyrinthine Tests.—In cases of suspected labyrinthine or acoustic nerve disease, tests have been designed to test the function of the labyrinth (Bárány's tests). They consist in observing the response to labyrinthine stimulation induced by rapid rotation, hot and cold water-irrigation of the ears, or a galvanic current applied to the mastoid process. Before making these tests evidence of *irritative* lesions of the labyrinth, cerebellum, or their connexions should be noted. The most important of these are nystagmus, a tendency to fall to one side, and pass-pointing, occurring spontaneously.

Full details of the tests will be found in neurological and otological text-books. As illustrations it may be noted that rotation normally produces nystagmus in the same direction and pass-pointing and falling in the opposite direction. Irrigation of the ear with cold water causes lateral nystagmus to the opposite side and pass-pointing and falling to the same side. If a destructive lesion is present on one side these responses will not be obtained.

The Ninth or Glossopharyngeal and Tenth or Vagus Nerves.—
ANATOMICAL CONSIDERATIONS.—The glossopharyngeal and vagus nerves are usually considered and examined together owing to their close association. They arise in medullary nuclei, and leave the base of the skull through the jugular foramina, where they are not uncommonly damaged. Bulbar affections also tend to involve the vagal nuclei.

The 9th nerve carries taste fibres from the posterior third of the tongue and innervates certain of the muscles concerned in swallowing, but in its motor function the nerve overlaps with the vagus.

The 10th nerve has a wide distribution and innervates many important organs, such as the heart, gastro-intestinal tract, etc. As a bilateral lesion of the vagus is uncommon and fatal, and a unilateral affection is compensated by the work of the other nerve, the examination of the vagus depends chiefly upon testing the function of the branches to the pharynx, soft palate, and larynx.

EXAMINATION.—

1. Test the sensation of taste on the posterior third of the tongue (*see* p. 328).

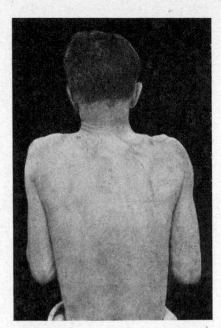

Fig. 251.—Paresis of the right trapezius in 11th nerve paralysis. The patient is shrugging the shoulders: the left moves upwards normally, but not the right: there is also wasting of other muscles of the shoulder girdle.

Fig. 252.—Paresis of the right sternomastoid in 11th nerve paralysis. The patient is turning his head to the left, but the sternomastoid does not stand out prominently as in the non-paralysed muscle on the left side.

Fig. 253.—Control. No paresis of the left sternomastoid, the belly of which stands out well on movement of the head to the right.

Fig. 251.

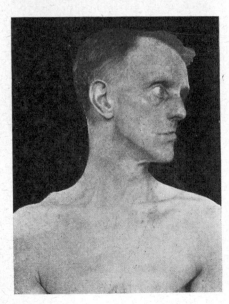

Fig. 252.

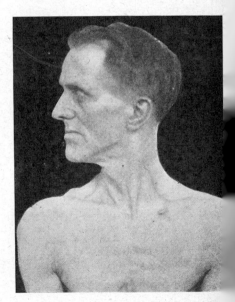

Fig. 253.

2. Test the pharyngeal reflex by tickling each side of the pharynx with a wooden spatula. Unilateral abolition of the reflex only results from organic lesions.

3. Ask the patient to say *ah*—. Normally the uvula moves backwards in the median plane, but in vagal paralysis it is deflected to the normal side. In supranuclear vagal lesions the movements are unaltered.

4. Note any difficulty in deglutition or speaking. In vagal paralysis regurgitation of food through the nose and a nasal voice often occur. These signs are most frequently seen in diphtheritic paralysis.

5. Hoarseness or aphonia calls for a *laryngoscopic examination*. The recurrent laryngeal branch of the vagus is often damaged by aneurysms and other mediastinal tumours, causing abductor paralysis, which when unilateral is symptomless and only discovered by routine use of the laryngoscope.

The Eleventh or Spinal Accessory Nerve.—The spinal accessory nerve supplies the sternomastoid and trapezius muscles. It emerges from the skull through the jugular foramen.

EXAMINATION.—The patient should be asked to shrug the shoulders, when the trapezii come into action, and then to rotate the head, in which act the sternomastoids are employed (*Figs.* 251–253). Sometimes in 11th nerve paralysis the vertebral border of the scapula stands out, rather like the 'winged scapula' of serratus magnus paralysis.

The Twelfth or Hypoglossal Nerve.—The hypoglossal nucleus is in the medulla and in intimate contact with the nuclei of the 7th nerve which control the orbicularis oris. Paralysis of the tongue and of the lips are therefore often found together

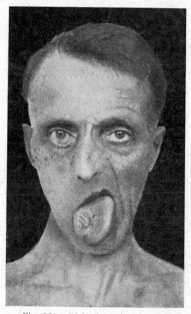

Fig. 254.—Right hypoglossal paralysis. Note the wasting and wrinkling of the right half of the tongue. There is also a 7th nerve palsy on the right side.

in medullary lesions, e.g., progressive bulbar paralysis. The 12th nerve leaves the skull by the anterior condyloid foramen and is subject to injury in its subsequent course in the neck.

EXAMINATION.—The patient should be asked to protrude the tongue. In lower neurone paralysis the affected side is wasted, wrinkled, and sometimes tremulous (*Fig.* 254). The tongue deviates to the affected side as in cases of facial paralysis, but in the latter the deviation can be rectified by straightening the corner of the mouth with the fingers. Dysarthria is often present.

THE DIAGNOSIS OF THE NEUROSES

Even the *definition* of the term neurosis is in a state of flux, but for the purpose of this elementary book it may be held to mean the appearance of symptoms or physical signs of disease in an individual whose organs and tissues, if examined post mortem by such methods as are now available, appear normal.   Clearly, certain conditions at present described as neuroses may be proved to be due to structural changes when our methods of examination both during life and after death become more accurate.

In turning to the *causation* of the neuroses we are on still more uncertain ground, and no attempt can be made here to apportion the blame for the development of neuroses to psychological, endocrine, molecular structural changes, or other suggested causes.   It must suffice to say that neuroses may imitate organic diseases in such minute detail as to make diagnosis extremely difficult, and occasionally impossible for a time.   The imitation only fails by the patient's lack of correct anatomical and physiological knowledge.   The more detailed this knowledge (acquired by observation of other patients, from the doctors' or nurses' conversation, etc.), the more closely is an organic condition simulated.

Symptoms in Neuroses.—Since the symptoms in neuroses arise principally from disturbances of the psychological processes, their name is necessarily legion.

The *hypochondriac* may declare that he has a cancer, that his bowels are stopped up, or that his liver is not working, statements without any foundation.

The *neurasthenic* frequently complains of a ' band round the head ', or a sense of weight on the vertex, of loss of sexual function, or of visceral disturbances such as palpitation, abdominal discomfort, etc.   He is easily fatigued both physically and mentally, and a history of masturbation is common.

The patient with an *anxiety neurosis* lives in a state of fear (phobia), sometimes of some well-defined condition such as heart disease or syphilis, sometimes of an ill-defined sense of calamity.

In *compulsion neuroses* the patient is subject to obsessions, to which all other features of his life are of secondary consideration.   He may be obsessed with the idea of killing, of stealing, of falling from a high building, to name a few examples.   In some cases these obsessional ideas are translated into action.   The person obsessed with the idea of personal uncleanliness may bathe many times daily.

The essential characteristics of *hysteria* is the appearance of *conversion* symptoms or signs.   By this is meant the expression in terms of disease of mental processes which for some reason cannot be allowed to enter the field of consciousness.   Thus grief or sexual emotion forcefully repressed may find expression in symptoms and signs such as pain, anæsthesia, or paralysis.   The symptoms are of every possible variety and combination, and what has been said of neuroses in general is especially true of hysteria, that the symptoms and signs are only limited by the patient's knowledge or lack of knowledge of disease processes. A point of great importance in hysterical manifestations is the suddenness with which they may appear and disappear.

Physical Signs in Neuroses.—It is only to be expected in view of the psychogenic origin of the neuroses that symptoms, e.g., phobias, obsessions, etc., are often present without physical signs. Nevertheless, physical signs are also found to support the diagnosis, especially in hysteria, in which they may be of extraordinary variety. They all differ, however, from the physical signs of organic disease in details which are only appreciated by the trained medical observer, and even to him may present problems of considerable difficulty. Some of the commoner physical signs of neurosis may be briefly considered.

Motor Signs.—*Fits* superficially imitating those of epilepsy may be seen. They rarely occur without an audience and do not have the definite sequence of true epilepsy. The convulsive movements have a struggling character and can often be modified (increased or diminished) by suggestion. Incontinence is uncommon, and the patient rarely injures herself.

Paralysis may be monoplegic, paraplegic, or hemiplegic as in organic disease, but the characteristic signs of upper or lower neurone paralysis are not to be found. Babinski's sign never occurs, nor true clonus, though the tendon reflexes may be exaggerated. Similarly, though the paralysis may be flaccid, the rapid wasting and electrical changes of lower neurone lesions are not present. The brisk response of the ' paralysed ' muscles to electrical stimulation may form most conclusive evidence of the functional nature of the condition. When the paralysis is limited, e.g., to certain movements of the arms, its functional character is often betrayed by lack of the adherence to anatomical detail which characterizes organic paralysis.

Paralyses are not confined to the limbs. A common variety is weakness of the adductors of the vocal cords, causing the popular hysterical symptom of *aphonia*, in which the patient speaks only in a whisper, though she may be able to sing. Ptoses, and weakness of half the tongue with consequent deviation to one side, are other illustrations.

Sensory Signs.—All types of anæsthesia may be found, but the ' glove ' and ' stocking ' varieties are especially characteristic. The sensory loss does not conform to a nerve or root distribution as in the case of organic disease, and when hemianæsthesia is present there is a sharp cleavage at the midline between the normal and the anæsthetic sides of the body, which makes no allowance for the normal cutaneous overlap.

Abnormalities of the Special Senses.—*Contraction of the visual field* is a common hysterical manifestation. Blindness is uncommon, and is usually limited to one eye. Photophobia may occur. Hysterical deafness, and derangements of the sense of smell or taste, are relatively uncommon.

Visceral Symptoms and Signs.—These are very common. *Constipation* is most frequent, though diarrhœa may occur. Hysterical *vomiting* may be associated with *anorexia* and cause emaciation. In the extreme

22

form of *anorexia nervosa* the patient may even die from emaciation. More commonly the vomiting does not interfere with the appetite, and though the symptom may persist for months, the general condition remains quite good.

Abdominal distension is another sign which may cause difficulty. In barren women the great desire for children may cause progressive distension of the abdomen simulating pregnancy—*pseudocyesis*.

The gastro-intestinal tract supplies most of the visceral signs in hysteria, but other systems may be selected. Retention of urine is common, incontinence less so. *Tachycardia* is occasionally present.

Occupational Neuroses.—These are closely allied to hysteria. The patient finds himself unable to perform the precise series of movements upon which his occupation depends. Such patients are usually of neurotic personality and their occupation requires the continual use of certain groups of muscles—e.g., players of stringed instruments, watchmakers, typists, and writers. The condition is seen most vividly in *writer's cramp*. The patient finds that the hand rapidly becomes fatigued, the writing shaky, and actual cramp-like pain may occur.

The Neurotic Personality.—In conclusion, a brief account of the type of individual in whom the symptoms and signs just described are commonly found will not be out of place. He is usually self-centred, pre-occupied with his own affairs, and in particular with his bodily health. His mental ability is often above normal, though in some cases of hysteria much below. Irritability, lack of concentration, and nervousness are common, especially in *neurasthenia*. In this condition also tremors of the hands and eyelids are usually noticeable, and the tendon reflexes are exaggerated.

Degenerate stigmata may be found in some cases, especially of *hysteria*. The lobes of the ears are ill formed and fused with the skin near the mastoid process, instead of hanging freely. The palate is often high and arched in Gothic style. The tongue may be unduly fissured and frothy. Anæsthesiæ of the pharynx or conjunctiva, though often described as stigmata, are really sensory manifestations of hysteria, and are not very commonly present.

SPECIAL INVESTIGATIONS

The more important special investigations in the examination of the nervous system include the chemical and microscopical examination of the cerebrospinal fluid, the employment of lumbar, cisternal, and ventricular puncture, lipiodol injections, encephalography and ventriculography, and the study of the electrical reactions. (*See* Chapters XII and XIV.)

CHAPTER X

FEVER

FEVER, or *pyrexia*, is present when the body temperature as taken in the rectum rises above 98·4° F. at any time in the twenty-four hours. It is a feature of many diseases in which other signs dominate the clinical picture, but sometimes it is the most prominent or even the sole abnormal physical sign for a period of time. The present chapter relates more especially to fever in such cases.

Use of the Thermometer.—The patient's temperature is almost invariably recorded in hospital by the nurse, but in private practice by the doctor, and the student should be quite familiar with the use of the clinical thermometer.

English thermometers are graduated in degrees Fahrenheit, ranging between 95° and 110°. An arrow points to the average normal temperature, 98·4°.

The temperature may be taken from the skin in the axilla, or groin in infants ; or from the mucous membranes, the mouth in adults and the rectum in infants.

The temperature in the mouth is approximately half a degree, and that in the rectum one degree, higher than in the axilla. Thermometers vary in the time taken to record the temperature, and it is a safe rule to allow longer than stated on the instrument, e.g., two minutes for a one-minute thermometer. The instrument should make close contact with the skin, and when used in the mouth should be gripped between the closed lips.

The normal temperature varies somewhat, and may be half a degree more or one degree less than 98·4° in perfectly healthy persons. Allowances should be made for trivial rises of temperature which may occur after meals, hot baths, and severe exertion. The evening temperature is normally about 1° higher than the morning. This variation is also noticeable in cases of fever, but occasionally an inverse type occurs—e.g., in some cases of phthisis, typhoid fever, and meningococcal infections.

The temperature may fall to 96° or 95° in cases of severe shock and collapse. Such a fall is described as a ' subnormal ' temperature. At the opposite extreme a rise of temperature to more than 105° is arbitrarily styled ' hyperpyrexia '.

TYPES OF FEVER

The type of fever, especially in cases of long duration, is often of great value in diagnosis. The temperature chart in cases of malaria, for example, may be almost pathognomonic. Characteristic features should be looked for in the rise, the course, and the fall of the temperature.

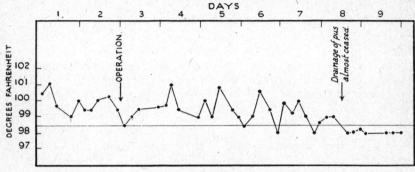

Fig. 255.—Remittent fever. Due to empyema. The temperature changes from a remittent to an intermittent form before it finally subsides.

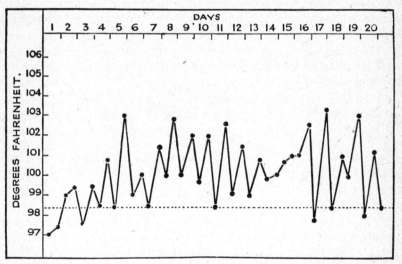

Fig. 256.—Remittent fever. Case of tuberculous peritonitis. Note that the temperature 'swings' between 99° and 103° F., but rarely reaches normal. (Figs. 256, 257 from the author's 'Text-book of Medicine for Nurses', Oxford University Press.)

The Rise.—The rise in some illnesses is abrupt, e.g., pneumonia and erysipelas, and quickly reaches 104° or 105°. In other conditions the rise is gradual, e.g., typhoid fever and miliary tuberculosis, taking several days to reach its maximum. In typhoid the temperature rises in a series of steps.

The Course.—The course of the temperature is classically described as continuous, remittent, or intermittent. The total duration is important, as the causes of fever of short duration differ from those of long duration.

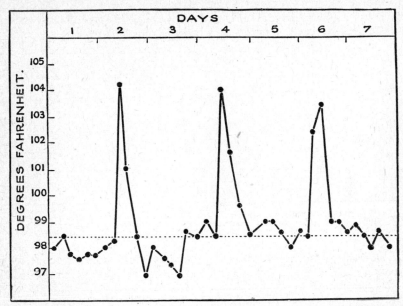

Fig. 257.—Intermittent fever. Case of malaria (benign tertian). Note that the temperature rises at approximately the same time each day, but falls below normal in the intervening periods.

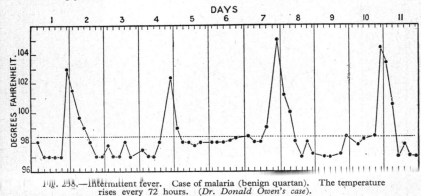

Fig. 258.—Intermittent fever. Case of malaria (benign quartan). The temperature rises every 72 hours. (*Dr. Donald Owen's case*).

The exanthemata form the most important group of initially obscure fevers of short duration.

Continuous Fever.—May continue for days or weeks. The difference between the morning and evening readings is comparatively small, usually $1°$ or $2°$. Examples are seen in lobar pneumonia (lasting seven days), typhoid fever in the second week, and erysipelas whilst the rash is spreading.

Remittent Fever.—Shows a considerable difference between the morning and evening temperature, usually between 2° and 4°, but the morning temperature does not reach normal (*Figs.* 255, 256). This type of fever is common in suppurative processes, especially deep-seated abscesses (e.g., appendix abscess and empyema) ; in tuberculosis, especially of the lungs ; and in many forms of septicæmia and pyæmia.

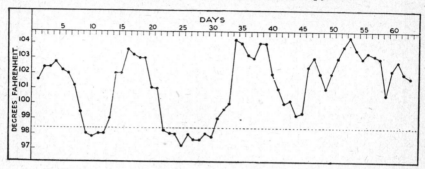

Fig. 259.—Pel-Ebstein phenomenon. The chart shows the maximum daily temperature over a period of 60 days. The characteristic alternation of pyrexia and apyrexia is present in the first 45 days, but the pyrexia is more continuous towards the end. (*Dr. Donald Owen's case.*)

Intermittent Fever.—In this type the temperature rises for a few hours, usually to 104° or 105°, and then falls to normal or below. It is classically

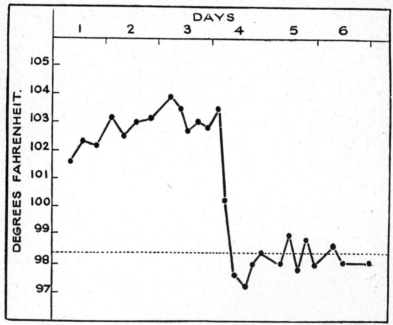

Fig. 260.—Case of lobar pneumonia ending by crisis. (*Figs.* 260, 261 *from the author's* 'Text-book of Medicine for Nurses', Oxford University Press.)

seen in the benign tertian and quartan fevers of malaria (*Figs.* 257, 258). In the former the temperature rises once in forty-eight hours, in the latter once in seventy-two hours.

Combination of these three types of fever are often found. In typhoid fever, for example, the temperature in the first week is slightly remittent, and often presents the *staircase phenomenon*, i.e., each day it is a little higher, although the morning remission may bring it below that of the previous evening. In the second week the fluctuations of temperature are slight and the fever is of the continuous type ; but in the third week the fluctuations are considerable (3° or 4°) and the fever is of a well-marked remittent variety.

Again in pneumonia the continuous fever of the first week may pass insidiously into a remittent fever if an empyema forms. This illustrates

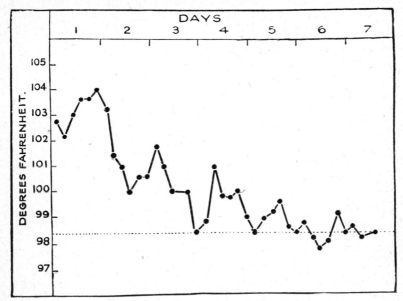

Fig. 261.—Case of broncho-pneumonia subsiding by lysis.

the *importance of a change in the form of the temperature curve*, which often indicates the presence of complications in the disease.

The course of a fever may be regular or irregular. Notable examples of *regular* fevers are seen in lobar pneumonia and the benign forms of malaria. *Irregular* fevers are commoner. Examples are found in bronchopneumonia, phthisis, sepsis, and so forth.

Sometimes the temperature is raised for a few days, to be followed by an apyrexial period. This occurs in an irregular manner in subacute infective endocarditis. A more regular alternation between pyrexia and apyrexia may occur in lymphadenoma, especially when deep-seated, and is known as the *Pel-Ebstein phenomenon* ; the temperature is raised for seven to ten days, after which it falls for about two weeks (*Fig.* 259). Of a similar type is undulant fever, due to infections with *B. abortus* and *B. melitensis.* True relapsing fever and rat-bite fever are rarer causes in this country.

The Fall.—The temperature may fall suddenly, reaching normal in 6 to 12 hours. This is known as a *crisis* (*Fig.* 260), and is generally accompanied by a simultaneous drop in the pulse-rate and an improvement in the patient's condition. A *protracted crisis* may take twenty-four hours for the temperature to reach normal. Crisis is well seen in pneumonia and erysipelas. Sometimes it is preceded by a sharp increase in the fever, known as the *pre-critical rise* ; in other cases by a fall, the *pseudo-crisis*, followed by another rise before the temperature becomes normal with the true crisis.

When the fever subsides gradually over several days the term *lysis* is used (*Fig.* 261). It is a commoner mode of termination than crisis, and is found in most fevers, e.g., exanthemata, broncho-pneumonia, typhoid, sepsis, etc.

SYMPTOMS AND SIGNS OF FEVER

Fever results from a disturbance of the heat-regulating apparatus of the body usually caused by bacteria or their toxins. For ordinary clinical purposes it can be taken, therefore, as a sign of infection, and its symptoms are similar whatever the nature of this may be. It is necessary, however, to note that the heat-regulating mechanism may be rendered unstable by causes other than infection. In patients convalescent from febrile and other serious illnesses, in neurotic individuals and addicts to alcohol and drugs, in profound anæmias, malignant disease, and metabolic disorders, transient pyrexia may occur, which has little clinical significance.

The more important symptoms and signs associated with fever are as follows :—

A *rigor*, or shivering attack, is common at the beginning of many fevers, especially those of an acute nature such as pneumonia and erysipelas. Repeated rigors may be of diagnostic value, suggesting the possibility of malarial fever if they occur at regular intervals, or of severe infections such as pyelitis, cholangitis, pyæmia, etc., when they occur irregularly.

Tachycardia is usual, but its degree varies much and may be a useful sign in differential diagnosis. For example, the pulse is unduly raised in scarlet fever and tuberculosis, but in typhoid is rarely above 110 in the second week, when the temperature may average 104°. Cerebral conditions with fever, e.g., meningitis and cerebral abscess, are accompanied by an unusually slow pulse due to the increased intracranial tension. In most fevers the heart-rate increases 8 beats per minute in an adult or 10 to 15 beats in a child for each degree rise in temperature.

The *appearance* of the patient is characteristic. The face is flushed and hot, the skin hot and dry, though sweating is characteristic of some fevers (e.g., rheumatic fever, sepsis) and occurs in most when the temperature falls.

Delirium is common, and may be of a low type with muttering and partial coma, or of an active violent type.

The *appetite* is diminished, but *thirst* is great. The *tongue* is furred, and, in prolonged pyrexia, dry and crusted. The *bowels* are usually constipated, though diarrhœa is a symptom in intestinal infections such as typhoid and cholera. The *urine* is diminished, of high colour owing to excess of urates, of high specific gravity, and may contain albumin. These changes result from loss of fluid by sweating and from the increased metabolism consequent on fever.

The *respiratory rate* is increased slightly in most fevers, but only respiratory infections (e.g., pneumonia, bronchitis) cause an increase of more than 2 respirations per minute for each degree of fever.

DIAGNOSIS OF DISEASES CHARACTERIZED BY FEVER

The diagnosis of scarlet fever with the rash developed, or of typhoid fever with characteristic symptoms and a positive Widal reaction, is simple, but without their special symptoms and signs they may present a very obscure picture in which fever is the only definite sign. How often is poor Dr. A denounced as a fool because he was unable to recognize a case of measles before the rash appeared, whilst clever Dr. B arriving on the fifth day instantly made a correct diagnosis ! Yet it must be frankly admitted that fever may remain the only symptom of a disease for days or weeks, and a diagnosis is not possible until other symptoms are forthcoming. In many instances, however, it is possible to make a provisional diagnosis by a careful consideration of the type of fever ; of the patient's history and environmental circumstances ; of any localizing symptoms and signs ; and of the results of special investigations.

The *type of fever* has already received attention.

The *history* may be important, especially in epidemic diseases, and inquiry should be made for any similar cases of fever in the household or district, or of any known case of typhoid, measles, scarlet fever, or other infectious disease. The purity of food and water is also of prime importance, and any contamination may have an important bearing on the case. Some diseases such as measles, scarlet fever, typhoid fever, and small pox confer immunity and only rarely affect the same individual twice. Others such as pneumonia, influenza, and rheumatic fever appear to predispose to subsequent attacks. This immunity from, or predisposition to, second attacks may be of value in difficult cases. Bites from rats and kittens may raise the possibility of rat-bite fever, and signs of inflammation may be still present around the region of the bite.

The *localizing symptoms and signs*, and the results of *special investigations*, require more detailed consideration.

LOCALIZING SYMPTOMS AND SIGNS

The symptoms and physical signs indicative of disease in individual systems or viscera are described elsewhere in this book. In the present section it must suffice to call attention to the importance of isolated and apparently trivial symptoms and signs in obscure cases of fever.

The Skin.—The skin should be inspected first. A rash may establish the diagnosis in the *exanthemata*—measles, small-pox, scarlet fever, etc.—but *repeated daily inspection* is necessary if the rash is not to be overlooked. *Petechial rashes* are important evidence of septicæmia, e.g., infective endocarditis and acute miliary tuberculosis. Many other febrile illnesses such as typhoid, typhus, and secondary syphilis have fleeting rashes at some part of their course, which may be useful diagnostic features.

The Face.—An area of relative whiteness round the mouth—circumoral pallor—can be seen in most fevers, but is especially prominent in scarlet fever. A miserable facies with coryza and conjunctival injection may suggest measles before the rash appears.

Herpes labialis has already been described (*see* p. 27). It is of diagnostic importance in pneumonia, malaria, and cerebrospinal fever, but occurs frequently with the common cold.

The diagnosis of *mumps*, an infectious form of parotitis, is made by inspection of the face. The parotid tumour forms a swelling in front of the ear, extending downwards and projecting backwards over the ramus of the mandible.

The Mouth and Throat.—An inspection of these is especially necessary in children. Small bluish white *Koplik spots* on the mucous membrane of the mouth may identity a case of measles before the rash has appeared. They appear usually on the second day of the illness. (*See Fig.* 43, p. 47.) The *strawberry tongue*, consisting of reddened papillæ projecting through a brownish fur, may be suggestive of scarlet fever, whilst in rheumatic fever the less pathognomonic thickly furred ' blanket tongue ' is often seen.

The clinical diagnosis of tonsillitis and diphtheria is made by inspection of the fauces. In *tonsillitis* the tonsils are enlarged, reddened, and dotted with a creamy yellow exudate which can be wiped off. The punctate character of the exudate may be lost if the patches fuse, and the exudate may then resemble that of diphtheria. The membrane of *diphtheria* is more continuous than that of tonsillitis, often covering the tonsils and uvula, and extending backwards into the pharynx. It is of a greyish appearance, and is not easily removed, leaving a bleeding surface behind if wiped. *Children with diphtheria frequently make no complaint of a sore throat*, and it is vital that the throat should be examined in all doubtful cases of pyrexia. It should be borne in mind also that tonsillitis is a common feature of other diseases, particularly of scarlet fever and rheumatic infections.

The Nose and Ears.—Infection of the *nasal sinuses*, antral, frontal, and ethmoidal, should be considered as a possibility in cases of fever with headache or facial pain. The diagnosis requires transillumination, X-ray examination, or proof puncture.

Earache generally calls attention to *ear infections*, which may cause fever and necessitate an examination of the ear-drums and mastoid processes.

The Respiratory System.—The symptoms and physical signs of respiratory disease are discussed in Chapter III. If any are present in a case of unexplained pyrexia, they should be given due consideration.

Early cases of *pneumonia* may prove very difficult to diagnose, but symptoms and signs such as increased respiratory rate, rusty sputum, and herpes are valuable leads to a correct diagnosis. Continued pyrexia after pneumonia should always raise the possibility of complications such as empyema, pulmonary abscess, pericarditis, etc.

The Cardio-vascular System.—The pyrexial disease of this system which causes most difficulty is *infective endocarditis*, especially in its sub-acute form, when for a long time pyrexia may be the only abnormal sign apart from evidence of a valvular lesion of the heart. Careful examination must be made daily for septicæmic signs (*see* p. 348), to support the diagnosis.

More rarely *rheumatic infections* (endocarditis, pericarditis, and myo-carditis) may cause difficulty, and other evidence of rheumatism, e.g., joint pains, nodules, or sore throat, must be sought.

The Digestive System.—The discovery of a focus of infection in the abdomen causing pyrexia is often very difficult. Deeply situated *abscesses*, e.g., from the appendix, kidney, or Fallopian tube, should always be contemplated, and the history and examination of the blood are of most value if the usual physical signs of abdominal disease are absent. Further consideration of these problems, however, would lead into surgical domains.

Typhoid and paratyphoid fevers are the most important medical diseases which cause pyrexia with abdominal symptoms. Typhoid, though less common in Great Britain than formerly, serves as a type of fever which illustrates many points in connexion with pyrexial diseases, and will repay a fuller study in a text-book of medicine. Here it is only necessary to draw attention to the difficulty of diagnosis when fever is the sole well-defined symptom. The insidious mode of onset (more sudden in para-typhoid infections) with epistaxis or bronchitis is suggestive. In the fully developed disease the semi-comatose condition of the patient, with low delirium and intestinal symptoms, are the principal diagnostic features. The intestinal symptoms include vague abdominal pain, with tenderness, tympanites, and either diarrhœa or constipation. The slow rise of tempera-ture by steps in the first week, the sustained fever of the second week, and the fall by lysis in the third week have already been mentioned. Septicæmic signs are the splenic enlargement and rash. Notable confirm-atory signs are a relatively slow pulse-rate, leucopenia, and a positive blood-culture or Widal reaction. Relapses are common in enteric infections.

The Hæmopoietic System.—Diseases of this system are rarely responsible for obscure pyrexia except in the case of lymphadenoma (*see*

Pel-Ebstein type of fever, p. 343). When diseases such as pernicious anæmia and acute leukæmia are responsible for pyrexia the other symptoms and signs make the diagnosis easy.

Under this system, however, *blood-stream infections* should be considered. Enlargement of the spleen (usually 1 to 2 in. below the costal margin), petechiæ, rigors, and sweating in cases of pyæmia, are the principal signs, but in low-grade septicæmias these signs may be absent and the diagnosis will rest upon special methods of examination. Pyæmia is further characterized by the formation of abscesses in different parts of the body.

The Genito-urinary System.—Frequency of micturition and dysuria should call attention to the possibility of urinary infection, and a full examination of the urine is then necessary.

Bacilluria may cause no fever, but if pyuria is also present, fever generally occurs, though it is less marked when the lower parts of the urinary tract (bladder and urethra) are affected. The accessory organs, prostate and seminal vesicles, should be examined for enlargement and tenderness.

In women, vaginal examination may be necessary to exclude inflammatory disease of the generative organs.

The Nervous System.—The full symptomatology of nervous diseases is considered in Chapters VIII and IX. Several infections of the nervous system may present difficulties in the early stages :—

Anterior poliomyelitis may be ushered in with fever and generalized pains, and is often thought to be an 'influenzal attack' until evidence of paralysis appears.

Acute myelitis may also present difficulties, but as a rule sensory and motor changes in the limbs and disturbances of micturition soon make a diagnosis possible.

Meningitis, especially the more insidious tuberculous variety, should be considered, particularly in children, as a possible cause of unexplained pyrexia. Photophobia, stiffness of the neck, and Kernig's sign should be looked for, but a lumbar puncture and examination of the cerebrospinal fluid is generally necessary to establish the diagnosis.

Encephalitis lethargica, a protean disease, also offers great difficulties. Mental symptoms, changes in sleep rhythm, and ocular paresis of a transient character should suggest the possibility of this disease.

Cerebral abscess may be suspected when signs of a cerebral tumour are associated with fever, especially if some focus of infection (e.g., otitis media, frontal sinusitis) exists from which infection may have spread into the brain.

The Muscles and Joints.—Diseases of these parts usually present no difficulty when they cause pyrexia, as other symptoms and signs point to the nature of the condition, e.g., *myositis*, and rheumatic and other forms of *arthritis*.

Deep-seated bone infections, especially *osteomyelitis*, may occasionally be responsible for obscure pyrexia. As in other forms of sepsis, the presence of leucocytosis is important (*see* p. 218).

SPECIAL INVESTIGATIONS

(For details *see* Chapter XIV.)

The special investigations are of particular importance in elucidating the problem of pyrexia of unknown origin. Amongst those of special value must be mentioned blood-culture in suspected septicæmias, agglutination reactions in enteric and abortus infections, leucocyte counts which may give a clue to the nature of the infection, and examination of pathological specimens—e.g., urine, fæces, and cerebrospinal fluid.

The *therapeutic test* may also be of great value. Few cases of rheumatic fever fail to respond to salicylates. Emetine is responsible for a rapid improvement in amœbic dysentery and sometimes in amœbic liver abscess. Paroxysms of malaria of the benign types can be abolished by a few suitable doses of quinine.

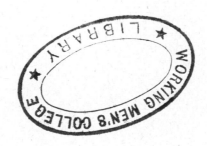

CHAPTER XI

THE EXAMINATION OF SICK CHILDREN

By NORMAN B. CAPON, M.D., F.R.C.P.

Professor of Child Health, University of Liverpool ; Hon. Physician, Royal Liverpool Children's Hospital ; Visiting Physician, Alder Hey Children's Hospital, Liverpool.

THE aims of this chapter are, first, to explain how best to lessen and overcome the difficulties which are so often met during the clinical examination of young patients ; and secondly, to give a short description of those findings which are encountered frequently during childhood, or which are more or less limited to children.* It will be necessary, also, to make reference to some clinical features which, although occurring at all ages, present peculiarities in the child.

The student who watches an efficient and experienced pædiatrician at work will quickly realize that his skill is the expression of much more than technical dexterity ; his clinical method, moulded to the practice of pædiatrics (though without loss of precision), and illuminated by the charity which comes of long contact with children, is so intimately a part of his nature that it may be considered to be a mode of living rather than an observational and experimental investigation. Years must pass before a like skill may be attained ; but the student should make a start as soon as possible, remembering that children form a large proportion of patients seen in general practice.

The following observations will be of help as a preliminary to the more detailed description :—

1. In general terms the established methods of clinical medicine are applicable to patients of all ages, though they require to be modified for children ; they should be used with common sense, accuracy, and gentleness. *To be a competent pædiatrician you must first be a competent physician.*

2. When the patient is a child, subjective symptomatology is often lacking, and the observer must try to make up for this by listening patiently to the mother's history and by unusual care, patience, and accuracy in the clinical examination. *You must take time, be patient, accurate, thoughtful, observant, and gentle when you are examining children.*

---

* For descriptive purposes it is often helpful to be able to indicate the particular portion of the childhood epoch to which one refers. The general significance of certain words used in this chapter is as follows :—
Newborn baby, a child who has not reached the 28th day of postnatal life.
Baby, a child under the age of 12 months.
Infant, a child in the second year of life.
Young child, a child between the ages of 2 and 6 years.
Older child, a child between the ages of 6 and 14 years.

3. Children are easily frightened, with the result that the clinical examination may be a failure. *You must learn a special dexterity and tact in handling children and their parents* ; but this will never be more than a technical facility unless honesty of purpose, humility, genuine sympathy, and interest combine in the undertaking. The clinician's character and personality are on trial each time he comes into professional contact with a child. He must not feign qualities which he does not possess, for a child quickly senses dishonesty.

4. It is important to learn about normal children and the physiological changes which take place in them from month to month and from year to year.

5. Finally, the student must learn to appreciate the breadth of pædiatrics. It is not, like gynæcology or dermatology, a comparatively small special subject bounded by anatomical limits ; nor is it, like obstetrics, concerned only with one physiological process and the pathological changes which may occur in or be associated with that process. Pædiatrics concerns the whole child in health and disease ; it includes the physical, mental, moral, educational, and spiritual aspects of childhood. Doctors are rightly consulted about many of the different problems, in addition to those associated with ordinary illness, which arise during childhood ; thus general management, hygiene, diet, and education are subjects upon which the physician should be qualified to give advice.

HISTORY OF THE PATIENT

The mother or nurse must be carefully questioned, and it is well to follow a set plan as far as possible. The most important details are :—

1. Family history, including the health of both parents and of all brothers and sisters. Information is not always volunteered about miscarriages, and it is well to put a definite question on this point.

2. The health of the mother during her pregnancy.

3. Obstetrical details of the labour, remembering that the rupture of membranes introduces the period of special danger to the fœtus:

4. The birth-weight, and a general outline of the subsquent growth in weight, height, and general physical, mental, and educational ability.

5. Exact details of feeding. This is particularly important when the patient is under the age of 2 years, and it may be necessary to see the spoons or measures in use before it is possible to be certain of the quantities of food which the child has received

6. Notes of important previous illnesses.

7. The possibility of recent contact with infection, including tuberculous adults.

8. The history of the present illness. The mother is generally a keen observer and it is seldom wise to cut short her description. She quickly recognizes slight changes in her child's behaviour, temperament, vitality, appetite, and appearance ; these facts are of great importance and fully compensate for the loss of time spent in listening to the theories which

she often brings forward to explain her observations. Furthermore, an observant clinician will learn much of the mother's temperament and of her ability in handling the child if he listens patiently to her remarks. Features of special importance, to be asked for if the information is not volunteered, are the following :—

a. Sleep : this should be of sufficient duration, and should be sound, peaceful, and unaccompanied by snoring.

b. Vitality and playfulness.

c. Appetite.

d. Temperament.

e. Bowel-actions : frequency and character of motions.

When the patient is a baby, the following further points require investigation :—

f. Cry : character and frequency. The strength of the cry may often be accepted as an indication of the child's vitality.

g. State of contentment.

h. Vomiting and colic.

CLINICAL EXAMINATION

The student's approach to a sick child should aim at winning the patient's confidence. Hurry, bustle, quick movements, and a loud voice all tend to alarm the patient. The observer should talk quietly to the mother or nurse and should seem scarcely to notice the child, who is thus given the opportunity of watching the physician and growing accustomed to him. To stare at a child may make him cry and prejudice the interview from its start. Put a toy in his hands and let him play with it while the history of the illness is described and recorded. Then approach the patient quietly and join him in playing with the toy ; in this way the child's fears may be overcome.

Well-meaning relatives frequently frighten a child by trying to assure him that the examination will be painless ; this difficulty may be lessened by having only one relative in the room during the consultation. Sometimes a child of speaking-age is interviewed most successfully when he is seen quite alone ; it may then be more easy to manage him, and he sometimes discloses valuable information about home conditions which he would not state in the presence of his parents.

The examination of older children may be carried out on the adult plan, taking system by system. Babies and infants, however, are seldom amenable to this method, and the description here given must be taken to apply especially to them.

If the child is lying quietly, asleep or awake, it is wise to note general features such as colour, state of nutrition, respiratory rate, attitude, and so forth before there is any likelihood of disturbance as a result of fear or temper. It may be possible to listen to the patient's heart before the clothes have been entirely removed and so hear the sounds clearly, free from the noise of crying. In any case it is always wise to leave the examination of certain parts, especially the throat, ears, and rectum (when this is necessary) until the end of the consultation.

The child should be stripped of all clothes except the napkin, and should lie wrapped loosely in a warm blanket on the lap of the mother or nurse. The observer, having washed his hands in warm water, sits facing the child, and it is well so to arrange the chairs that the light comes from behind the physician, and falls upon the patient. An electric radiator placed beside the physician may be used by him to warm his hands during the examination, and may be so directed that its beam falls also upon the child. A clean receptacle for urine (chamber or small basin) should be nearby, in order to obtain a specimen of urine if the bladder is emptied during the examination. Many children over the age of 6 months cry if they are made to lie down, and it is often better to begin the examination with the patient sitting up. A crying infant may sometimes be pacified by giving him a feed or by allowing him to suck a dummy-teat.

The student will probably experience more difficulty in forming an accurate opinion of the child's general condition than he will in recognizing some local disability, such as paralysis of one limb. This is one way in which pædiatrics differs from 'adult' medicine, for even a layman of average intelligence can recognize when a man or woman is desperately ill, though he may not know the nature of the illness. Not so with children ; long experience may be required to detect even serious states of disablement, such as loss of consciousness, blindness, or mental defect, in a baby.

For this reason, and also because infectious illnesses are common in childhood, the student should always ask two questions of himself while he is examining the patient : (1) Is the child seriously ill or seriously deformed, either physically or mentally ? and (2) Has the child a contagious or infectious illness ? The evidence which must be weighed up in answering the first question is dealt with in the following pages of this chapter. In regard to infection and contagion, the entire skin-area and the interior of the mouth should be examined for a rash ; the ears and nose for any discharge ; the fauces and umbilicus for diphtheritic membrane ; the vulva and eyes for gonorrhœa ; and the hair and scalp for parasites of various kinds. When an infectious or contagious disease is diagnosed, it must be remembered that the illness of the patient is not necessarily explained by it, for the infection may be a chance finding.

General Examination. The following are the most important features which require investigation : (1) Weight and height ; (2) Cardiac and respiratory rates ; (3) Temperature ; (4) Consciousness ; (5) Vitality and playfulness ; (6) Tissue-turgor ; (7) Colour ; (8) Muscle tonus and stance ; (9) Sleep ; (10) The sucking reflex ; (11) The voice ; (12) The skull ; (13) The face ; (14) The neck.

1. *Weight and Height.*—Babies should be weighed naked, on a blanket of known weight. A simple weighing machine, with pan and weights, is excellent for the purpose, being more accurate than the small

23

spring-balance. The mean of two weighings should be taken, the longitudinal position of the baby being reversed between the two readings.

The height or length of babies and infants is generally of less value than the weight, but in some circumstances (e.g., cœliac disease and infantilism) it is of great importance. The crown-heel measurement is usually employed, care being taken to ensure that the hips and knees are not flexed.

There are various types of bodily configuration in childhood as in adult life, and it is not possible to lay down any absolute standards of weight and height at different ages. The following figures give average findings, and are of value in determining whether a child is materially above or below the normal.

The birth-weight at full term is about 7 lb. ; during the first week of postnatal life there is usually a loss of about 8 oz., but the birth-weight is regained by the 10th to 12th day, and thereafter there should be a steady but gradually decreasing gain of 5 to 8 oz. a week. Hence at 3 months the child weighs $11\frac{1}{2}$ to 12 lb. ; at 5 months 14 lb. (double the birth-weight) ; at 6 months $15\frac{1}{2}$ lb. ; at one year 20–21 lb. (treble the birth-weight). The child of 2 years weighs about 27–28 lb., at 6 years he reaches 42–44 lb., and at 14 years about 84 lb.

It is not always remembered that gain in weight *at a satisfactory rate* is as normal a feature of healthy childhood as maintenance of flesh is a feature of normal adult life ; hence a child that is gaining weight at less than the average normal rate is equivalent to the adult who is losing weight. This statement may require modification if the period of time under consideration is short, because growth is not absolutely regular month after month and year after year : there are periods when the rate of growth is reduced, and other periods when it is considerably accelerated.

Big and rapid variations of weight during infancy generally indicate loss or gain of tissue-fluids rather than of flesh. Malnutrition accompanies all severe and chronic illness, and is often found when there is serious deformity, such as a congenital lesion of the heart. Its most important forms, however, are met with in prematurity, in under-feeding, in defective feeding, and in alimentary and parenteral infections. Wrinkling of the skin (especially over the buttocks and thighs), lack of subcutaneous fat, loss of tissue-turgor, and muscular atony are usually obvious in such cases.

Excessive weight may be due to various causes, such as familial or racial tendency, over-eating, preponderance of carbohydrate in the diet, and various ductless gland disorders, such as giantism and dystrophia adiposo-genitalis.

Observation of the weight is one of the best means of measuring a fluctuating œdema in nephritis.

The length of a full-term baby is 19–20 in. ; at one year the infant is 27–28 in. long, and thereafter a gain of $3\frac{1}{2}$ in. a year is noted up to the 5th year, followed by an annual gain of 2 in. up to the 15th year.

2. *Cardiac and Respiratory Rates.*—Whenever possible the cardiac and respiratory rates should be counted during sleep, for nervousness often causes a temporary but misleading quickening of both. This advice has been emphasized particularly in rheumatic children, for the heart-rate may be one of the most important indications of cardiac involvement.

At birth, the pulse-rate is usually 120–140 per minute, and the respiratory rate 30–40 per minute. By the age of one year, they have diminished to 100–110 and 25 respectively, with a further decrease to 100 and 20 by the age of 5. Thereafter there is a gradual diminution to the adult rates, which are reached between the 12th and 15th years.

The radial pulse is frequently difficult to feel in babies, and the tension of the anterior fontanelle is generally found to be a better guide than the pulse-volume in estimating such states as dehydration and vasomotor collapse.

Sinus arrhythmia is frequently noted and is of no special significance. The other forms of cardiac irregularity are uncommon in childhood.

Healthy infants frequently breathe irregularly from time to time—a state which is the more readily observed because abdominal respiration is the rule in young children. One often notes an inverted form of respiration, in which the long pause occurs between inspiration and expiration, while the interval between expiration and inspiration is comparatively short. It is surprising for how long a period an infant may hold his breath without showing evidence of discomfort.

Dyspnœa and cyanosis should suggest, in addition to pneumonia, the possibility of an inhaled foreign body, of laryngeal diphtheria, and of congenital cardiac deformity. Infantile paralysis affecting the abdominal muscles or diaphragm may produce characteristic respiratory difficulties.

3. *Temperature.*—The temperature of older children may be taken under the tongue, but for younger children it is better to use either the groin or rectum. The latter is the most accurate method, and special thermometers which are safe against the danger of breakage may be obtained for this purpose.

The younger the child, the more unstable is the heat-regulating mechanism ; even comparatively slight changes in environment, such as an additional blanket, may cause pyrexia in the premature baby. Not infrequently newly born babies develop fever (inanition fever of the newborn) lasting a few days during the first week of life. Intracranial birth-trauma and infection are other fairly common causes of pyrexia during the neonatal period, but the absence of fever is small evidence against the presence of inflammation in the early weeks of life.

It is imperative to examine the throat, ears, and urine of every child who has fever ; and in regard to the nasopharynx, it must be remembered that a moderate pyrexia lasting days or weeks may be caused by a low-grade infection in the nose and postnasal pharynx.

An unexplained fever should always arouse the suspicion of pneumonia, because the pulmonary signs of this disease may not appear until the child has been ill for several days ; other pyrexial conditions which may be puzzling are paratyphoid fever, abortus infection, sinus infection, tuberculous adenitis in chest or abdomen, and atropine fever.

Although fever unusually indicates organic disease, it must be remembered that some children of nervous constitution may show an evening rise of temperature to 99.5° or 100° for weeks—a state of affairs which is likely to continue as long as there is anxiety in the home regarding the child's condition. Some normal children show a rectal temperature of 100° or higher after exercise, but it quickly returns to normal on resting.

A low temperature is observed frequently in premature babies, and may be quickly fatal if treatment is not given ; hence a special low-reading thermometer should be used for these infants.

4. *Consciousness.*—Attention has already been drawn to the difficulty which may be experienced in deciding whether a baby or infant is conscious ; and, if the evidence indicates that he is not fully conscious, in deciding whether the condition is due to delayed mental progress (mental defect) or whether it indicates active disease of a serious nature—e.g., pneumonia, severe anæmia, etc. A conscious infant reacts readily to his environment by smiling if he is pleased, or by crying if he is frightened or annoyed. He reaches an average age-standard in the efficiency of his response to stimuli striking upon his sense organs—e.g., a conscious child aged 3 months will follow with his eyes and head the movements of a light, and often hold out his hands as if to grasp it ; he responds to pain-stimuli, such as light pin-pricks, by drawing away the part stimulated and by crying.

With tests such as these, and by a careful clinical examination to discover any illness which might cause diminution or loss of consciousness, the observer will be able to form some opinion ; but with added experience it is found that more and more stress comes to be laid on the facies as a valuable addition to the evidence noted above. Although certain definite features such as lack of expression, dropping of the lower jaw, or staring of the eyes may be very obvious, experienced observers rely mainly on the diminution of lively interest, either friendly or hostile, which characterizes the semi-conscious child. The student is therefore recommended to take every opportunity of observing the facial appearance of normal children of all ages, in order that average standards may become engraved on his mind.

5. *Vitality and Playfulness.*—Acute illness quickly lessens a child's normal vitality and destroys his natural interest in toys. Slight ailments often make him unwilling to run about, though he may still show an interest in playthings. At all periods of childhood smiling is an important feature of good health, and it is seldom that a child who is seriously ill gives a natural smile ; the commonest exception to this rule is the patient with some congenital malformation—e.g., a seriously deformed heart— who, while lying quietly without strain upon his reserve cardiac power, may behave like a normal child and smile happily.

6. *Tissue-turgor.*—The student should accustom himself to the ' feel ' of healthy flesh, especially that on the inner side of the thigh ; it is

comparatively solid, firm, and resistant to pressure, and the overlying skin and subcutaneous tissues have a characteristic elasticity which is often lost in debility, in dehydration, and in many serious illnesses.

7. *Colour.*—The normal colour of children is rosy-pink, and any pallor, tinge of blueness, or jaundice, should not be overlooked. It is to be remembered that a baby of healthy colour when awake may appear to be definitely pale when asleep. Sometimes the extremities of newborn babies are of bluish colour for some days after birth, yet without serious significance. On the other hand, either pallor or cyanosis during the neonatal period may indicate atelectasis (frequently observed in prematures), birth-asphyxia, infection or intracranial birth-trauma.

Anæmia gravis of the newborn is infrequent, but sometimes a marked anæmia is noted in a baby recovering from hæmolytic disease of the newborn. Syphilis may be a cause of anæmia in infancy, but rickets, nutritional disturbances, scurvy, and the von Jaksch type of anæmia are more common.

When a child is definitely anæmic special search should be made for jaundice, hæmorrhages, and enlargement of the lymphatic glands, spleen, and thymus. The ' dark ring around the eyes ' frequently noted by mothers is generally an indication of indigestion.

Jaundice in the neonatal period is usually of the so-called physiological type ; the other types, such as icterus gravis (hæmolytic disease of the newborn), syphilitic icterus, septic icterus, and congenital obliteration of the bile-channels, are comparatively uncommon.

8. *Muscle Tonus and Stance.*—The muscle tone of normal infants is well marked, and many states of disease, such as rickets, general debility, and malnutrition, cause a noticeable softness of muscles and flaccidity of joints. Increase of tone occurs in a variety of conditions : tetanus, tetany, meningitis, and many cerebral lesions may be cited as examples. In children of walking age a diminution of muscle tone is recognized by the stance, which becomes drooping, the shoulder girdles seeming to slip down upon the thorax and to rotate in such a way that the inferior angle of the scapula becomes unduly prominent. At the same time there is an obvious lordosis with flattening of the chest, prominence of the lower abdomen, a tendency to genu recurvatum, and flattening of the foot-arches. Orthostatic albuminuria is often found in these debilitated children.

9. *Sleep.*—The sleep of normal children is long, deep, and undisturbed by restless movement, crying, or bad dreams. There should be no stertor, snuffling, or snoring.

In the neonatal period sleep is almost continuous, and is scarcely interrupted except for feeding, and for the short periods of crying which serve to expand the lungs. Undue somnolence, which is recognized by the failure of the child to wake properly for these important functions, is often an indication of intracranial trauma during birth.

Disturbed sleep in infancy is frequently due to indigestion, rickets, or scurvy, though there are, of course, many other causes.

Encephalitis lethargica in older children sometimes causes a reversal of normal conditions, the child sleeping in the daytime but remaining awake at night.

10. *The Sucking Reflex.*—This reflex is remarkably strong in healthy infants, and may be stimulated by light contact of any object with the baby's lips. Diminution or disappearance of the reflex in small babies may indicate a diseased or deformed condition of the child's mouth or upper respiratory passages (e.g., rhinitis, cleft palate, and hare-lip), but more often the disability suggests a severe general cause, such as acute illness, atelectasis, intracranial birth-trauma, or mental defect.

11. *The Voice.*—Any alteration of phonation in older children is quickly noticed by hoarseness of the voice, which usually indicates laryngitis, either simple or diphtheritic, or a retropharyngeal abscess ; the presence of coincident stridor or dysphagia should be considered.

A similar disability occurring before the speaking age can be recognized by listening to the child's cry. It is not possible to describe in words the normal cry of infants, but certainly it should not be whining, shrieking, moaning, or fretful. When the baby's cry is hoarse, one must consider, in addition to simple and diphtheritic laryngitis, the following lesions : laryngismus stridulus, congenital laryngeal stridor, congenital syphilis, laryngeal polyp, and croup (laryngitis stridulosa).

During the early weeks of life crying is an important factor in causing full expansion of the lungs ; under normal conditions this cry is strong and loud, but lasts only about one or two minutes at a time. The baby who cries too much or too little may be suffering with an intracranial lesion associated with birth, or a severe general illness.

12. *The Skull.*—Observation gives an indication of the size and shape of the skull, and severe examples of hydrocephalus and microcephalus may be recognized at a glance.

The circumference of the skull should be measured, the tape passing over the frontal and occipital eminences ; the following figures represent average normal findings (Still) :—

At birth	..	.. ..	$13-13\frac{1}{2}$ in.
3 months	..	.. ..	15 ,,
5 ,,	..	.. ..	16 ,,
9 ,,	..	.. ..	17 ,,
12 ,,	..	.. ..	18 ,,
3 years	..	.. ..	19 ,,
7 ,,	..	.. ..	20 ,,
13 ,,	..	.. ..	21 ,,

The skull bones and sutures are now carefully palpated, and it will be noted that the full-term baby has firm though elastic bones which are well and uniformly ossified. It is not unusual to feel a small soft area of parietal bone adjacent to the sagittal suture, towards the posterior part of the bone ; this represents the parietal foramen and speedily disappears.

In premature infants the bones feel definitely soft, especially along the edges of the sutures, and may resemble firm parchment to the touch.

Occasionally one meets with a circular or oval opening in the midline of the occipital bone or immediately above the bridge of the nose : this is a congenital malformation and may give exit to a hernia of the brain or meninges. Craniotabes due to rickets is most often found near the lambdoidal suture from the third month onwards.

The anterior fontanelle is inconstant in size, but its diagonal measurement should not be more than 1 in. at nine months ; it usually closes between the eighteenth and twentieth months. Delay in closure indicates rickets in most cases, but may also be caused by hydrocephalus and hypothyroidism. The student must learn to gauge the tension of the anterior fontanelle by gentle palpation ; there may be a visible bulging, with increased tension, in intracranial birth-trauma, hydrocephalus, meningitis, brain tumour, and other conditions causing an increase of intracranial pressure.

A lowering of the fontanelle tension is of grave significance, especially if severe enough to cause visible retraction when the child is held in the sitting position. Dehydration as a result of severe illness (e.g., gastroenteritis) is the commonest cause.

In rickets the skull may be absolutely or relatively increased in size ; it is frequently flat on top, and there may be bossing of the frontal and parietal bones causing the so-called natiform deformity.

Premature babies frequently show a relative enlargement of the skull (megacephalus) between the second and twelfth months.

Flattening of the occipital region is seen in mongoloid defectives, the skull appearing to be small, soft, and brachycephalic. Infants who are forced by disease or deformity to remain in the lying position for long periods may develop flattening of the occipital bone or of one of the parietal bones.

Oxycephaly is characterized by elevation of the vertex, the frontal bone sloping upwards and backwards to a great height ; there may be early union of the sutures.

Percussion and auscultation of the skull are of less value than observation and palpation, but a distinctive note—which defies description in words—is often to be obtained on percussion of the hydrocephalic head. A systolic murmur is sometimes audible at the anterior fontanelle even in healthy infants.

The caput succedaneum is a sero-sanguinolent effusion into the scalp tissues of newlyborn babies, and is usually absorbed by the end of the first week ; it may conceal a linear or depressed fracture of bone.

Cephalhæmatomata are seldom seen until the second or third day after birth ; the hæmorrhage lies between the bone and its outer periosteal covering, and therefore the edge of the effusion never oversteps a suture. These swellings are tense, and quickly develop an elevated, hard edge adjacent to which, by the second or third week, one may be able to palpate a thin parchment-like membrane. A cephalhæmatoma usually remains obvious for about three months, and is gradually absorbed.

13. *The Face.*—Many diseases cause more or less characteristic changes

in the facial appearance, and it is scarcely necessary to mention pneumonia, nephritis, whooping-cough, adenoid obstruction, facial paralysis (*Fig.* 262),

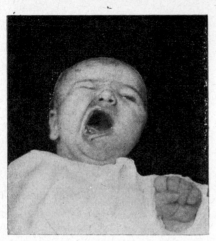

Fig. 262.—Left facial paralysis (forceps delivery).

and measles in this connexion. Other examples, perhaps not so readily recognized, are infantile tetany, causing a puckering and protrusion of the pursed-up lips (' carp-mouth ') ; dehydration, with sunken staring eyes, open mouth, and shrunken cheeks ; pink disease, with melancholia, photophobia, a bluish-red colour of the nose and cheeks, and carious teeth ; and congenital syphilis, characterized by sunken bridge of nose, scars around the mouth, frontal bossing, and, in older children, by Hutchinsonian teeth and interstitial keratitis.

Mongoloid defectiveness (*Fig.* 263) and hypothyroidism (cretinism) seldom present diagnostic difficulty to the student who has seen a well-marked case of each, though the slighter degrees of both these disabilities may be perplexing. The chief features of the mongoloid defective are softness of the skull bones ; brachycephaly ; palpebral apertures which slope downwards towards the midline of the face ; delicate skin and soft silky hair ; protruding tongue ; muscular hypotonicity ; incurving little fingers ; wide separation between the first and second digits of the feet (*Fig.* 264).

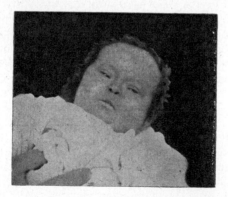

Fig. 263.—Mongoloid defective.

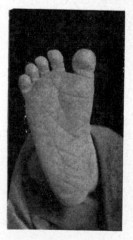

Fig. 264.—Foot of mongoloid defective.

The cretin, on the other hand, has a coarse dry skin with gelatinous subcutaneous tissue, scanty dry hair, large tongue, thick lips, stunted stature, low temperature, slow pulse, and a tendency to constipation. (*Figs.* 265, 266.)

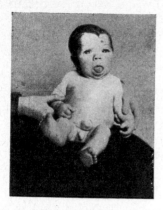

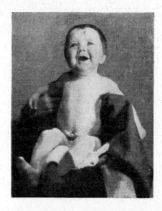

Fig. 265.—Cretin. Note coarse ' pot-belly ' with umbilical hernia. Protuberant tongue.

Fig. 266.—Same case after 5 months' treatment with thyroid extract. (*Figs.* 265, 266 *by kind permission of Dr. J. D. Hay.*)

Hare-lip is recognizable at a glance, and congenital ptosis of one or both upper eyelids should not present difficulty (*Fig.* 267). The sucking pad often causes an obvious swelling of the cheeks in infantile atrophy.

Eczema of infancy is seen with special frequency on the cheeks, chin, forehead, and scalp. Photophobia with blepharospasm usually indicates corneal ulceration.

In many cases it is wise to postpone examination of the eyelids and eyes until later in the interview, lest the child be frightened. When purulent ophthalmia is found in the newlyborn infant one must remember the possibility of gonorrhœal infection, and take precautions to protect oneself and others against contagion.

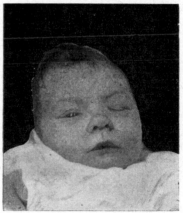

Fig. 267.—Congenital ptosis.

A fixed stare in infancy suggests the possibility of blindness, especially when a rapid movement of the observer's hand towards the patient's face does not cause blinking. Subconjunctival hæmorrhage in newborn babies is usually an indication of birth-trauma ; while in infancy and young children it is commonly a result of whooping-cough paroxysms. Hæmorrhage into the eyelids, with proptosis, occurs in suprarenal tumours and scurvy.

14. *The Neck.*—In the newlyborn a sternomastoid hæmatoma may be found as a small hard swelling in the muscle, usually about the mid-point ; the

tumour disappears gradually and is seldom followed by torticollis. The clavicles should be palpated carefully for fracture—a lesion which often causes little pain or disability. Thyroid enlargements in neonatal life may be due to vascular engorgement of the gland, especially after breech delivery ; or to hereditary predisposition, the mother herself having enlargement of the gland ; or to an embryonic tumour. Simple goitre may be seen in childhood, especially at puberty.

Lymphangioma of the neck or axillæ may be recognized as a fairly soft diffuse swelling which tends to increase in size.

Rigidity of the neck is recognized with ease when it is well marked and is accompanied by opisthotonos, as in posterior basic and tuberculous meningitis. Slighter degrees, though of great clinical importance, may be more difficult to demonstrate, for many sick children resist forcible attempts to flex the head upon the chest. The observer's hand should be passed gently behind the patient's occiput, and after waiting a few moments the child's head should be raised gently from the pillow ; in this way one can usually detect the presence of any cervical rigidity. In older children it is sometimes useful to let the patient sit on the side of the bed, and ask him to flex his spine sufficiently to enable his face to touch his knees ; by this test it may be possible to recognize the early stages of anterior poliomyelitis (meningeal type) and serious meningitis.

Common causes of cervical rigidity are meningitis, meningismus of pneumonia and pyelitis, and spastic diplegia ; tetanus and infections in the spinal bones and joints are less frequently responsible. It is noteworthy that tonsillitis, cervical adenitis, otitis, retropharyngeal abscess, acute glaucoma, sinus thrombosis, and acute rheumatism may cause marked cervical rigidity in childhood.

Enlargement of the cervical lymphatic glands may be found at any age ; it is generally an indication of septic absorption from mouth (cheeks, tongue, floor of mouth, teeth, jaw bones), tonsils, pharynx, ears, sinuses, or skin, often simple in nature, sometimes tuberculous. Less often these glandular enlargements indicate a general infection (e.g., rubella, glandular fever, or syphilis), or a blood disorder such as lymphadenoma or leukæmia. After examining the lymphatic glands of the neck it is usually convenient to pass at once to those of the elbow regions, axillæ, and groins.

The Limbs.—After the general investigation the limbs are examined. Abnormal features may be at once obvious. For instance : cyanosis and coldness of the extremities, frequently found in premature and atelectatic infants, in children who have a congenitally poor circulation, in indigestion, in pink disease, in paralysis of the arms, and in congenital cardiac lesions ; œdema, which may be due to nutritional disturbances and tetany in addition to the well-recognized causes such as nephritis and cardiac failure ; and finger-clubbing, which is generally associated with either congenital cardiac malformation or bronchiectasis.

The examination of a limb which is relatively immobile should be carried out gently, because it may be affected by a painful lesion such as scurvy, which causes swelling and tenderness of the legs with hæmorrhages around erupting teeth ; septic osteomyelitis periostitis, and epiphysitis (frequently streptococcal or staphylococcal) ; infective arthritis and peri-arthritis ; acute articular rheumatism ; or syphilitic epiphysitis and periostitis, more often affecting the upper than the lower limbs, and causing a painful swelling with immobility, generally in the region of the elbow-joint. Fracture of a limb or other physical damage such as separation of an epiphysis is usually suggested to the observer by a history of trauma, but in the newborn baby a fracture of clavicle or humerus, or separation of the upper humeral epiphysis, may be overlooked unless a careful examination is made.

Some of the causes of local swelling and deformity have already been mentioned, but reference must be made also to rickets, which produces some enlargement of the ends of the long bones, and a ' beaded ' appearance of the fingers, as well as deformities such as genu valgum and coxa vara ; to Still's disease (rheumatoid arthritis of children), causing characteristic deformity affecting especially the small joints of the wrists, hands, and feet ; to hæmorrhage into a joint in hæmophilia ; and to tuberculous dactylitis and tuberculous disease of the hip-joint. It is well to remember that a deformity may be overlooked if a child is not seen in the standing position as well as lying down, and this is especially true of the bone deformities which accompany many cases of renal infantilism ; genu valgum is the most common of these, and its presence in a child over the age of 5 or 6 years should indicate the desirability of making examination for polyuria, proteinuria, azotæmia, and cardiac hypertrophy. Congenital dislocation of the hip may not be suspected until the waddling type of gait is observed.

Syphilis may cause a variety of lesions ; reference has already been made to syphilitic epiphysitis, but in addition one may see dactylitis, periostitis (' sabre tibia '—*Fig.* 32, p. 37), or bilateral arthritis of the knee-joints.

The deformity of tetany (carpopedal spasm) may usually be recognized at a glance, but when the subject is a young infant the thumb is often held fully flexed in the palm and gripped by the fingers, which are acutely flexed at the metacarpo-phalangeal joints. Œdema of the dorsal aspects of hands and feet, ' carp mouth ', facial irritability, laryngismus stridulus, diminished blood-calcium, and a tendency to convulsions should be sought as additional signs.

Whenever rheumatism is suspected, careful search should be made for rheumatic nodules, especially over the extensor surface of the elbow-joint, the anterior aspect of the knee joints, and both sides of the ankles. Rheumatic nodules are small fibrotic masses lying in the subcutaneous tissues, sometimes no bigger than the head of a pin ; they may be adherent to bone or to tendons, and are best seen when the underlying joint is flexed in order to stretch the tissues over the nodule.

The two main types of paralysis, flaccid and spastic, may usually be differentiated without difficulty by noting the posture of the limb and by moving it passively. Spastic paralysis is frequently diplegic in distribution, and is then commonly due to imperfect development of the cortical cells of the brain ; when it is hemiplegic the cause is more often encephalitis or vascular damage by birth-injury or by hæmorrhage or embolism. Spinal caries is a fairly common cause of spastic paralysis of the legs.

The most common cause of flaccid paralysis is acute anterior poliomyelitis, and muscular atrophy usually occurs rapidly. Sometimes a diphtheritic neuritis is responsible, but spinal birth-injury, myelitis, and spina bifida are comparatively uncommon causes. Rickets may cause marked weakness of all the limbs, to a degree that paralysis is suspected. Damage to the brachial plexus during birth generally causes a lesion of the 5th and 6th cervical roots (upper-arm or Erb's paralysis) resulting in a characteristic posture of the limb : the arm lies at the side of the body and is internally rotated, with pronation of the forearm, the palm of the hand being directed backwards and outwards (*Fig.* 268). It may be accompanied by, or confused with, separation of the upper humeral epiphysis.

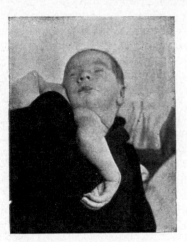

Fig. 268.—Erb's paralysis.

The lower-arm type of brachial plexus injury (Klumpke's paralysis), in which the 7th and 8th cervical and 1st thoracic nerves are injured, is much less common than Erb's type. The hand muscles are paralysed, and owing to simultaneous sympathetic involvement there may be miosis and narrowing of the palpebral aperture on the affected side.

Flaccid paralysis of the limbs may indicate one of the various forms of myopathy ; the affected muscles are usually smaller than normal in bulk, though this wasting may be concealed by the subcutaneous fat. A radiograph, using soft X rays, is useful to show the muscle-outline in this type of case.

In the pseudohypertrophic form of myopathy, the affected muscles (especially those of the buttocks, thighs, and calves) are larger than normal in bulk during the earlier stages of the disease and fibrous nodules may be felt in them.

Involuntary movements of the limbs usually indicate chorea, especially when they vary in type from moment to moment, and are accompanied by weakness and ataxia. In some cases of chorea the weakness is the most obvious feature, and prolonged observation may be necessary before the involuntary movements are seen.

A habit spasm is usually a very obvious action which is repeated time after time, and possesses purposive qualities—e.g., sniffing ; shrugging the shoulders.

The Chest.—The front of the chest is examined while the child is lying on his back, but whenever possible the chest should also be viewed with the child sitting and standing. In young and seriously-ill children, a nurse should support the child in the sitting position while the back of his chest is examined ; it is important to see that the patient's body is held evenly, the spinal column being vertical.

Disease may cause thoracic deformity with surprising rapidity in children. Hence one may observe bulging of the præcordium when there is cardiac hypertrophy ; indrawing of the costal cartilages and lower ribs as a result of adenoid and tonsillar obstruction ; splaying-out of the lower ribs due to hepatic and splenic enlargement ; and collapse of one-half of the chest, accompanied by scoliosis, in the presence of pulmonary fibrosis. Rachitic pigeon-breast, with enlargement of the costo-chondral junctions, is fairly frequent.

Cough, tachypnœa, dyspnœa, cyanosis, overaction of the accessory muscles of respiration (e.g., alæ nasi), and stridor are important features of many respiratory affections. In regard to cough, one must remember that indigestion, rhinitis and pharyngitis, tonsillar and adenoid hypertrophy, or nervousness may be the cause ; while whooping-cough, measles, and simple tracheitis and bronchitis must always receive consideration. In childhood, cough is seldom accompanied by expectoration, *for any secretion coming up through the larynx is usually swallowed.*

In young infants the normal respiratory rate is usually about 35 per minute, becoming gradually slower month by month until the adult rate of 18 per minute is reached about the twelfth year. Respiration is mainly abdominal in type, and therefore the physical signs revealed by auscultation may be missed unless the patient is breathing forcibly, as in crying. Infrequent, sighing respirations may indicate a serious intracranial lesion, such as tuberculous meningitis ; and in some cases of encephalitis the rate and depth of respiration waxes and wanes in cycles. Many normal babies breathe quite irregularly, breaking into short bouts of rapid shallow respiration and then reverting to the more usual rhythm.

After a careful inspection, one compares, as well as possible, the respiratory movements of the two halves of the thorax, and then proceeds to auscultation, using a stethoscope with a small chest-piece. The breath-sounds in childhood are harsh (puerile breathing), and the student may mistake this character for bronchial or tubular breathing, especially when a lesion causing collapse and diminished air-entry to the other lung accentuates the difference between the two sides ; in this way arises the mistake of diagnosing pneumonia on the wrong side. As previously noted, the breath-sounds may be so shallow and feeble that no abnormality, such as tubular quality or presence of crepitations, may be heard until the deep respiration of crying occurs.

Auscultatory signs at first suggestive of cavitation—e.g., amphoric breath-sounds with crepitations—more often indicate a patch of consolidated lung adjacent to a bronchus. Great care must be taken to auscultate the axillary regions, for it is here that the signs of a central pneumonia are usually heard first.

The breath-sounds may be clearly audible over a pleuritic effusion, and their presence should not be considered to weigh against this diagnosis.

Percussion is likely to be more distressing to a child than auscultation, and for this reason the order of the adult method of examination is reversed. It should be employed *very lightly* and carefully, not only because a heavy stroke may cause the child to cry when this is not desired, but because small superficial areas of consolidation may be overlooked when the percussion is not gentle. Comparison between the two sides is not permissible unless the stroke is made at the same phase of the respiratory cycle. Percussion during crying frequently causes a marked ' cracked pot ' sound.

A peculiar type of boxy tympany may be obtained over an early pneumonic patch ; it may be difficult to show definite pulmonary physical signs in some cases of broncho-pneumonia, and the general features (pyrexia, dyspnœa, cyanosis, movements of alæ nasi) may be more important than the local signs in the chest.

The flat resistant note of pleural effusion is of the greatest importance, far outweighing all other signs in the diagnosis of this condition.

The inspiration of a foreign body must be considered as a possible cause of pulmonary signs in childhood, especially when a right-sided bronchostenosis with pulmonary collapse is found. Dyspnœa is a common feature, but it is not invariable.

Tuberculosis seldom causes the apical signs of consolidation and caseation found in adults. Enlargement of the lymphatic glands surrounding the bifurcation of the trachea is probably the commonest form in childhood, and in these cases there is usually a pulmonary lesion which is too small to be shown by clinical signs, though it may be revealed on X-ray examination. Caseous pneumonia, miliary tuberculosis, and tuberculous infiltration passing outwards from the lung root are other types which may occur.

The Cardio-vascular System.—The radial pulse may be difficult to palpate in babies, young infants, and fat children, but there is no excuse for the omission of this examination. The tension of the anterior fontanelle gives information comparable to the pulse-volume.

At birth the heart-rate is usually about 120 beats per minute, and there is a gradual slowing during childhood, the adult rate of about 72 beats per minute being reached at the age of 12 years. Nervousness is a frequent cause of temporary tachycardia during medical examination ; the cardiac rate should be recorded during sleep when this is possible.

Sinus arrhythmia and premature systoles are the only common types of irregular cardiac action met with in childhood ; the former occurs frequently and may be marked in degree.

A sphygmomanometer provided with a small cuff is used for recording the blood-pressure, but the results are not likely to be of value in young children until the test has been repeated a number of times and the patient has grown accustomed to the sensation of constriction. Average readings are as follows (Feer) :—

				SYSTOLIC		DIASTOLIC
1 year	..	..	..	75–80 mm. Hg		60 mm.
6 years	..	..	..	85–90 ,,		65 ,,
10–12 years	..	..	..	100 ,,		70 ,,

The præcordium should be observed carefully, noting the presence of deformity and the characteristics of the apex-beat. Pericardial adhesions, with ventricular hypertrophy, are especially prone to cause bulging of the præcordium and a diffuse, wavy, forcible cardiac impulse which varies little in position when the child is moved from dorsal to lateral decubitus.

The younger the patient, the higher is the position of the apex-beat ; and before the age of 6 or 7 years the cardiac thrust may be normally outside the nipple line. Displacement of the heart by disease above or below the diaphragm (e.g., pleural effusion, pulmonary fibrosis, ascites, enlargement of liver and spleen) occurs more easily in children than in adults. The student should learn the quality of the normal apex-beat in order that he may recognize with certainty the comparatively forceful thrust produced by even slight left ventricular hypertrophy ; this point is one of considerable importance in helping to differentiate the organic murmur of mitral regurgitation from a functional bruit.

The younger the child, the more ' tic-tac ' are the cardiac sounds ; close attention should be paid in particular to the first mitral and second pulmonary sounds.

It is often unwise to give a definite opinion regarding the nature of a cardiac bruit on the findings noted at one examination only. A persistent and loud murmur in a child under the age of 5 years frequently indicates a congenital cardiac lesion, but in some infants, especially if premature or immature, a bruit of this type may disappear after several days' duration.

The absence of a definite rheumatic history (pains, tonsillitis, chorea, etc.) should not be taken as evidence against rheumatic endocarditis in a child over the age of 5 or 6 years who shows a persistent apical systolic murmur of blowing character with diminution or disappearance of the first mitral sound, accentuation of the second pulmonary sound, and even a suspicion of left ventricular hypertrophy.

Cardiac dilatation may occur with great rapidity and to marked degree in childhood ; the differential diagnosis from pericarditis with effusion is often difficult in these cases.

Every attempt to assess prognosis in the cardiac affections of childhood should include a careful estimate of general functional impairment, with special attention to cyanosis, finger-clubbing, dyspnœa on exertion, state of nutrition, desire and ability to participate in games, and so forth. It is quite wrong to condemn a child to invalid life because he has, say, a harsh systolic murmur indicative of a mild interventricular patency which does not lessen the functional ability of the heart.

Cardiac failure in childhood may not cause the gross general objective signs seen in adult life (œdema, venous congestion, etc.) until its terminal stages. For this reason great emphasis should be placed on persistent tachycardia and poor cardiac response.

The Abdomen.—The abdomen in young children is relatively larger and more prominent than in adult life. Inspection and palpation are the most valuable methods of examination, but percussion is also of help, especially when ascites is suspected. The clinician's hand should be warm, and relaxation of the abdominal muscles may often be obtained by engaging the child's attention with simple conversation, or, in the case of infants, by offering a feeding-bottle. This is especially valuable when pyloric stenosis is suspected, for it is of the greatest importance to see peristaltic waves passing along the stomach and to feel the pyloric tumour.

It is sometimes possible to feel the lower border of the liver and spleen in normal infants, but the finding should usually be taken to indicate enlargement or displacement of these organs. The younger the child, the higher the position of the bladder, and in the newborn baby this organ is located in the abdomen rather than the pelvis.

Tuberculous peritonitis is comparatively frequent in childhood, but care should be taken to differentiate the abdominal distension of rickets and of cœliac disease from this disorder. Palpation for enlarged abdominal glands requires patience and should be thorough ; fæcal accumulations may be misleading, and it is frequently wise to refrain from a definite diagnosis until the effect of an enema has been observed ; sometimes the employment of special tests, such as radiography, is of assistance.

An acute abdominal crisis in childhood is often a most perplexing problem to elucidate ; it is not proposed to discuss the subject fully in this chapter, but the observer must bear in mind the comparative frequency of appendicitis, with secondary peritonitis. Alternative diagnoses of fairly common occurrence are intussusception with melæna and a palpable tumour ; pneumococcal peritonitis, often accompanied by diarrhœa, herpes labialis, and acute febrile reaction ; acute pyelitis ; Henoch's purpura ; and acute enterocolitis. Acute pleuro-pneumonia is a fairly frequent imitator of the ' acute abdomen ' in children.

A swelling deeply situated in the abdomen should always suggest the possibility of tuberculous spinal disease which has given rise to a cold abscess.

The Anus and Rectum.—It is generally possible to recognize an imperforate anus by inspection of the part, but sometimes the occluding diaphragm is situate about half an inch from the surface, and in doubtful cases a digital examination should be made. The examiner's little finger, well lubricated, should be used for this purpose. Condylomata may be found at the anal margin.

Prolapse of the rectum occurs with special frequency in wasted children who suffer with a severe cough (e.g., whooping-cough) or diarrhœa.

The Spine.—Deformity of the spine may be seen in a variety of conditions, of which the commonest are diffuse kyphosis of rickets, seen best when the child is sitting ; angular kyphosis of tuberculous vertebral disease ; and spina bifida. The last-mentioned may be so slight that radiography is necessary to reveal it, but any pigmentation, abnormal hairiness, or wart-formation in the lumbosacral region should suggest the possibility of this deformity.

The range of spinal movement is easily tested, extension being investigated by placing the child face downwards and lifting the lower limbs up from the bed. This test provides a simple means of differentiating the kyphosis of rickets from that of spinal caries, for in the latter disease angulation does not disappear when the spine is extended.

Scoliosis with kyphosis is sometimes a congenital malformation, but more often it is due to infantile paralysis, or to intrathoracic disease such as pleuro-pulmonary fibrosis.

Lordosis is frequently seen in the debilitated and nervous child, and is often accompanied by genu recurvatum, flattening of the feet, and orthostatic albuminuria. A more severe grade of lordosis may be caused by congenital dislocation of the hips, rickets, dwarfism, and some of the myopathies.

The Genito-urinary System.—The genitalia should be carefully examined, and, as a precautionary measure, any vaginal or vulval discharge should be regarded as gonococcal until the result of bacteriological examination has been obtained. Lack of ordinary cleanliness is, however, the most common cause of genital infection. In older children the possibility of a foreign body in the vagina must be considered.

A milky-white mucoid vaginal discharge is frequently seen during the neonatal period ; and ' menstruation of the newborn ' is a well-recognized condition.

Phimosis is seldom so severe as to impede the passage of urine. Balanitis, vulvitis, or vaginitis may be the cause of pyuria ; and a meatal ulcer may cause a sharp pain, sometimes with slight bleeding, on micturition.

The testicles are exceptionally mobile in babies ; even exposure to cold air, or handling while removing a napkin, may cause them to be retracted out of the scrotum.

The daily volume of urine passed by children is variable, and only approximate standards can be given. At 3, 6, and 12 months the volume is 12, 14, and 16 oz. respectively ; thereafter a gradual increase is noted, reaching 30 oz. at 7 years and 40 oz. at 12 years. Alarm may be caused when the newborn baby does not pass urine for, say, twenty-four hours after birth, but there is generally no abdominal evidence of bladder distension, and the explanation of this oliguria lies partly in the fact that micturition has occurred during delivery, and partly in lack of fluid intake during the hours immediately after birth

The frequency of micturition varies much with the age of the child ; in infancy the urine may be passed every two or three hours during the daytime, but adult standards are usually reached by the tenth or twelfth year. The healthy child of $2\frac{1}{2}$ years should have control of the bladder both by day and by night.

The urine may cause a brownish-red (' brick-dust ') staining of the napkin in the first ten days of life ; hæmorrhage is suspected, but the discoloration is usually caused by a deposit of urates.

24

A skilful nurse can generally obtain a specimen of urine for examination, and it is not always necessary to resort to appliances for its collection. Exposure to cold air, or the application of a sponge over the pubic region is frequently a sufficient stimulus to micturition ; whenever possible the genitalia should be bathed and dried before the urine is passed.

When necessary, a test-tube may be applied over the penis, by adhesive plaster, for the collection of a specimen ; and for girls, a wide-mouthed flask, or bird's drinking fountain, may be used in the same way. It is most important to avoid any contamination of the urine with fæces.

Catheterization should only be used as a last resort, and it is seldom necessary when the nursing staff is efficient.

The Nervous System.—The examination of the nervous system differs little from the routine for adults, but is more difficult in childhood because the patient's co-operation is frequently lacking, and great patience is required of the examiner before results of real value can be obtained.

Reference has already been made to sleep in childhood (p. 357), and to the state of consciousness (p. 356). Headache may be difficult to diagnose, but is suggested when crying is of screeching type, and when the child frowns, pulls at the hair or ears, and moves the head restlessly. The presence of facial irritability should be sought by gentle tapping over the branches of the facial nerve while the patient's attention is diverted. Photophobia occurs most frequently in the following conditions ; corneal ulceration, measles, tuberculous meningitis, pink disease, teething, and oxaluria.

It is often impossible to recognize sensory changes unless they are very definite.

Most infants under the age of 2 years give an extensor response to the plantar reflex.

The nervous system of a child reacts markedly to many general illnesses, especially when they are febrile, or when the alimentary system is disturbed. Hence a state of irritability, or the onset of convulsions, may be caused by any feverish illness, or by indigestion, gastro-enteritis, etc.

Teething and infestation with parasities should not be regarded as an adequate explanation of nervous phenomena unless other causes have been excluded as fully as possible.

Mental Development.—The mental development of a young child is difficult to gauge accurately, though it is often a comparatively easy matter to say that a patient is definitely backward. In the early months and years one must be guided first by the physical appearance of the child (e.g., microcephalus, hydrocephalus, mongoloid defectiveness, hypothyrodism), and secondly by the rate of progress in achievement. Thus the normal baby shows the following attainments approximately at the ages stated :—

Co-ordinated movements of the eyes directed upon
    a moving object—e.g., bright light   .. 4 to 6 weeks

Smiling }
Voluntary sounds emitted }   ..   .. 6 to 8 weeks

Taking notice of surroundings
Gradual development of co-ordination in hands } 3 months
    and arms (grasping objects)
Turning of head towards a sound }
Lifting head from pillow   ..   3rd to 4th month
Beginning to sit up   ..   ..   .. 6th month
Sitting up alone   ..   .. }
Obvious interest in surroundings } ..   .. by 7th to 9th month
Recognition of a few words   )
Standing, holding side of cot |
Beginning to say simple words | ..   .. 9th to 12th month
Speaking simple sentences }
Walking a few steps   }   ..   .. 18 months

It must be remembered that individual children show considerable variation in the rate of developmental progress, and that this is especially true of speech. A general opinion should be formed in each case, and no child should be diagnosed as mentally backward because there is delay in one attainment only. It will be realized that impairment of physical health—e.g., by severe illness at an early age, or by a sensory abnormality such as congenital deafness—may cause developmental delay comparable to that seen in mental disease or deformity.

The intelligence of older children is tested by 'intelligence tests' (Binet-Simon) ; for a description of these the special literature must be consulted.

The Mouth.—The examination of the mouth and throat of a sick child is of great importance and should never be omitted, even though local symptoms would appear to be absent. Many children object to the examination, which should be deferred, therefore, until the end of the interview. A young child must be held securely lest a sudden movement of the head causes the spatula to damage mucous membrane or teeth. Older children often respond to sympathetic handling and will allow a thorough examination to be made without difficulty.

Chronic rhinitis may cause an inflamed and sometimes septic condition of the upper lip. Herpes labialis, impetigo, and syphilitic rhagades with subsequent scarring do not present any special difficulty in diagnosis. Angular stomatitis and cheilosis may point to hyporiboflavinosis.

The breath may have an offensive smell in many conditions, of which constipation, indigestion, septic teeth and tonsils, and bronchiectasis are the most important. The sweet and fruity smell of acetone in the breath is easily recognizable with a little experience.

The state of the tongue is at least as important in childhood as it is in adult life ; many conditions of ill health cause it to be coated, and careful attention should be paid to any hyperæmia, dryness, atrophy, or ulceration of its mucous membrane. A white tongue dotted with red hyperæmic papillæ is characteristic of one stage of scarlet fever. Many mongoloid defectives develop a rough crevassed tongue which seems too large for the mouth. An ulcer of the frænum of the tongue is suggestive of whooping-cough.

The inner surface of the cheeks and the soft palate may show petechiæ or the rash of an infective fever. Koplik's spots are white or bluish-white punctæ on an inflamed base, seen most often opposite the lower molars : they appear early in the development of measles, before the rash appears, and are of great diagnostic importance (see Fig. 43, p. 47). The opening of Stensen's duct, opposite the second upper bicuspid tooth, is frequently inflamed and protuberant in mumps.

Thrush may be recognized as a discrete white punctate deposit on the tongue, soft palate, and inner surface of the cheeks in delicate infants : the patches enlarge and tend to fuse. Aphthous stomatitis, which affects the same area, produces small greyish-yellow ulcers with surrounding inflammation, local tenderness, and profuse salivation.

The teeth are cut at approximately the following dates :—

Milk or Temporary Set (20 teeth).—

Lower central incisors (2)	6–8 months
Upper central incisors (2)	7–9 ,,
Upper and lower lateral incisors (4)	9–12 ,,
First molars (4)	12–18 ,,
Canines (4)	18–20 ,,
Second molars (4)	24–28 ,,

Permanent Set (32 teeth).—

First molars (4)	6 years
Incisors (8)	7–8 ,,
Premolars or bicuspids (8)	9–10 ,,
Canines (4)	12–14 ,,
Second molars (4)	12 ,,
Third molars (4)	17–25 ,,

Delayed dentition is frequently due to rickets or malnutrition, and rachitic defects of the enamel are commonly seen. Dental caries, which often causes alveolar abscess formation, should be noted. Congenital syphilis may reveal itself in the second dentition (Hutchinsonian teeth).

A spongy hæmorrhagic condition of the gum, especially surrounding an erupting primary tooth, frequently indicates infantile scurvy, and may occur also in leukæmia.

The tonsils are small structures before the age of two or three years, but inflammatory enlargement of the post-nasal adenoid mass is fairly common at this early age ; it is frequently accompanied by rhinitis, and there is snuffling, nasal obstruction, enlargement of the cervical lymphatic glands, and general ill health.

Tonsillitis and tonsillar diphtheria are common in childhood, but no special description is required in this chapter.

The Sputum.—Young children usually swallow any discharge coughed up from the respiratory tract, and there may be difficulty in obtaining a specimen for microscopical examination. Sometimes some of the discharge may be swabbed from the pharynx immediately after the patient has coughed, but a more certain method is to wash out the stomach with normal saline in the early morning before food has been taken. The washings contain masses of respiratory secretion, which may be removed with ease and examined microscopically or by animal inoculation.

The Ears.—The general practitioner must be able to diagnose otitis media, and it is remarkable that this condition may cause little pain and local tenderness surrounding the ear ; the affection must be sought not only by careful examination for œdema and tenderness of the mastoid area, and for enlargement of the cervical, post-auricular, and pre-auricular glands, but also by examination of the tympanic membrane. An electric auriscope is valuable for this purpose, and the appearance of normal and abnormal tympanic membranes must be learnt. Otitis media occurs even in young infants, and is frequently a complication of pharyngitis and upper respiratory infection in general. Sometimes the lesion is tuberculous, and this possibility should be suspected especially when facial paralysis occurs early in the illness.

Deafness may be congenital, and is then accompanied by mutism. Other causes of deafness are chronic infection of the ears, congenital syphilis, and meningitis.

The Fæces.—The character of the fæces constitutes an important indication of health in childhood, and especially in infancy.

During the early days of life the newborn baby passes tenacious motions of a dark green colour (meconium) ; but as the mother's breast-milk becomes more plentiful the stools change in appearance and are soon found to be of mustard-yellow colour, smooth in consistency and acid in reaction.

The fæces of artificially-fed babies are usually alkaline, fairly solid in consistency, and the colour is pale-yellow or greyish.

In the early months of life the motions are passed from two to four times daily ; they gradually become less frequent, and formed stools of a brown colour are generally noted after the second year.

When an infant is underfed or vomits the food, the motions become small in quantity, brown or green in colour, and frequently mucus is visible (" starvation stools "). Their number may be increased, and if the wrong diagnosis of enterocolitis be made, the infant's feeds may be still further reduced in strength and volume.

Infective enteritis causes frequent green evacuations which are watery ; they often contain much mucus and blood, and the patient's buttocks rapidly become excoriated.

Blood in the motions may be due, as noted above, to infective conditions of the alimentary tract, to intussusception, to the hæmorrhagic disease of the newborn, and sometimes to scurvy or one of the blood diatheses, e.g., purpura hæmorrhagica. A constipated motion showing streaks of bright-red blood on its surface usually indicates no more than a slight physical trauma of the intestinal mucous membrane.

Excess of carbohydrate in the diet causes gaseous, irritating, acid motions ; while an excess of fat in the fæces produces a pale, bulky, and offensive stool somewhat resembling porridge in appearance (cœliac disease ; defective pancreatic and hepatic function).

The presence of parasites, especially threadworms, should be carefully noted.

CHAPTER XII

MEDICAL OPERATIONS AND INSTRUMENTAL INVESTIGATIONS

IN this chapter the technical details of some of the commoner medical operations and instrumental investigations are described. When the actual performance of the operation or the use of the instrument is such that the student or practising doctor is unlikely to be responsible for it, the technical details have been omitted, and only the value of the method mentioned (e.g., bronchoscopy, electrocardiography).

THE RESPIRATORY SYSTEM

PARACENTESIS PLEURÆ

Fluid may be withdrawn from the pleural cavity for two purposes : (1) Relief of symptoms and as a method of drainage of purulent effusions ; (2) Diagnosis.

The area of the chest to be explored should be rendered aseptic by cleaning the skin with ether or alcohol and then painting with iodine or picric acid.

Aspiration can be made with a Record syringe and the fluid removed for diagnostic purposes, or a two-way syringe or Potain's aspirator (*Fig.* 269) can be used if it is desired to remove large quantities for therapeutic purposes. The needle should be of *wide bore* if there is any possibility of the fluid being purulent, as a fine needle is easily blocked by thick pus.

Local anæthesia is desirable. The skin may be sprayed with ethyl chloride, or, better, the skin and intercostal muscles in the operation area should be infiltrated with 1 per cent novocain. The needle should then be pushed steadily and firmly through the intercostal muscles and pleura and the fluid withdrawn. If no fluid is obtained, the needle may be withdrawn slightly and pushed in a different direction, before trying another intercostal space. The area of maximum dullness should be chosen as the site for exploration, but the surface markings of the pleura should always be borne in mind, and care taken not to insert the needle too low. When aspirating from the back, the needle is generally entered through the 8th or 9th intercostal space in the mid-scapular line, or in the 6th or 7th space in the mid-axillary line.

The removal of large quantities of fluid should be carried out slowly and discontinued if there are signs of collapse. The patient should be warned that slight hæmoptysis may occur after the operation, owing to relaxation of the lung tissue.

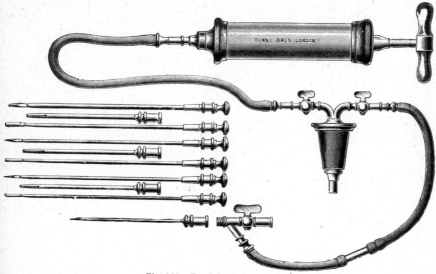

Fig. 269.—Potain's aspirator.

LIPIODOL INJECTIONS INTO THE BRONCHI

It frequently falls to the lot of the house physician to inject lipiodol into the bronchi before radiological examination. This procedure is employed to outline the bronchial tree and give information as to any obstruction or dilatation of its branches.

Lipiodol and similar preparations are heavy oils containing a high percentage of iodine which is opaque to X rays. It may be given by several routes, two of which are described here.

1. **Through the Nose.**—One nostril and the entrance to the nasopharynx are sprayed with 2 per cent cocaine until anæsthetic. The larynx is similarly dealt with by spraying directly through a syringe with a curved nozzle inserted over the depressed tongue.

The patient is placed in a good light in the sitting posture—preferably on a chair—and a No. 5 catheter lubricated with sterile paraffin is passed through the anæsthetized nostril into the nasopharynx. The head should be tilted slightly backward until the catheter is visible about the level of the fauces. Care should be taken that the catheter does not coil forwards into the mouth. The head must now be put quite vertical and the catheter gently pushed forward until it encounters a slight resistance at the entrance of the glottis. The patient is then instructed to take a deep breath and the catheter passes easily into the larynx. To determine that it is not in the œophagus, the patient should be asked to speak, when it will be noted that phonation is interfered with if the larynx has been entered. Another simple method is to get the patient to breathe out with the catheter held under water, when air-bubbles will escape if the catheter has been correctly inserted.

The lipiodol may now be injected by means of a 100-c.c. syringe attached to the catheter. About 10 to 20 c.c. of warm (body temperature) oil should be used for each lung. To ensure that the lipiodol passes into the side required, the patient should be tilted about 30° from the vertical, and should maintain this posture for a short time after the injection. X-ray examination should be made within a few minutes to obtain the best results, as the bronchi tend to empty the lipiodol into the alveoli after a short time.

2. **Through the Cricothyroid Membrane.**—The skin over the cricothyroid region is anæthetized by infiltration with 1 per cent novocain. The membrane is then perforated with a hypodermic needle and 1 per cent cocaine injected into the larynx to prevent the coughing which would otherwise ensue when the lipiodol is injected. Finally the membrane is again perforated by a fine needle attached at a 10-c.c. syringe containing warm lipiodol. The oil is injected slowly and the patient tilted as in the nasal route to the side into which it is desired the oil should pass.

OTHER SPECIAL INVESTIGATIONS

Laryngoscopy.—Examination of the larynx is necessary when laryngeal symptoms such as hoarseness, aphonia, or laryngeal pain are present. It should be employed when stridor or unusual types of cough (bovine and brassy) suggest possible affections of the vocal cords. In pulmonary tuberculosis the discovery of laryngeal involvement is important in prognosis.

Bronchoscopy.—The bronchoscope is playing an increasingly important role in the diagnosis of respiratory diseases. Apart from its use for the discovery and removal of foreign bodies it is of value in discovering new growths in the bronchi, evidence of bronchial stenosis, and in ascertaining the condition of the bronchial wall.

It should be employed particularly if any signs of bronchial obstruction remain unexplained, and in cases of hæmoptysis in which tuberculosis is unlikely.

Examination of the Nasal Sinuses.—The nasal sinuses—frontal, ethmoidal, and maxillary—are so frequently the source of infection in respiratory disease that they may need special investigation by transillumination, proof puncture, or X rays.

Radiological Examination.—This is undoubtedly the most valuable accessory method employed in examination of the lungs. There are cases of pulmonary disease almost impossible of diagnosis by the usual clinical examination, but on which X-ray examinations throw much light. This is particularly so in some cases of phthisis, especially when the signs of this disease are obscured by others, such as those of emphysema. Deep-seated pneumonia or pulmonary abscesses, small areas of fibrosis, or pleural effusions may similarly be shown up for the first time by X rays.

An *X-ray examination should, therefore, be employed in all cases of doubt,* and, if possible, in all cases of serious respiratory disease. But it is equally important to remember that clinical examination may show abnormal signs which are not suggested by X-ray examination, and the clinical approach usually gives more indication of the activity and progress of any disease present. *Repeated* X-ray examinations are of more value than single ones. It is important to emphasize the *necessity for combined study of the clinical and radiological findings.* (*See* Chapter XIII.)

THE CARDIO-VASCULAR SYSTEM
Paracentesis Pericardii

This measure is employed in cardiac tamponade (great dyspnœa, fall in venous pressure, etc.). The best site for puncture is in the fifth interspace just internal to the maximum cardiac dullness. The needle should be inserted upwards, backwards, and inwards. Alternative routes include puncture to the right of the sternum, especially if the effusion appears to be great in that position. Puncture may also be made at the episternal notch directing the needle upwards parallel to the sternum.

Graphic methods have been responsible for a much better understanding of the normal mechanism of the heart's contraction, and the disorders which may befall it. When the student has had an opportunity of comparing them with ordinary clinical methods, he will have gained knowledge which on many occasions will allow him to dispense with the graphic methods and rely solely on his unaided senses. In some cases, however, especially in arrhythmias, diagnosis is scarcely possible without the use of the electrocardiograph or polygraph.

THE SPHYGMOGRAPH

Pulse tracings can be taken quite simply by the use of this instrument (*Fig.* 270), which does not need as much skill as the use of the polygraph.

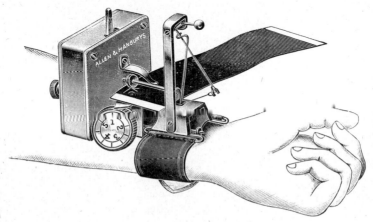

Fig. 270.—Dudgeon's sphygmograph.

It is convenient to mark the position of the radial artery with a skin pencil, taking care not to displace the skin in doing so. The button of the instrument should then be placed carefully on the blue line and the straps tightened *until the maximum excursion* of the needle is obtained. The roller carrying the paper may then be released.

The sphygmograph records the pulse-wave graphically so that its form can be studied more accurately than it can be appreciated with the fingers.

THE POLYGRAPH

By means of this instrument tracings can be taken simultaneously from the jugular bulb, representing auricular activity, and from the carotid artery, representing ventricular activity. The use of the polygraph requires attention to detail and some practice before the results obtained are of value, and much of the information it gives (e.g., on arrhythmias) can be more accurately secured with the electrocardiograph. To the student or practitioner who is particularly interested in heart disease, however, the instrument will prove of great service and interest, and is considerably less expensive than the electrocardiograph.

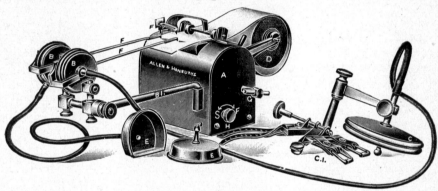

Fig. 271.—Mackenzie's polygraph. A, Clockwork motor, with time recorder (⅕ sec.) ; B, Writing tambours with supporting bar (B.I.) ; C, Wrist tambour, with attachment for wrist (C.I.) ; D, Paper holder ; E, Cup-shaped receivers ; F, Tambour and time-marking pens ; G, Winding key for paper-rolling mechanism ; H, Key for regulating speed of paper, direction for fast or slow being indicated by letters F and S.

Fig. 271 shows the parts of the instrument. The receiver should be placed in the position shown in *Fig.* 272 so as to cover simultaneously the jugular bulb and carotid artery. The excursions of the pointer carrying the pen should be observed, to note the most favourable movement, before allowing the pen to write. Too small an excursion gives a record difficult to read ; too great movement may carry the pen off the roll of paper. The magnitude of the excursion depends chiefly on the pressure exerted by the receiver, and the optimum pressure can only be found by experiment.

On the same strip of paper it is usual to record the polygram, a sphygmogram (a sphygmograph is an integral part of most polygraphs), and a time tracing marking each fifth of a second.

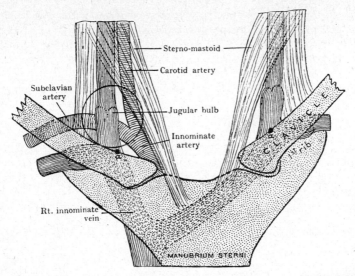

Fig. 272.—Shows the relation of the internal jugular vein to the carotid and subclavian arteries and to the sternomastoid muscle. The circle represents the position of the receiver in taking a tracing, and is seen to cover not only the jugular vein but also portions of the carotid and subclavian arteries. The spot at a is 1 in. from the internal end of the clavicle. (Keith.) (From Mackenzie's 'Diseases of the Heart', Oxford Medical Publications.)

THE ELECTROCARDIOGRAPH

This instrument yields most important information on the rhythm of the heart, and on the path of conduction taken by the excitatory wave as it passes from the sino-auricular node to its final distribution in the ventricles. The instrument consists of a string galvanometer, the fibre of which forms part of the electrical circuit, in which the patient is included. The changes in potential coincident with the heart's contractions pass through the fibre and cause it to be deflected. These deflections are magnified and recorded on a moving plate. Electrocardiographs on wireless-valve and oscillograph principles are also in use.

The electrocardiograph should be employed in all doubtful cases of arrhythmia, and in cases where myocardial disease is suspected. In the latter, defects in conductivity or abnormalities in the final ventricular wave (T wave) may be present in cases in which no abnormal clinical signs have been found.

Principles of Interpretation of the Electrocardiogram.—A clinical electrocardiogram (Fig. 273) usually consists of three separate records taken through three 'leads'. In Lead I, the patient is connected to the electrocardiograph by electrodes applied to his left and right arms; in Lead II, the electrodes are from the right arm and left leg; in Lead III, from the left arm and left leg. The records obtained are similar in many respects, but a comparison of the variations in the three leads sometimes reveals important data. Thus when the R wave is most prominent in

Lead I, and the S in Lead III, left ventricular preponderance is indicated. Right ventricular preponderance is similarly recognized by a prominent S in Lead I and a prominent R in Lead III. Ventricular preponderance means that one ventricle is relatively heavier than the other, so that

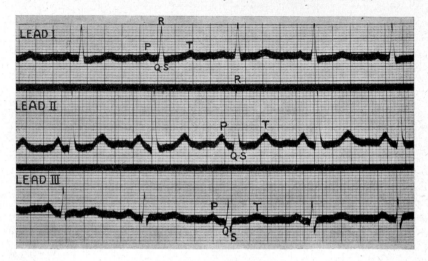

Fig. 273.—Normal electrocardiogram.

the normal balance between the right and left sides of the heart is disturbed. A fourth lead is commonly employed when coronary thrombosis is suspected, but not revealed by changes in Leads I, II, and III. This fourth lead requires a chest electrode and another placed on the right arm or left leg (Leads IV R and IV F).

The waves produced by the heart's contractions are arbitrarily named P, Q, R, S, and T.

The P wave : P represents auricular contraction. It is therefore absent in auricular fibrillation, in which the auricles are paralysed, and occurs more frequently than the ventricular waves in auricular flutter and heart block, in which the auricular rate is greater than the ventricular. Normally the P wave is upright, but it is inverted in true dextrocardia and commonly in conditions in which the cardiac pacemaker is not in the sino-auricular node (e.g., paroxysmal auricular or nodal tachycardia and auricular flutter). P is followed by the ventricular events Q, R, S, and T. The P–R interval is normally 0·14 to 0·18 sec. and represents the time taken by the excitatory wave to pass from the auricle to the ventricle. The P–R interval is increased (more than 0·2 sec. is generally considered pathological) when the bundle of His loses its conductile power. This may merely indicate some temporary effect, e.g., digitalis poisoning, or may be a permanent condition in heart block, in which all grades of defective conductivity are found from slight prolongation of the P–R interval to complete auriculo-ventricular dissociation—complete heart block. In the last case the auricular P waves bear no relationship to the ventricular events Q, R, S and T. The P waves occur at a normal rate of 72 (approximately) per minute ; the $Q R S T$ only at about 30 per minute.

The $Q R S$ complex : Q is usually a small downward deflection forming a relatively unimportant part of the ' $Q R S$ complex ', waves which correspond with the initial parts of ventricular contraction. R is the main deflection in the ' $Q R S$ complex ' ; it is normally upright in all leads, and occurs as a tall spike, rarely slightly notched even in health. S is normally a small wave directed downwards. $Q R S$ together occupy no more than 0·1 sec. $Q R S$ ' spread '—i.e., when the deflections occupy more than 0·1 sec.—indicates some impairment in conductivity through the branches of the bundle of His or their final arborization in the ventricular muscle. It is thus seen in bundle branch block and ' arborization block '. In these cases the $Q R S$ is usually notched and bizarre in shape. Extrasystoles produce a large $Q R S$ complex with the final deflection in an opposite direction to the initial.

The T wave : T represents the final electrical change coincident with ventricular contraction. It is upright and slightly rounded in Lead I, but frequently inverted (negative) in Lead III in normal subjects. Persistent negativity of the T wave in Leads I and II is found in myocardial disease and disease of the coronary arteries.

Sometimes the S-T interval is modified. Instead of a flat portion, it may become curved or modified into the so-called Pardee curve (*see Fig.* 284). Such changes in the S-T interval are suggestive of coronary thrombosis.

Reference to the illustrative electrocardiograms (*Figs.* 274–286) and their accompanying legends will explain some of the commoner electrocardiographic changes.

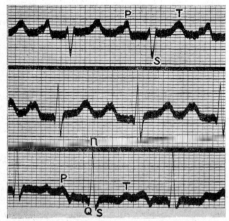

Fig. 274.—Right ventricular preponderance. Note prominent S in Lead I and prominent R in Lead III, i.e., the main deflection is downwards in Lead I and upwards in Lead III. These are the characteristics of right ventricular preponderance. There is also a split P wave in Lead II, common in mitral stenosis, and a prolonged P-R interval.

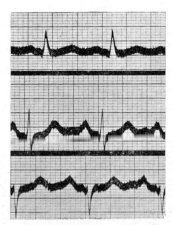

Fig. 275.—Left ventricular preponderance. Prominent R in Lead I and prominent S in Lead III, i.e., the main deflection is upwards in Lead I and downwards in Lead III.

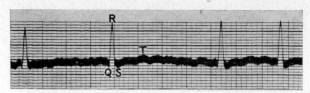

Fig. 276.—Auricular fibrillation (fine type). Complete irregularity and absent P waves.

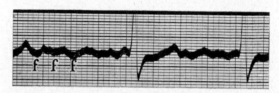

Fig. 277.—Auricular fibrillation (coarse type). Note complete irregularity and absent P waves. f = fibrillations.

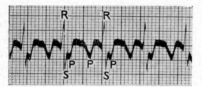

Fig. 278.—Auricular flutter. 2 : 1 rhythm ; P waves inverted. (*Dr. Cunningham's case.*)

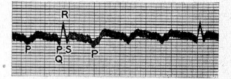

Fig. 279.—Auricular flutter. 4 : 1 rhythm ; inverted P waves, of which one is submerged in the Q R S complex.

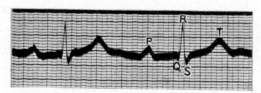

Fig. 280.—Early heart-block. P-R interval prolonged to 0·29. No dropped beats.

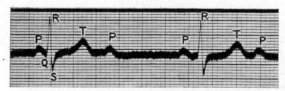

Fig. 281.—Complete heart block. The ventricular complexes (Q, R, S, and T) occur independently of, and at a different rate from, the auricular complexes (P).

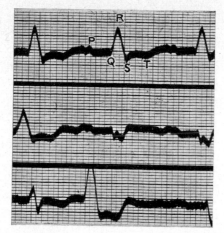

Fig. 282.—Bundle branch block. Q R S spread, with T waves in opposite direction to the R waves. The main deflections in Leads I and III are also opposite.

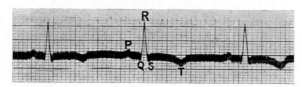

Fig. 283.—Inverted T wave. Commonly found in myocardial and coronary artery disease. Also produced by digitalis poisoning.

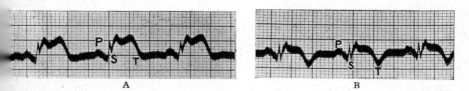

A   B

Fig. 284.—Coronary thrombosis. A, So-called Pardee curve ; note S T deviation with the high "take-off" of the S–T interval. B, One week later, S T deviation diminishing ; T waves negative. One of the most important points in favour of coronary thrombosis is a changing electrocardiogram.

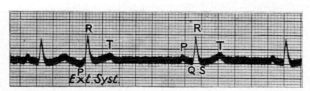

Fig. 285.—Auricular extrasystoles. The P wave is inverted and the following Q R S complex is of normal form.

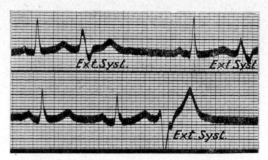

Fig. 286.—Ventricular extrasystoles. Note variation in form from the normal complexes. The extrasystole tends to give a diphasic Q R S complex larger than normal. No P waves precede the premature beat.

X-RAY EXAMINATION

In the estimation of the size of the heart and great vessels it has already been pointed out that inspection, palpation, and percussion are methods adequate on many occasions, but sometimes inaccurate and sometimes not applicable. This is especially so in fat persons and in cases of emphysema. In these a *teleradiogram* (an X-ray taken at a fixed distance, usually 2 m. from the patient, to avoid divergence of the rays) gives an accurate outline of the heart and great vessels.

Even greater accuracy may be attained by use of the *orthodiagraph*, in which the central rays are allowed to move round the heart margin, which is then drawn on thin paper placed over the screen. The resulting orthodiagram furnishes actual measurements of various parts of the heart and great vessels. Whilst screening the patient before making an ortho-diagram, the *pulsations* of the heart and vessels may also be observed.

X-ray examination not only gives relatively accurate data on the size of the heart, but also enables the shape of the heart and great vessels to be ascertained. Abnormalities of shape may be of great diagnostic value in cases of valvular disease. (*See* Chapter XIII.)

THE URINARY SYSTEM

X Rays.—X-ray examination may show the presence of an enlarged kidney or of stones in any part of the urinary tract (kidney, pelvis, ureter, bladder, or urethra), and should therefore be employed when these con-ditions are suspected. The shape and size of the kidney pelvis and the ureter may be shown up radiologically by the intravenous use of certain chemical substances (e.g., *uroselectan*) which are excreted through the kidney and are opaque to X rays. The method is of considerable value in suspected cases of hydronephrosis, kidney tumours, etc. (*See* Chapter XIII.)

Cystoscopy.—Examination of the bladder and of the orifices of the ureters may be made through the cystoscope. This method is of particular use when inflammatory or neoplastic conditions of the bladder are suspected, but may also be employed to discover the presence of stones and to see whether urinary secretion through the two ureters is normal. In order to simplify the latter observation a dye, such as methylene blue, is given intravenously and the urine may then be seen to enter the bladder in blue spurts.

Ureteric Catheterization.—By means of a cystoscope it is also possible to pass very fine catheters into the ureters and collect samples of urine from each kidney in turn. By the same method opaque substances may also be injected into the pelvis of the kidney, and the shape and size of the renal pelvis then ascertained by X-ray examination (*pyelography*). Pyelography is of use in similar cases to those in which uroselectan is employed.

THE DIGESTIVE SYSTEM

THE ŒSOPHAGUS

Radiology is so essential in the diagnosis of œsophageal diseases that it has already been mentioned on p. 162 as a routine method of examination. Further details are given in Chapter XIII.

Œsophagoscopy allows of the inspection of the œsophagus from its junction with the pharynx down to the cardia. In skilled hands it may be valuable in showing the presence of ulcers, diverticula, and growths, but it should not be used until the question of extrinsic pressure by aneurysms and other tumours has been excluded, and in the case of malignant disease great care must be exercised to prevent perforation of the growth.

Bougies.—Œsophageal bougies are occasionally used to localize the position of an obstruction.

THE STOMACH AND DUODENUM
Radiology
(*See also* Chapter XIII)

The outline of the stomach and first part of the duodenum can be shown by radiological examination after a meal containing barium. The degree of motility of the stomach can be observed and the length of time the meal remains in it before passing into the duodenum. It is not within the scope of this book to discuss all the various radiological changes which may be seen after a barium meal, but as X-ray examination takes a more prominent part in the diagnosis of gastro intestinal diseases than in most other types of disease, a few of the more important points demonstrated by X-ray examination may be summarized.

1. **Shape.**—This varies considerably in health ; various types are seen in *Figs.* 138–144 on pp. 175, 176, and in *Fig.* 293. Abnormalities in shape may be seen in mechanical deformities such as hour-glass stomach and in grosser irregularities of malignant disease.

2. **Position.**—Our ideas of the position of the stomach have undergone a great change since the introduction of X-ray examination. It is now

25

recognized that in health the stomach may extend well below the epigastrium, often into the pelvis. Moreover, the organ changes a great deal in position according to the posture of the patient, the general state of health at the time of examination, and the type of meal which has been taken.

3. **Motility.**—The tonicity of the stomach is demonstrated by its position and shape in the abdomen, and by the number and size of the contractions passing along the lesser curvature to the pylorus. The *hypertonic* stomach (*Fig.* 296) is placed high in the abdomen, tends to be more transverse, and shows an increased number of contractions. Increased size of the contractions is seen in the early stages of pyloric stenosis, when the contractions are at first strong and the stomach tonic, but finally the stomach becomes completely atonic. The *atonic* stomach is low in the abdomen, tends to be vertical, and shows small sluggish contractions. It is known that hypertonus is often associated with hyperchlorhydria and with gastric and duodenal ulcers, whilst hypotonus is frequently seen in debilitating illnesses, in visceroptosis, and in carcinoma of the stomach.

The stomach usually empties within three to six hours of the barium meal, but in exceptional cases may take longer without any pathological lesion. In cases of pyloric obstruction great delay in emptying may be present (8–48 hours). Slight delay (6–8 hours) is also found in visceroptosis, and in reflex spasm of the pyloris due to such causes as appendicitis and cholecystitis.

4. **Filling Defects.**—In cases of gastric and duodenal ulcer and in carcinoma of the stomach of an ulcerative type, the barium lodges in the ulcer and usually produces a projection on the stomach wall in some *constant* position. The constancy serves to distinguish it from irregularities due to the normal peristaltic waves (incisuræ). Further, the pocket of barium often remains in the ulcer crater after the stomach has emptied itself of the remainder of the meal (*Figs.* 295, 297). Ulcer craters are often associated with spasm, particularly in the first part of the duodenum, and sometimes in the stomach with an hour-glass contraction.

5. **Deformities of the Duodenal Cap.**—The duodenal cap—i.e., the first part of the duodenum—may be persistently deformed in cases of ulceration near the pylorus, especially, of course, on the duodenal side (*Fig.* 298), but too much importance should not be attached to a defect in the duodenal cap which is not present in *all* the X-ray photographs. Inconstant defects are more often due to acute cholecystitis, old cholecystitis with adhesions, or chonic appendicitis. In all such cases there is, of course, no ulcer crater.

Gastroscopy

Great advances have been made recently in the use of the flexible gastroscope. With this instrument it is possible to inspect the gastric mucosa and determine the presence of various forms of gastritis, apart from the actual presence of ulcers. Neoplasm is sometimes, though more rarely, recognized, when other methods have failed to reveal it.

THE INTESTINES

Radiology.—X-ray examination is chiefly of value in lesions of the large intestine. In chronic obstructive lesions, especially those produced by neoplasm, the barium meal may be held up at some constant point in the large intestine, and in such cases it is advisable to employ a barium enema which rapidly outlines the whole of the large intestine and demonstrates any narrowing of its lumen. The position and length of the appendix should also be noted, and whether it fills and empties in a normal manner. Similarly, diverticula of the colon may be revealed by the small masses of barium which collect in them.

Duodenal Intubation.—It is possible to reach the duodenal contents and aspirate them for chemical analysis by using a specially long tube of smaller calibre than the Rehfuss tube. Although not of the same general importance as the fractional test-meal, this method may give important data on duodenal digestion and on the secretion of bile. If an analysis of bile is desirable Lyon's method is useful. This consists in putting through the duodenal tube a concentrated solution of magnesium sulphate (20 c.c. of a 25 per cent solution), which produces a reflex emptying of the gall-bladder.

Sigmoidoscopy.—For examination of the rectum and sigmoid flexure of the colon, a sigmoidoscope may usefully be employed. The lower bowel is first washed out by enemata and the sigmoidoscope gently inserted as far as it will go. The patient should be in the left lateral or knee-elbow position. If the investigation is carried out under anæsthesia the lithotomy position may be used. Sigmoidoscopy is of value in cases where ulceration, diverticula, or malignant disease of the bowel is suspected. If the examination is confined to the rectum the term *proctoscopy* is used, and a shorter instrument may be employed.

THE GALL-BLADDER AND BILE-DUCTS

Radiology.—X-ray examination is necessary in all doubtful cases of gall-bladder disease. A *direct* X-ray may demonstrate gall-stones, but a negative result does not exclude their presence. By *Graham's method* the size, shape, position, and function of the gall-bladder can be investigated. The method consists in the administration by mouth or intravenously of a dye, tetra-iodo-phenolphthalein, which is excreted by the liver into the bile and forms an opaque shadow in the radiograph conforming with the shape of the gall-bladder. If the gall-bladder function is normal, a well-defined shadow appears and concentrates in 18 to 24 hours, and disappears after a fatty meal (*Figs.* 304, 305). In disease of the wall of the gall-bladder the shadow may be small, irregular, or in many cases absent. (*See also* Chapter XIII.)

THE NERVOUS SYSTEM

LUMBAR PUNCTURE

This operation consists in tapping the cerebrospinal fluid in the lower lumbar region by introducing a special needle (8 cm. in length) through the spinal theca.

The spinal cord ends in the adult on a level with the first lumbar vertebra, so that a needle can be introduced below this level with safety. The spaces between the third and fourth or between the fourth and fifth lumbar vertebræ are generally chosen, as they are the widest and easiest to penetrate.

In the performance of lumbar puncture, the position of choice is with the patient sitting across a bed or chair, bending well forwards so as to increase the width of the interlaminal spaces (*Fig.* 287). If the patient is too ill to assume this position the lateral must be adopted ; the head and shoulders should be well bent forward and the knees drawn up so as to be on a level with the chest.

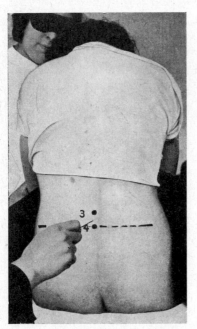

The head should be supported by pillows so that it is in the same horizontal plane as the sacrum.

The skin is prepared as in PARA-CENTESIS (p. 374), and the skin and deeper tissues infiltrated with 2 per cent procaine ; the needle is directed obliquely and pushed firmly and steadily through the tissues until it encounters a different sense of resistance (the theca), which the practised hand soon learns to appreciate. Slightly more pressure is needed at this point to penetrate the meninges. The stylet is then withdrawn and the cerebrospinal fluid allowed to drip into sterile tubes in sufficient amount for diagnostic or therapeutic purposes as the case may be. If no fluid escapes, the needle may be withdrawn very slightly, its axis twisted, and the stylet reinserted to clear any possible obstruction (e.g., blood or thick cerebrospinal fluid).

Fig. 287.—Lumbar puncture. The needle is inserted obliquely midway between the spines of the 3rd and 4th, or 4th and 5th, lumbar vertebræ.

The *pressure* of the cerebrospinal fluid can be measured easily by attaching one limb of a special lumbar puncture needle to a manometer. The normal pressure is taken as 100 to 150 mm. of water, and must be recorded with the *patient lying on the side.*

The free *communication between the fluid in the lumbar region and that in the cerebral cisterns* may be tested either by making the patient cough or by compressing the jugular veins (Queckenstedt's test). The result in each case is an increase in the pressure of the cerebrospinal fluid. This increase will not occur in lesions obstructing the free movements of the fluid up and down the spinal canal. It is absent, for example, in some cases of spinal tumour.

LIPIODOL INJECTION

The introduction of the radiological opaque oil lipiodol into the spinal theca by means of cistern or lumbar puncture is a useful method of localizing exactly the level of compressive lesions of the spinal cord, e.g., spinal tumour. From a cistern injection the oil sinks down to the upper level of the tumour. If it is necessary to localize the lower level also, the lipiodol can be introduced by lumbar puncture ; if the patient is then partially inverted (exaggerated Trendelenburg position) the oil runs upwards to the point of obstruction.

ENCEPHALOGRAPHY AND VENTRICULOGRAPHY

By these methods air is introduced into the cerebral cisterns and ventricles. The air may enter through lumbar puncture or by puncture of the ventricle through the skull. The skull is then X-rayed and the contour and size of the ventricles and cisterns studied. Valuable data are afforded in cases of cerebral tumour, obstruction to the subarachnoid space and cisterns, etc. (*See* Chapter XIII.)

ELECTRO-ENCEPHALOGRAPHY

The cells of the brain produce action currents which can be recorded in graph form by the electro-encephalograph. Disturbance of these action currents have been recorded in a number of nervous diseases, e.g., epilepsy, cerebral tumour, psychosis, etc. Fuller details are available in neurological monographs.

ELECTRICAL REACTIONS

The electrical excitability of muscles and their nerves is tested by the use of faradic and galvanic stimulation. Faradic currents can only evoke a response when the nerve is not too degenerated to allow of the passage of the current. The current is applied over a motor point, i.e., where the nerve enters the muscle. Variations of the electrical reactions are found in lower neurone lesions, myopathies, and other rare conditions. They *do not occur in upper motor neurone lesions.*

Galvanic stimulation produces responses which normally vary with polarity. The term ' closing contraction ' is used to describe the completion of the electrical circuit, ' opening contraction ' to describe its interruption. Normally kathodal closing contraction is greater than anodal closing contraction. Both are greater than anodal opening contraction, which is itself greater than kathodal opening contraction. Briefly expressed :—

$$K.C.C. > A.C.C. > A.O.C. > K.O.C.$$

These normal responses are disturbed in certain nervous diseases, especially of the lower neurone, in which the reaction of degeneration (R.D.) takes place usually after the lesion has been present ten to fourteen days. Before this stage there is often a preliminary increase in the electrical excitability.

Reaction of Degeneration.—The characteristics of this response are :—
1. Loss of response to faradism.
2. Sluggish response to galvanism.
3. Altered polar responses—
$$A.C.C. > K.C.C.$$
Many grades of this reaction are seen, varying from diminished response to faradism with no change in the galvanic reaction, to complete absence of any response to faradism and galvanism (complete R.D.).

Special Electrical Responses.—Brief mention may be made of the following peculiar reactions :—

In *myopathies* the electrical reactions are quantitatively diminished without any alteration in qualitative reaction.

The *myasthenic reaction* occurs in myasthenia gravis. It is a rapid failure of the muscle to contract to the faradic current, after a few initial contractions. After a brief rest the muscles recover, but fatigue again on repetition of the stimuli. This phenomenon is analogous to the rapid fatigue which occurs in certain muscles on voluntary movement.

Similarly in *myotonia congenita* there is an electrical counterpart to the clinical characteristic in which contracting muscles fail to relax normally. With electrical stimulation the contraction induced likewise continues longer than normal.

In *tetany* a state of increased electrical excitability occurs.

HÆMOPOIETIC SYSTEM

Sternal Puncture.—The technique of this procedure is quite simple. An area of the subcutaneous tissue over the manubrium sterni should be infiltrated with procaine, 2 per cent, about half-an-inch above the angle of Louis. The infiltration should be carried down to the bone. A specially constructed needle of the Sahli type, guarded so as to allow limited penetration of about a quarter of an inch, should now be firmly pressed through the sternum. The trocar of the needle is then removed and a syringe used to withdraw about $\frac{1}{4}$ c.c. of bone-marrow. Films should be made on similar lines to ordinary blood-films. In sensitive or nervous individuals, $\frac{1}{4}$ gr. morphine may be given half-an-hour before the procedure.

CHAPTER XIII

RADIOLOGY

By P. H. WHITAKER, M.B., M.R.C.S., D.M.R.E. (L'pool).

Assistant Lecturer in Radiology, University of Liverpool ; Honorary Assistant Radiologist, Royal Infirmary, Liverpool ; Visiting Radiologist to the Liverpool City Hospitals.

To appreciate the value of radiology in clinical diagnosis it is necessary to understand the method by which a radiograph is obtained. X rays, which are generated by a vacuum tube, are absorbed selectively by materials and tissues in direct proportion to their density. The rays also cause changes to take place in a photographic emulsion placed in their path, and the blackness of the film depends on the intensity of radiation to which the emulsion is submitted. Therefore, if a beam of radiation is allowed to pass through a series of varying densities (i.e., the body of a patient), before reaching a film coated with photographic emulsion, the resultant image will, after chemical development, represent the tissues through which the rays have passed. The fluids of the body, e.g., blood in the heart, will absorb more rays than will the lungs which are less dense, and will in consequence show a denser shadow. In this way the tissues of the body can be recognized on the film in contrast to each other.

Bones, on account of their greater density than soft tissues, will tend to predominate on the radiograph, and abnormal or pathological changes in the bones and pathological calcification in the organs can therefore easily be recognized. To a less degree the renal and liver outlines can be seen against the abdominal musculature. This direct visualization of the tissues in the radiograph is of value in the appreciation of the renal outline and size and the presence of calculus, in the diagnosis of lesions of the lungs, and in the appearances of the bones ; but to demonstrate the gastro-intestinal tract, bronchial tree, or the function of the liver, kidneys, and gall-bladder, it is necessary to introduce opaque media into the organs either by mouth or the blood stream. Generally speaking, pathological conditions, owing to their increased blood-supply, will increase the density of the tissue and cause a corresponding increase in the density of the shadow. For example, pneumonic consolidation shows as a denser shadow than the surrounding lung.

Direct radiography is used in examination of the bones (*Figs.* 288–290), the chest, the renal tract (for size and position of the kidneys and for calculus), and for examination of the soft tissues. The use of opaque media is necessary for examination of the gastro-intestinal tract, the bronchial tree, the Fallopian tubes, the spinal canal, and the function of the gall-bladder and renal tract.

X rays also cause fluorescence in a prepared screen and it is thus possible to examine the movements of organs through a fluorescent screen in a darkened room.

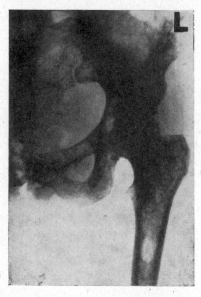

Fig. 288.—Secondary carcinoma of bone. Multiple small areas of translucency throughout the bone (osteolytic).

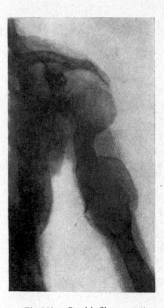

Fig. 289.—Osteitis fibrosa cystica. Expansion of the bone with cystic formation and increased trabeculation.

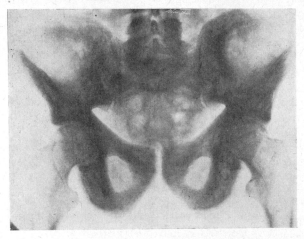

Fig. 290.—The pelvis in Paget's disease. Irregular increase of density of the bone, with increased width of cortex and irregular increase of trabeculation.

INTERPRETATION OF THE NORMAL RADIOGRAPH

Interpretation of a radiograph depends entirely upon the possession of accurate knowledge of the normal anatomy of the part radiographed and of the radiographic anatomy of the parts through which the rays have passed. The student must therefore be aware of normal radiographic features and how far these identify various anatomical structures. For this purpose he is advised to collect a full set of normal radiographs.

With the normal in mind, abnormalities can be determined and their significance appreciated by comparing them with known pathological processes. For example, in a radiograph of the chest, opacity of even character might be noted in the lung field involving the whole of one lobe but not causing any pulmonary collapse. Such an opacity is found to be associated with simple pulmonary consolidation, as might be expected from the increased density which would result from pneumonic consolidation in a lung or one of its lobes. The anatomical distribution of the consolidation, confining itself strictly to the lobe boundaries, would suggest pneumonia rather than other forms of pulmonary consolidation.

In the examination of a radiograph, the whole film, from the centre to the periphery, should be examined and the main anatomical landmarks identified. Attention should then be directed to any features which are not considered to be within the limits of the normal.

In lesions of the bones the normal architecture of the bone should be considered. Alteration in the density of the bone with disturbance of the normal architecture will denote the presence of a pathological process.

Fractures are distinguished from normal anatomical markings and vascular grooves by their clarity of outline, and by the fact that they do not follow the anatomical lines. Diseases of the joints are shown by alteration in the joint spacing and associated swelling of the soft tissues.

In chest radiographs it is helpful to compare one side of the chest with the other as both sides are anatomically similar. In examining the film attention is first directed to the heart and mediastinal shadows, then the lung root and hilar shadows are examined and their type and extent noted, and any lesion in the substance of the lung identified. Finally the framework of the chest, i.e., the ribs, is examined.

In radiographs of the abdomen the renal outlines should be identified and their size and position compared with the normal anatomical size and position. In pyelography the calices should be identified and their distribution defined and the sharpness and clarity of their cupping noted. Abnormal calcification should be noted and its position identified in relation to the gall-bladder and renal outlines.

In gastro-intestinal examinations after ingestion of an opaque meal the outline of the œsophagus should be noted, also the various indurations from extrinsic organs. The size and shape of the stomach should be observed together with the haustration and position of the small bowel and colon.

Finally, in every clinical case examined which has been radiographed the student would be well advised always to compare the radiological findings with the clinical features of the case.   In this way he will learn to assess the value of his findings.   Advantage should always be taken of the opportunity to examine the maximum number of radiographs and so obtain a complete knowledge of the features which may be regarded as normal in various types of physique.

THE GASTRO-INTESTINAL TRACT

Examination of this part is carried out by the administration of barium into the tract by means of a suspension of barium and a cereal in the form of a meal, or for examination of the colon only by the introduction of barium in solution in the form of an enema.

Barium is a fine metallic powder which is easily emulsified and which passes through the tract unchanged.   On account of its density it is opaque to X rays and shows up the outline of the tract.   The meal may be watched through the pharynx, down the œsophagus, and on its course through the thorax, and defects and deformities of these organs can be noticed on screen examination.   (*Figs.* 291, 292.)

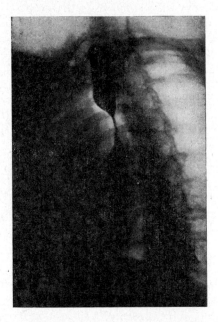
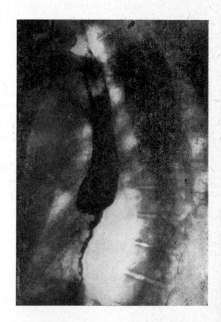

Fig. 291.—Syphilitic stricture of œsophagus.   Note even stricture in upper part of œsophagus.   Little dilatation above stricture and normal œsophagus below.

Fig. 292.—Malignant stricture of œsophagus.   Note ragged filling defect in lower part of œsophagus with considerable dilatation of œsophagus above.

When the meal reaches the stomach the outline of this organ can be seen, its tone and muscular contractions noted, together with its emptying rate, and mobility on palpation and changes of posture (*Fig.* 293).   By examination at intervals the meal can be watched through the small bowel and colon. Examinations, in addition to the one immediately after taking the meal, are usually made three, six, twenty-four, and forty-eight hours after ingestion of the meal. (*See also Figs.* 138–144, pp. 175, 176.)

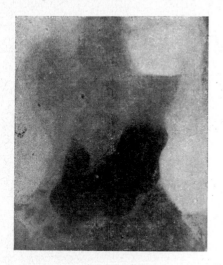

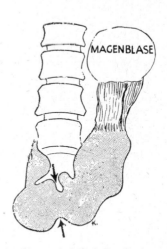

Fig. 293.—Normal stomach (tonic or sthenic type). The stomach is J-shaped. A normal incisura (i.e., an indentation due to contraction) is indicated by the arrows. The duodenal cap is well formed.

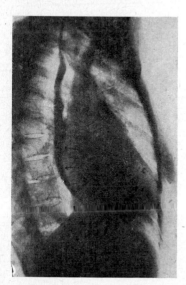

Fig. 294.—Oblique view of heart demonstrating displacement of the œsophagus in the lower third due to an enlarged left auricle.

Lesions of the œophagus either cause local deformity, i.e., filling defects of the lumen with consequent obstruction due to stricture (which may be simple or malignant), or protrusion from the lumen as in the formation of ' pouches ' or diverticula. In cardiac lesions the œsophagus is displaced and distorted by enlargement of the posterior border of the heart (*Fig.* 294). Displacements are also noted in mediastinal enlargement and in diaphragmatic lesions.

Malignancy of the stomach or colon is seen as a filling defect which is fixed and is constant in position, and which will cause obstruction to the passage of the opaque meal or enema (*Fig.* 295). Ulcers are seen as ' puckerings ' of the mucous membrane and protrusion of barium from the lumen of the stomach (*Figs.* 296–301), just as diverticula will show up as protrusions from the lumen of the colon (*Fig.* 302).

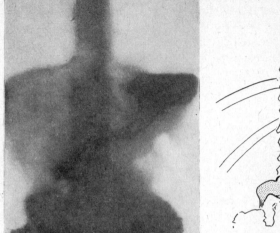
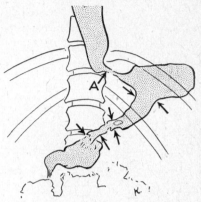

Fig. 295.—Malignant disease of the stomach.   Shows extensive filling defects involving both curvatures (see arrows).   Note also the œsophageal delay (A).

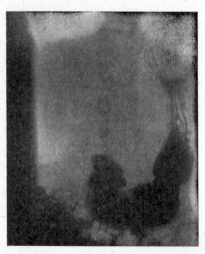
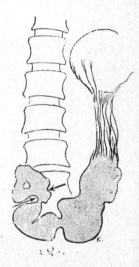

Fig. 296.—Duodenal ulcer (hypertonic stomach).   Note the deep incisuræ in the stomach, and more significantly in the duodenal cap.

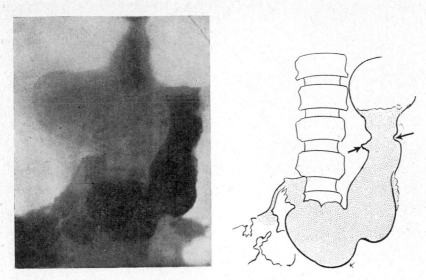

Fig. 297.—Gastric ulcer. An ulcer crater is seen high on the lesser curvature, with an incisura opposite on the greater curvature (*see* arrows).

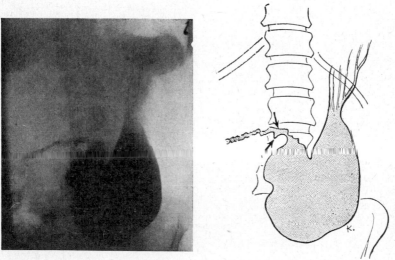

Fig. 298.—Duodenal ulcer. Note the ill-formed duodenal cap with an ulcer crater in the base (*see* arrows).

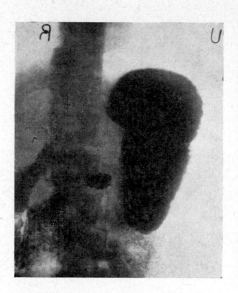

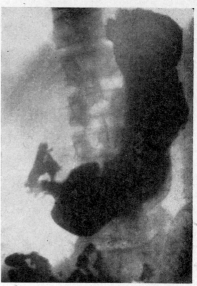

Fig. 299.—Gastric ulcer. Stomach after barium meal. Ulcer on posterior wall filled with barium. Rugæ running towards the area.

Fig. 300.—Duodenal ulcer. Stomach after barium meal. Deformity of duodenal cap. Showing ulcer.

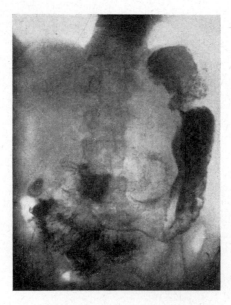

Fig. 301.—Gastric ulcer. Stomach after barium meal. Small ulcer on lesser curvature shown by protrusion from the stomach. Partial spasm pointing to ulcer.

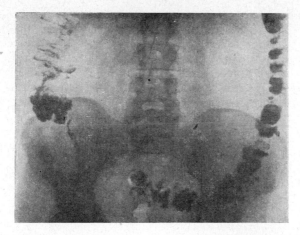

Fig. 302.—Diverticulosis. Radiograph of descending and pelvic colon after barium enema, showing bud-like projections from the haustral segmentation of the colon.

The appendix, if it is seen filled, can be palpated, and its tenderness, mobility, and emptying rate noted. Deformity and displacement of the tract due to extrinsic abdominal lesions can be outlined and localized to their organ of origin.

THE LIVER AND GALL-BLADDER

Under suitable conditions it is possible to visualize the liver margin in a direct radiograph, and also to demonstrate the presence of calculi in the gall-bladder. Calculi in this situation are seen as rounded shadows in the right upper abdomen (*Fig.* 303). The function of the gall-bladder can be demonstrated by means of an opaque dye derived from a compound of tetraiodo-phenolpthalein such as ' Opuuol ' which is given by mouth. This dye is absorbed through the liver, excreted through the bile-ducts, and concentrated by the gall-bladder twelve to fifteen hours after ingestion. In cases where it is impossible to give the dye by mouth it may be given intravenously.

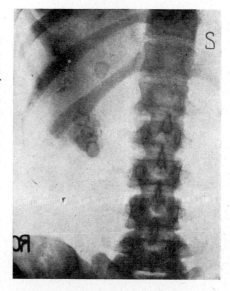

Fig. 303.—Gall-stones. Rounded shadows in the right abdomen. Stones in the gall-bladder. The higher shadow is due to a stone impacted in the cystic duct.

Non-function and occlusion of the gall-bladder is demonstrated by the fact that the dye, although present in the bowel, is not seen in the gall-bladder. Sub-normal function and the presence of non-opaque gall-stones can also be demonstrated, by lack of the usual density of the shadow of the dye in the gall-bladder in the former case, and by the presence of translucent shadows in the outline of the gall-bladder in the latter. The test naturally depends on good liver function and is of course not satisfactory when jaundice or liver damage is present. (*Figs.* 304, 305.)

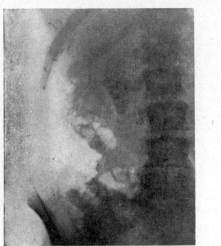
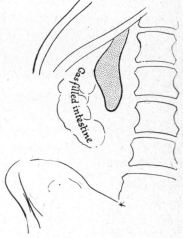

Fig. 304.—Normal gall-bladder. The gall-bladder is shown as a shadow placed beneath the costal margin.

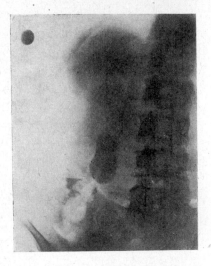
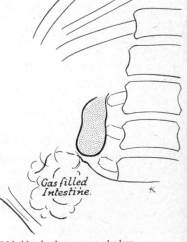

Fig. 305.—Normal gall-bladder. The gall-bladder is shown as a shadow placed just above the crest of the ilium.

THE UTERUS AND FALLOPIAN TUBES

The outline of the uterus and Fallopian tubes may be seen on a radiograph taken after the introduction of lipiodol into the uterus. This test, which demonstrates the passage of lipiodol into the peritoneal cavity if the tubes are patent, will also demonstrate the anatomy of the uterus and tubes.

SALIVARY GLANDS, SUPERFICIAL SINUSES, AND EMPYEMA CAVITIES ·

These can be demonstrated after the introduction of lipiodol, and after screen examination radiographs can be taken to record their anatomy.

THE NERVOUS SYSTEM

The outlines of the brain and spinal cord cannot be demonstrated in a direct radiograph as they are surrounded by ' bony cages.' It is possible, however, to introduce air into the ventricular system via a trephine, and resultant radiographs will show the anatomy of the ventricular system. Tumours may deform and displace the outline of the ventricles (*Figs.* 306–309), or may cause interference with the flow of cerebrospinal fluid and will cause dilatation of the ventricles. This is particularly noted in tumours of the base of the skull.

Air may be injected by the spinal route. This method of examination is known as ' encephalography.' Spinal fluid is removed and replacement by air carried out. Radiographs taken after this procedure will show up the cortical markings and, if the basal foramina are patent, will also show up the ventricles.

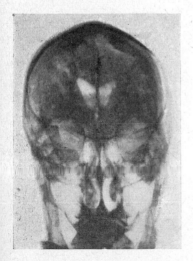

Fig. 306. — Normal encephalogram. Subject lying on back. Anterior horns filled symmetrically. Third ventricle lies below the anterior horns in the midline.

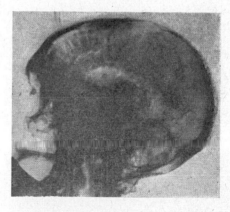

Fig. 307.—Normal encephalogram. Latera view. Ventricles are normal in shape, slightly enlarged. Air is seen in the cortical markings.

26

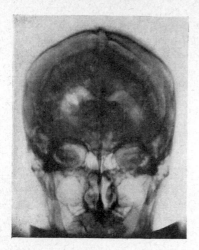 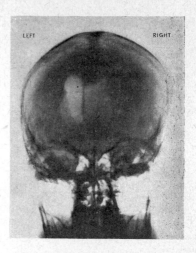

Fig. 308.—Normal encephalogram. Face down. Showing posterior horns of ventricles.

Fig. 309.—Ventriculogram showing dilated anterior horns and a dilated third ventricle which is displaced to the left side by a tumour of the right temporal area.

Similarly, lipiodol injected into the spinal theca will demonstrate any blockage due to the presence of a tumour mass, and if the lipiodol is allowed to flow up and down the spinal canal by tilting the table upon which the patient lies at varying angles, protrusion of the intervertebral disk into the spinal space can be demonstrated as a filling defect.

THE RENAL TRACT

The renal outlines can be demonstrated in contrast to the abdominal viscera, and their position noted. Owing to their calcium content calculi in the kidneys, bladder, and ureters can be clearly seen. (*Figs.* 310, 311.)

In order to examine the function of the kidneys an intravenous injection of an organic dye is administered. This dye, made up in ampoules of 20 c.c., contains in aqueous solution 15 g. of the sodium salt of 3 : 5-di-iodo-4-pyridoxyl-N-methyl-2 : 6-dicarboxylic acid. The iodine in this preparation renders it opaque to X rays. It is known pharmaceutically as iodoxyl (B.P.) (proprietary names—uroselectan, pyelectan).

The dye is excreted unchanged by the kidneys, and radiographs taken within a few minutes of its injection will show the outline of the renal pelves and also the ureteric and bladder outlines (*Fig.* 312). Non-function, blockage of the ureters, hydronephrosis, and filling defects due to tuberculosis and carcinoma can thus be demonstrated. (*Figs.* 313, 314.) In cases where there is non-function of the kidney the pelvis and ureter may be explored by cystoscopy and the passage of a catheter up the ureter followed by the injection of iodoxyl into the pelvis of the kidney. A radiograph taken immediately after this has been done will show the nature of the lesion present.

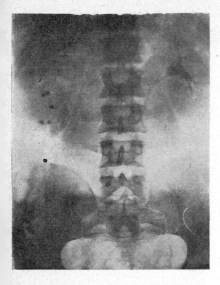

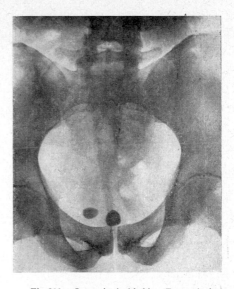

Fig. 310.—Renal calculi. The renal tract 20 minutes after giving uroselectan. The left kidney shows a normal pyelogram. Dense shadows due to calculi are seen in the right kidney, and also in the right ureter. The dye is not excreted by the right kidney.

Fig. 311.—Stones in the bladder. Dense shadows of bladder calculi are seen in the pelvis.

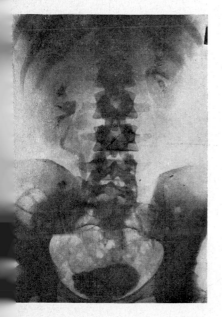

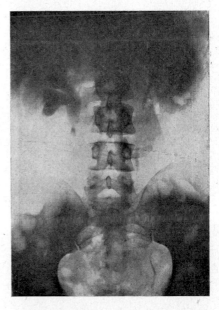

Fig. 312.—Normal pyelogram, 20 minutes after administration of uroselectan. There is ptosis of the right kidney.

Fig. 313.—Hydronephrosis. Pyelogram after uroselectan. Stone in the upper right ureter causing hydronephosis of the kidney. Dilated pelvis with blunting of calices.

Examination of the bladder and ureters and kidneys can also be made by retrograde pyelography, i.e., by simple injection of solution of sodium bromide into these organs (*Fig.* 315).

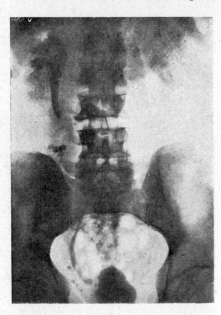

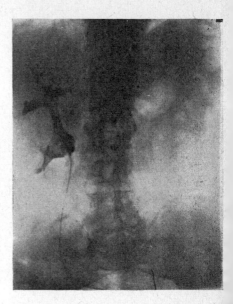

Fig. 314.—Renal tuberculosis. Pyelogram taken 5 minutes after injection of uroselectan. Small contracted bladder. Impaired function of left kidney ; poor visualization. Early dilatation of right ureter and right renal pelvis.

Fig. 315. — Renal neoplasm. Retrograde pyelogram of right kidney showing deformity due to neoplasm.

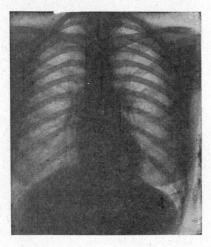

Fig. 316.—Radiograph of normal lungs.

THE CHEST

The mediastinal contents and lungs are examined for their general outline, and screen examination is made to view their mobility and expansion. The degree of diaphragmatic movement and lung expansion can be compared, and unusual pulsation of the heart and aorta is noted in this way. The detail of the lungs has to be examined in the radiograph taken (*Fig.* 316). The lung trabecular markings can be outlined and clearly distinguished. In pneumothorax the absence of lung markings is noted together with any displacement of the mediastinum (*Fig.* 317). The changes with pleural effusion are similar, but the translucency is replaced by opacity due to the fluid (which absorbs the radiation) (*Fig.* 318). In lesions of the parenchyma of the lungs consolidation is demonstrated by an even opacity of the lungs which is localized to the lobes (*Figs.* 319, 320). Its resolution is noted by an increase in the translucency and recession of the shadow.

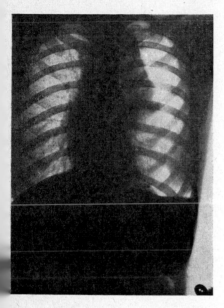

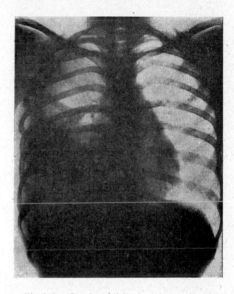

Fig. 318.—Opacity of right chest due to pleural effusion.

Fig. 317.—Partial pneumothorax of the left chest. The margin of the collapsed lung is clearly seen.

Tuberculous infiltration is demonstrated as a ' cotton-wool ' type of mottling which tends to coalesce and break down into cavity formation. (*Figs.* 321–323.)

Carcinoma, if of the bronchial type, by causing obstruction of the bronchus, will be demonstrated as consolidation and lack of movement of the part affected, and later as an atelectasis. (*Fig.* 324.) Introduction of lipiodol will outline the defect in the bronchus. If of the hilar type there will be an absolute opacity infiltrating the lung substance, and in extreme cases showing displacement of the mediastinum, but pleural effusion usually follows rapidly and obscures the underlying pathology. Secondary growths are noted by their circular outline and multiplicity.

Silicosis causes discrete mottling of an even density which is of a fan-shaped distribution and is associated with increased fibrosis of the lung roots and increased density of the hilar shadows.

The greater part of the mediastinum is made up of the heart and thoracic aorta. The heart is placed obliquely in the thorax and the outline

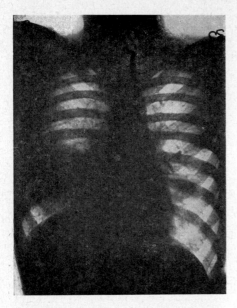

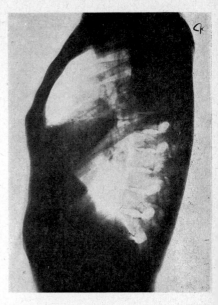

Fig. 319.—Pneumonia. Consolidation of the right middle lobe of the lung, showing a localized and clearly demarcated even opacity.

Fig. 320.—Pneumonia, lateral view. Consolidation of the right middle lobe, clearly outlined by the interlobar pleural fissures.

of the left side of the heart is made up mainly by the left ventricle, pulmonary artery, and the arch of the aorta. The right outline is made up of the right auricle and the great vessels, and this side is placed mainly anteriorly.

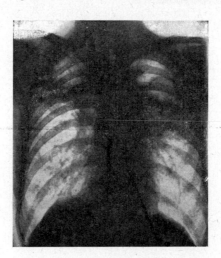

Fig. 321.—Radiograph showing large cavities. At each apex is a large cavity surrounded by dense fibrous tissue.

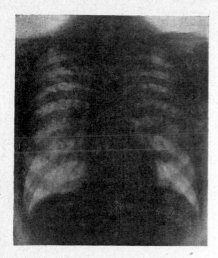

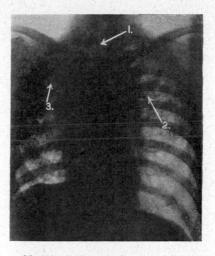

Fig. 322.—Radiograph of bilateral active phthisis. Diffuse 'cotton-wool' type of mottling, widely distributed, characteristic of early phthisis.

Fig. 323.—Radiograph of extensive bilateral phthisis. 1, Trachea displaced to right ; 2, Punctate mottling characteristic of active phthisis ; 3, Dense mottling with darker strands indicative of fibrosis.

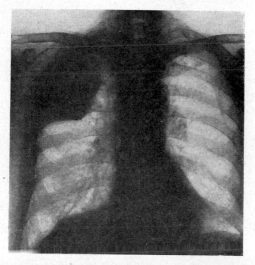

Fig. 324.—Peripheral carcinoma of the chest. Dense shadow in the periphery of the lung field, base to the surface and obliterating the lung substance. Rounded margin.

Enlargement of the particular parts is shown as prominence of the part and by alteration of the outline from the normal. In left ventricular hypertrophy the cardiac outline is enlarged to the left side and the heart appears to be 'boot-shaped' (Fig. 325). In mitral stenosis (Fig. 326) the outline tends to become quadrilateral. The aortic knuckle protrudes to the left of the midline, and diffuse or aneurysmal enlargements are clearly seen in the anteroposterior position (*Fig.* 327) and even better in oblique positions (*Fig.* 328).

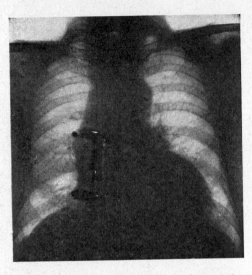

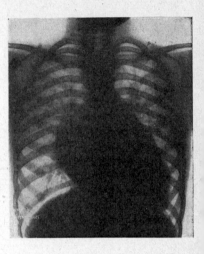

Fig. 326.—Cardiac enlargement due to mitral stenosis. Right-sided enlargement (quadrilateral-shaped heart), with prominent pulmonary artery (left side).

Fig. 325.—Cardiac hyperthrophy. Left ventricular enlargement (boot-shaped heart), with diffuse dilatation of the aorta.

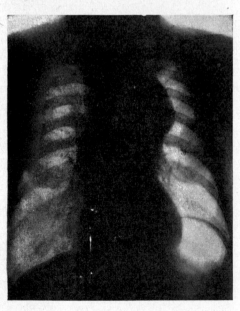

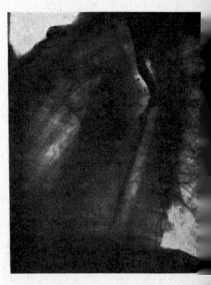

Fig. 328.—Oblique view (left posterior oblique) of chest demonstrating indentation of œsophagus in the upper third due to an enlarged arch of the aorta.

Fig. 327.—Aneurysm of the arch of the aorta. Rounded shadow to the left of the sternum.

Lipiodol can be introduced into the bronchial tree either directly down the larynx through a catheter (inserted under local anæsthesia) or by means of a bronchoscope. The outlines of the bronchi and alveoli are clearly seen and the presence of dilated alveoli in bronchiectasis is demonstrated (*Figs.* 329, 330.)

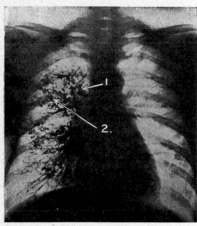

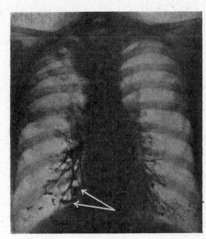

FIG. 329. FIG. 330.

Fig. 329.—Radiograph of normal bronchial tree. 1, Bronchus outlined with lipiodol; 2, Alveoli filled with lipiodol.

Fig. 330.—Radiograph of bronchiectasis. Small bronchiectatic cavities are seen partially filled with lipiodol, giving the characteristic 'bird's-nest' appearance (indicated by the arrows). In each cavity an air-filled space is seen above the fluid level.

CHAPTER XIV

CLINICAL PATHOLOGY AND BIOCHEMISTRY

ONLY such simple laboratory procedures have been included here as may be reasonably undertaken by the student in the clinic room, or by the practitioner in his surgery. Investigations requiring special knowledge or constant practice for their accuracy are advisedly left in the hands of the pathologist or biochemist.

MICROSCOPICAL EXAMINATION OF SPUTUM

The patient should rinse the mouth with sterile water before collecting the sputum, which should preferably be the first morning specimen. This should be expectorated straight into a sterile vessel. Care should be taken that the specimen is not entirely saliva or muco-pus from the nasopharynx. A small amount of the most purulent portion is then taken on a platinum loop and placed on a glass slide. For examination of an unstained specimen, a cover-slip may be placed on top. If a stained preparation of the sputum is required, some of the purulent material is teased out on a slide to make an even, but not too thick, film. The preparation is gently dried over the flame of a bunsen or spirit lamp and finally fixed by passing rapidly through the flame two or three times. Any charring of the material makes the preparation valueless. For general examination methylene blue is a suitable stain.

The following constituents should then be carefully looked for in the specimen :—

1. Red corpuscles.
2. Pus cells.
3. Epithelial cells (nearly always abundant). These cells are usually in a state of partial disintegration.
4. Elastic fibres—representing lung destruction, e.g., in tuberculosis, bronchiestasis.
5. Charcot-Leyden crystals—octahedral crystals found in cases of asthma—not very important.
6. Curschmann's spirals, consisting of a central core with a delicate network around. These are common in asthma uncomplicated by much bronchitis.
7. Casts of the bronchi, found on rare occasions in bronchitis and pneumonia.
8. Organisms. These require special stains for their identification, and frequently cultural methods (see STAINING FOR BACTERIA, p. 435);

expert bacteriological advice is often necessary. An examination for tubercle bacilli, pneumococci, and streptococci should, however, be possible to every student and practitioner.

EXAMINATION OF PLEURAL, PERICARDIAL, AND ASCITIC PERITONEAL FLUIDS

Pleural Fluids.—

Macroscopical Examination.—In empyema the pus varies from a slightly turbid fluid to thick creamy pus. With a thin turbid fluid microscopical examination is necessary to confirm the presence of pus cells. The fluid in other conditions, e.g., transudates in renal disease and cardiac failure, and exudates in tuberculosis or 'rheumatic' pleural effusion, is usually clear and of light yellow colour. Blood-stained effusions are less common, and are seen most frequently in malignant disease of the lungs, pleura, or mediastinal tissues, in tuberculosis of the pleura, or in trauma.

Microscopical Examination.—A film may be made in a similar manner to a blood smear. In the majority of fluids encountered it is necessary to concentrate the solid constituents by centrifuging, and to make films from the deposit. The fluid is examined chiefly for its cellular and bacterial content. To demonstrate the cells Leishman's stain is appropriate. The principal cells found are endothelial cells, polymorphonuclear leucocytes, and small lymphocytes. Neoplastic cells are practically never recognized in ordinary films, requiring for their identification special methods of preparation and staining. Eosinophils are found rarely in parasitic infections.

Endothelial cells are large, with pale blue cytoplasm, frequently vacuolated. They are present in the pleural transudates of cardiac failure, renal disease, or neoplasm.

Polymorphonuclear leucocytes are present in acute pleural infections, especially of coccal origin. The fluid in which they are found may be clear when the polymorphs are few in number, turbid when they are moderately numerous, or definitely purulent (empyema) when the numbers are great. Bacteria (especially pneumococci or streptococci) are generally found in association with them.

Small lymphocytes are found in excess in chronic inflammatory lesions of the pleura, especially tuberculosis, and rarely in syphilis or Hodgkin's disease.

The examination of the fluid for micro-organisms requires the technique described for different bacteria (*see* p. 435). When tuberculosis is suspected but no tubercle bacilli are discoverable, it is usual to inject the fluid into a guinea-pig, which develops signs of generalized tuberculosis within a few weeks.

Pericardial and Ascitic Peritoneal Fluids.—These are examined in a similar way to pleural fluids, by naked-eye inspection and microscopy. The effusions are generally clear, though occasionally purulent, and the cellular and bacterial content should be noted. The milky appearance of the fluid in chylous ascites, though rarely encountered, is typical.

TESTS FOR LIVER FUNCTION

Careful observation has shown that no single test of liver function is reliable as indicative of liver disease, but when several tests suggest impairment, they may be useful in confirmation of a clinical diagnosis. Even more important is the assessment of prognosis, for as in the case of renal disease, clinical manifestations may be similar in cases having a very differing outlook. Two cases of hepatitis for example may be shown by liver efficiency tests to vary greatly in prognosis according to the functional capacity of the liver, one likely to recover, the other to die.

The more important tests include excretion estimations—hippuric acid and lævulose, and blood chemical examinations which have the advantage that they can be carried out on a single specimen of blood.

Lævulose Index.—This is based upon the estimation of the blood-lævulose after administration of 100 g. of sucrose (comparable with a glucose tolerance test in diabetes). The normal figure is about 11 and rises up to 13 may occur in non-liver diseases. In hepatic disease, figures from 20-30 may be found.

Hippuric Acid Excretion.—Benzoic acid is given by mouth and is followed by excretion of hippuric acid, which is estimated at 2- and 4-hour intervals. Figures of 60 per cent at 2 hours and over 80 per cent at 4 hours are normally found, and may fall to 35 per cent and 60 per cent respectively in liver disease.

Plasma Bilirubin.—The reactions of bilirubin to Ehrlich's diazo reagent in the van den Bergh reaction are discussed on p. 171, and it need only be emphasized that this qualitative reaction is of value in distinguishing various types of jaundice.

Bilirubin may, however, also be estimated quantitatively and when found in excess taken as evidence of liver damage. Normal figures are given as 0·1 to 1 mg. per 100 c.c. serum, but most commonly the figure is about 0·5 mg. In liver disease an increase to as much as 20 mg. may be found, the higher results occurring when jaundice is present.

Icterus Index.—This is a colorimetric method of estimating the serum bilirubin. Normal figures are 1 to 5 units (5 units = 1 mg. per 100 c.c.).

The amount may rise to 10 or 15 units in cases of latent jaundice, in which the pigment is insufficient to stain the skin, or to much higher figures (40-50) when obstructive jaundice is present.

Plasma Phosphatase.—This enzyme is found in considerable amounts in the liver; in blood-plasma it is usually present in amounts of 6-10 units and may rise in liver disease to 20, 50, or more units.

Plasma Proteins.—In liver diseases there is a tendency for the plasma albumin to fall and the globulin to rise. Normal plasma protein content ranges from about 4·5 to 4·7 g. of albumin per cent, and 2 to 2·4 g. of globulin per cent. In liver diseases the albumin may fall to nearer 3 per cent and the globulin rise to 3 per cent. Lesser alterations in the albumin content are found in certain other diseases.

TESTS FOR PANCREATIC FUNCTION

As in the case of the liver, serious disease of the pancreas may exist without gross alteration in its function. In some cases, however, the existence of disease may be indicated by signs of pancreatic insufficiency. The more important tests used for the detection of this condition are :—

1. Examination of the Stools for Steatorrhœa (the presence of excess of fats).—The fats are neutral, as they are not split into fatty acids and glycerol owing to the deficiency of lipase. The stools should also be searched for striated muscle-fibres, *creatorrhœa*, indicating defective protein digestion owing to the lack of trypsin.

2. Examination of the Urine.—High values in the urinary *diastase*, e.g., 200 or more units, may be found in cases of acute pancreatitis. The normal figures range between 7 and 33 units, but the disturbance of diastase contained is of very little value in the diagnosis of chronic pancreatic disease. It is possible for diseases of the pancreas to destroy the islets of Langerhans resulting in deficient secretion of insulin and the production of *glycosuria* and *hyperglycæmia*. It is, however, possible to have very grave diseases of the pancreas without any such effects.

EXAMINATION OF STOMACH CONTENTS

The detailed analysis of the specimens obtained in a fractional test-meal (*see below*) is best left to laboratory workers whose technique is made perfect by constant practice. Two simple tests are included here which are applicable to isolated specimens of stomach contents obtained by spontaneous vomiting or by removal with a stomach pump. (*See also* Chapter VI, p. 202.)

Test for Free Hydrochloric Acid (*Günzburg's reagent*).—The reagent is phloroglucin-vanillin in alcoholic solution, a few drops of which are gently heated with two drops of the filtered stomach contents in a small evaporating dish. If hydrochloric acid is present a delicate pink colour develops.

Test for Organic Acids (*Uffelmann's reagent*).—The gastric contents frequently have a sour or rancid odour when an excess of organic acids is present. Lactic acid gives a bright yellow colour when $\frac{1}{2}$ c.c. of the filtered stomach contents is added to 3 c.c. of Uffelmann's reagent (consisting of 1-20 carbolic acid and a dilute ferric chloride solution in equal parts).

Test Meal.—After X-ray examination a fractional test meal forms the most reliable accessory method of examining the stomach functions. Although it is open to the criticisms that the artificial conditions imposed by the nature of the meal and the discomfort to which the patient is subjected may alter the composition of the gastric juice, much useful information can generally be obtained.

The *quantity of gastric contents from the fasting stomach*, the ' resting juice', may be measured, and its chemical properties compared with specimens derived from a stomach in active function. These specimens are obtained by giving the patient a special ' test meal', consisting usually of weak gruel. The specimens are drawn up from the stomach through a thin rubber tube at intervals of fifteen minutes up to about two and a half hours from the time the meal was taken. In this way portions of the meal can be examined at various stages of digestion.

The amount of free hydrochloric acid and of *total acids* is estimated in each specimen, and the curves formed by plotting the figures for these amounts are singularly constant in the majority of persons.

Apart from acid, the specimens are examined for the presence of *bile, mucus, blood, starch*, and other rarer constituents.

The following findings based on the observations of Ryle can be taken as a standard. The fasting juice varies between 10 and 150 c.c., averaging 50 c.c. Bile is present in about 40 per cent of cases. The range of free acidity, in the majority of cases, varies between 0 and 22 per cent. The total acidity ranges from 4 to 38 per cent. In many cases absence of acid (*achlorhydria*) and excess of acid (*hyperchlorhydria*) are found in normal persons, and they cannot be regarded as pathological when they occur as isolated signs, though if associated with other evidence of disease they may be valuable confirmatory facts—e.g., the achlorhydria of pernicious anæmia and the hyperchlorhydria of duodenal ulcer (*Figs.* 331–334).

Traces of blood may be found in some of the specimens if there has been injury to the œsophagus or stomach in passing the tube, but the *persistent presence of blood, particularly when altered, is nearly always due to organic disease*, especially ulcer and cancer of the stomach.

Two of the commonest pathological findings in a fractional test meal are great *excess of free hydrochloric acid in duodenal ulcer*, less constantly

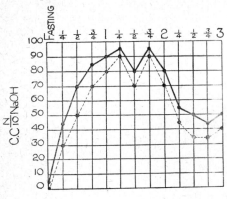

Fig. 331.—Curve showing hyperchlorhydria such as may occur with duodenal ulcer.

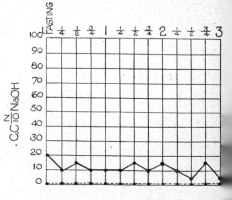

Fig. 332.—Complete achlorhydria with low total acidity. Such a curve is usual in pernicious anæmia, though it may occur in a certain percentage of normal people.

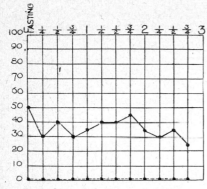

Fig. 333.—Achlorhydria with high total acidity in carcinoma ventriculi.

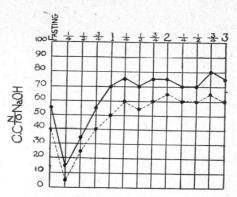

Fig. 334.—Plateau curve in pyloric obstruction.

in gastric ulcer, and *deficiency of free acid in carcinoma*, especially in that affecting the stomach itself. In the latter case there is often a relatively *large amount of organic acids* owing to fermentative changes. The resting juice in carcinoma may be characteristically foul, and contain starch and blood. Pyloric obstruction may be indicated by delayed emptying and persistent high concentration of free hydrochloric acid, resulting in a ' plateau ' type of course.

In *pernicious anæmia and subacute combined degeneration, achlorhydria is also pronounced*, but in contrast with cancer of the stomach there is deficiency of both organic and inorganic acids. Further points of distinction may be rapid emptying of starch as compared with delay, and the absence of blood. The powerful gastric stimulant histamine is sometimes given to confirm the presence of an absolute achlorhydria and achylia.

These important examples by no means complete the list of diseases in which alterations are found in the chemistry of the gastric contents, but further discussion of this is outside the scope of the present work.

EXAMINATION OF THE FÆCES

Macroscopical Examination.—The naked-eye inspection of the fæces has already been partially considered in Chapter VI. When foreign bodies such as gall-stones and intestinal worms are anticipated, the stool should be washed repeatedly through muslin or a fine sieve.

Chemical Examination.—The most important chemical test applicable in the clinic room is that for *occult blood*, by which small amounts of blood may be recognized. This is of great value when slight continual bleeding occurs from ulceration or carcinoma of the stomach or intestine.

Benzidine Test for Occult Blood : *Technique.*—The patient should be on a farinaceous diet for forty-eight hours previously.

Mix a small portion of fæces in water in a test-tube. Boil to inactivate enzymes, and cool. In another test-tube make a saturated solution of benzidine in 2 c.c. of glacial acetic acid, and add 2 c.c. of hydrogen peroxide (10 vol.). Add some of the emulsion of fæces to this latter mixture. A blue colour develops in the presence of blood.

This reaction is a very delicate one for blood, and care should be taken in its performance. Solutions of benzidine are affected by light and should be freshly prepared each time the test is performed. It is essential to use scrupulously clean glassware. A control should be made concurrently to see that no blue colour develops without the addition of the blood extract.

Wagner slide modification : Take a little of the solid stool on a match-stick, smear it on a clean slide, and pour freshly prepared reagent over it. It turns blue if blood is present and there is no misleading green tint from fluid. Make the solution as follows : Add a knife-tip of benzidine to 2 c.c. of glacial acetic acid, and then add 20 drops of a 3 per cent solution of hydrogen peroxide.

By this technique soiling of the fingers is avoided and the sensitivity is not impaired, as compared with the ' wet ' reaction.

Microscopical Examination.—The fæces should be mixed evenly with a little normal saline and a drop of the suspension placed on a glass slide with a cover-glass. If mucus or blood is present in the stool, a portion should be chosen which contains these.

To the inexperienced eye the normal constituents are so abundant as to obscure the abnormal.

ABNORMAL CONSTITUENTS.—The more important are pus cells, red blood-corpuscles, ova, and pathological bacteria.

Pus Cells.—These are similar in character to those found elsewhere, but may need staining to demonstrate them. They may be demonstrable by the microscope in ulcerative conditions of the bowel, although not present to the naked eye.

Red Corpuscles.—Red corpuscles may be recognized in the stools when hæmorrhage has taken place fairly low in the large intestine although it may not have been sufficiently large to cause the appearance of blood visible to the naked eye.

Ova and Bacteria.—The distinction of various types of ova, parasites, and pathological bacteria usually requires the opinion of a skilled pathologist and will not be dealt with here.

NORMAL CONSTITUENTS. These are mainly derived from the digestion of food and the desquamation of intestinal epithelium. The character of the diet naturally makes a considerable difference to these constituents and must be taken into consideration in every case.

Muscle-fibres.—Found in meat eaters, but when striated fibres appear in large numbers some failure of protein digestion or excessive intake of protein may be suspected. They appear as small yellow bodies.

Fat Globules.—Recognized as rounded refractile bodies. They should not appear unless the patient is taking excess of fats or has had an oily enema.

Fat Crystals and Soaps.—Common in normal fæces. The soaps dissolve on warming and are coarsely crystalline. The fatty acids appear as sheaves.

Starch Granules.—A few of these may be present in normal fæces, and are easily demonstrated by introducing a little iodine solution beneath the cover-slip. The starch granules turn blue. Excess usually indicates some error in carbohydrate digestion.

Vegetable Debris.—The disintegration products of the digestion of fruit and vegetables result in many varied-shaped bodies in the normal fæces. Spiral-shaped masses and cellular structures are particularly common.

Parasites in Fæces.—Many parasites may be found in the stools, but most of them fortunately are uncommon in Great Britain, and on the rare occasions in which they are suspected the opinion of a pathologist is usually advisable (*see* EXAMINATION FOR TROPICAL PARASITES, p. 437). Three varieties are, however, not uncommon and are deserving of brief mention here, viz., tapeworms, roundworms, and threadworms.

Tapeworms.—Roundworms, threadworms, and segments of tapeworms may be obvious to the patient or examiner when the stools are inspected. Should the last be found a search for the head is advisable, though it must be admitted that this is often unsuccessful. For the diagnosis the student will frequently have to rely on the characters of the segments. The main characteristics of the common tapeworms are as follows :—

Tænia solium is about 10 ft. long. Each segment (proglottis) is 10 mm. long and 5 to 6 mm. broad, and the genital pores are laterally placed. The uterus has about ten lateral, coarsely arranged branches. The head is about the size of that of a large pin, and is recognized by its four suckers and two rows of hooklets on the rostellum. *Tænia solium* is found in its immature forms in infected pork (especially in Germany), but occasionally occurs in this form in man (cysticercus). More usually it is found in the mature form, the characteristics of which have just been described.

Tænia saginata may attain a length of 20 to 25 ft. The segments are comparatively large (16 mm. long × 5 mm. broad) when ripe. The uterus has 20 to 25 fine branches, and the genital pore is laterally placed. The head is larger than that of *Tænia solium* and has four suckers but *no hooklets*. This parasite is derived from infected beef, and only occurs in man in the mature form.

Tænia echinococcus is not found in the adult form in man. In its intermediary form of hydatid cysts it may occur in most parts of the body. The diagnosis rests on clinical evidence, on Casoni's skin test, or on a complement deviation or precipitin test. It is inadvisable to needle the cysts owing to the great risk of spreading infection.

Roundworms (Ascaris lumbricoides).—These may be recognized by their resemblance to the common earth-worm. They are several inches in length, the female longer than the male. Often only the ova are found in the stools.

Threadworms (Enterobius vermicularis).—The name of these parasites is a sufficient description. They appear like minute strands of white cotton,

27

5 to 10 mm. in length, and occur in large numbers. They are particularly common in children of the poorer classes, and may be seen in active movement in a recent specimen of fæces. The ova can be found only by obtaining scrapings or swabbings from the peri-anal skin where they are deposited. The N.I.H. swab, a glass rod covered with cellophane held in position by an elastic band, has proved of the greatest value in diagnosing oxyuriasis. After swabbing, the cellophane is opened out, moistened, and spread on a slide, and examined microscopically for eggs after covering with a slip.

EXAMINATION OF THE CEREBROSPINAL FLUID

No neurological diagnosis can be considered complete without the examination of the cerebrospinal fluid. Elaborate chemical and microscopical methods are now available which are of great help in many cases and frequently essential. These are best carried out by the laboratory worker, but there remain certain preliminary and valuable observations which can be made by the student or practitioner. The more important of these are :—

Colour and Consistency.—Normal cerebrospinal fluid is clear and water-like, and it retains these characteristics in many diseases of the nervous system (e.g., disseminated sclerosis, G.P.I., etc.). In meningeal infection (especially by cocci), it may be turbid or definitely purulent. When hæmorrhage occurs into the subarachnoid space (e.g., ventricular hæmor: hage, leakage of cerebral aneurysms, and basal fractures) the fluid is *evenly* blood-stained, and remains yellow (*xanthochromia*) after centrifugalization. This must be distinguished from blood-stained fluid produced by trauma. Here the blood and spinal fluid are less intimately mixed, and the fluid becomes clearer as more drips away. After centrifaging a specimen of this kind the supernatant liquid is clear (colourless).

Chemical Reactions.—

Protein.—Shake up the fluid. Excessive frothiness which takes more than a few minutes to disappear is to be noted when there is an increased protein content. Occasionally the cerebrospinal fluid contains such enormous amounts of protein that spontaneous coagulation occurs. When this is combined with xanthochromia it receives the name of Froin's syndrome, and is most commonly to be seen in compression of the spinal cord.

Add a few drops of 2 per cent salicylsulphonic acid solution. A white precipitate occurs in the presence of excess of protein. A normal fluid gives a precipitate with stronger solutions of the reagent.

Pandy's reaction for globulin consists in adding a few drops of cerebrospinal fluid to 1 c.c. of Pandy's reagent (10 per cent aqueous solution of phenol). Normal fluid usually remains clear or rarely gives a faint haze. Excess of globulin varies from a cloud to a flocculent precipitate.

Other important constituents, particularly sugar and chlorides, require laboratory methods for their estimation.

SIGNIFICANCE OF CHEMICAL CHANGES.—

Protein Content.—The normal cerebrospinal fluid contains 20 to 30 mg. protein per cent. Moderate increase occurs in most conditions in which the cell-count is increased, especially inflammatory processes such as cerebral and spinal meningitis, meningo-vascular syphilis, etc.

Sugar Content.—Glucose occurs in normal cerebrospinal fluid in rather smaller amounts than in blood, viz., 50 to 80 mg. per cent. It is notably *decreased in meningitis* of all types, and may be entirely absent. This is a useful sign in distinguishing meningitis, and to a lesser extent poliomyelitis, from *encephalitis lethargica*, in which an *increase* is sometimes found, never a decrease.

Chloride Content.—Chlorides are present in amounts of 700 to 760 mg. per cent in normal cerebrospinal fluid. A diminution occurs in *meningitis* (600 to 650 mg. per cent) and may help in distinguishing meningitis from cerebral abscess. The diminution is most pronounced in tuberculous meningitis.

Microscopical Examination.—The fluid should be centrifuged, the supernatant liquid decanted, and a loopful of the deposit taken up on a platinum wire and put on a glass slide, as in making a preparation of a urinary deposit. It is fixed by gentle heat or merely allowed to dry in the air. It may then be stained with methylene blue or a special stain such as Gram's stain or Ziehl-Neelsen carbol-fuchsin.

The preparation is examined for (1) its cellular content, (2) bacteria.

Cellular Content.—Normally when examined under the oil immersion lens there should not be more than 2 or 3 lymphocytes in the field, and no polymorphonuclear leucocytes. If there is an excess of cells note should be taken whether these are mononuclear or polynuclear. An exact count may be made before centrifuging in a special counting chamber, similar to that used for blood-counts.

SIGNIFICANCE OF THE CELL-COUNT.—In *acute inflammatory lesions* of the brain and meninges, especially meningitis, a great *increase in polymorphonuclear leucocytes* occurs. This is especially so when the invading organisms are cocci, though bacillary infections (e.g. tuberculous meningitis) may be accompanied by a polymorphonuclear increase if the intensity of the infection and the reaction of the patient is great. If the inflammatory lesion is localized (cerebral abscess) this polymorph response is not found to a marked extent.

In *subacute and chronic inflammatory lesions of the brain and meninges* the increased cell-count is mainly made up of *small lymphocytes*, with a smaller number of large mononuclear cells. This lymphocytosis is particularly characteristic of parenchymatous cerebrospinal syphilis (*tabes* and *general paralysis of the insane*), but occurs in tuberculous meningitis and also in other less common conditions.

Not infrequently mixtures of polymorphs and lymphocytes are found in the same case (for example, in acute anterior poliomyelitis), or one ty of cell may give place to the other. This happens in acute inflamma ₁c lesions which become more chronic as the disease progresses. For example, in tuberculous meningitis the onset may be acute and the increased cellular content chiefly polymorphs ; later the disease becomes more chronic and lymphocytes predominate.

Bacteria.—The staining methods used are those described on pp. 435 et seq. The most important organisms to be demonstrated are the Gram-positive pneumococci and streptococci and the Gram-negative *intracellular* meningococci. Tubercle bacilli may be found in many cases of tuberculous meningitis, but require patient search. They are most abundant in the fine coagulum which separates in a few hours from a tuberculous cerebrospinal fluid and which looks like a fine thread suspended in the centre of the test-tube.

OTHER SPECIAL INVESTIGATIONS

Colloid Gold Reaction (*Lange's Test*).—This test depends upon the precipitation of colloidal suspensions of gold by cerebrospinal fluid containing abnormal amounts and proportions of protein. The cerebrospinal fluid is added to the gold suspension in 10 dilutions (1 : 10, 1 : 20, 1 : 40, 1 : 80, 1 : 160, etc.). The reaction with normal cerebrospinal fluid is negative—i.e., there is no precipitation of the gold, which remains in suspension in the presence of that amount of protein normally contained in the healthy spinal fluid. This is expressed as 0 0 0 0 0 0 0 0 0 0. If the amount of protein in the fluid is increased, precipitation occurs, but may not occur if the increase is above a certain level. In diseased states in which the protein content is increased, precipitation is most pronounced at certain dilutions, and the degree of precipitation is judged by colour reactions which are graded from 1 to 5, 5 representing complete precipitation. The results may be expressed in figures, or graphically in ' curves '. The more important pathological results may be summarized :—

Luetic or Syphilitic Curve.—Numerically an average case reads as 0 1 2 3 3 1 0 0 0 0. Such a curve is found in *tabes* and other types of cerebrospinal syphilis. It may also occur in *disseminated sclerosis* (but here the Wassermann reaction is negative and the cell-count normal).

Paretic Curve.—Represented by the figures 5 5 5 5 4 3 1 0 0. It is characteristic of *general paralysis of the insane.*

Meningitic Curve.—The curve is not specific, and occurs in various types of meningitis. It will be represented by some such figures as 0 0 0 1 3 4 4 2 1 0.

It is important to secure the spinal fluid free from blood, the addition of which causes precipitation of gold.

Wassermann Reaction.—The reaction is always positive in cases of general paralysis, in most cases of tabes, and in a smaller number of cases of meningo-vascular syphilis. When positive in the spinal fluid it is usually positive in the blood, though exceptions occur. The reverse, however, is not necessarily true, and neurosyphilis cannot be established on a positive blood Wassermann alone, even though signs of a nervous lesion are present.

EXAMINATION OF THE BLOOD

Blood-counts.—The blood may be taken from the *lobe of the ear* or from a finger, either on its dorsal aspect just above the nail or from the finger-tip on its palmar aspect. The skin should be partially sterilized by wiping with ether-soaked wool, and pricked with a Hagedorn or triangular needle. The prick must be sufficiently deep to cause bleeding without *squeezing* the part, several pricks being made if necessary.

RED CORPUSCLES.—For counting the red corpuscles the *Thoma-Zeiss hæmacytometer* is generally employed. The special pipette (*Fig.* 335) has two marks on the stem, 0.5 and 1. The bulb above the stem terminates with a graduation mark 101, the capacity of the bulb being 100 times that of the stem. There is a glass bead in the bulb to help mix the blood and diluent. Blood is sucked into the pipette up to the 0.5 or 1 mark. The special diluting fluid is then drawn up until it fills the bulb to the mark 101. The blood will then be diluted 1–200 or 1–100 according to whether the 0.5 or 1 mark was chosen.

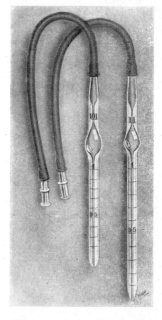

Fig. 335.—Pipettes for blood-count. The pipette for red cells is graduated to 101, that for white cells to 11.

All blood must be removed from the outside of the pipette, by wiping it with filter paper, and the *blood must be thoroughly mixed with the diluting fluid*, by rolling the pipette between fingers and thumbs, followed by gentle shaking with the fingers closing each end of the pipette.

Two or three drops should be expelled from the pipette in order to ensure that the contents of the stem are not used, and one drop is then placed on the central platform of the counting chamber. A little practice soon determines the optimum size for the drop, which must not overflow the platform ; care must also be taken to avoid air-bubbles The cover-slip is placed over the fluid, and the preparation allowed to settle for a few minutes. The cover-slip may be gently pressed until Newton's rings appear. These consist of coloured rings between the cover-glass and the outer platforms of the slide, and are best seen by looking obliquely at the slide. Their appearance is a guide to whether the cover-slip is pressed down sufficiently to give the correct depth to the fluid.

The microscope used for counting should be fitted with low-power (2/3-in.) and high-power (1/6-in.) objectives, mechanical stage, and a diaphragm.

Preliminary examination under the low power is of value in finding the lines marking the squares of the counting chamber. These are best seen when the diaphragm is stopped down. When they are found the 1/6 objective must be used for counting the corpuscles.

The ruled area will be seen to consist of sixteen large squares each bounded from its neighbours by two lines enclosing rectangular spaces, not to be confused with the squares. The large squares are subdivided into sixteen small squares, making in all 256 small squares.

In cases of slight or moderate anæmia it is convenient to count the corpuscles in 5 large squares, i.e., eighty small squares, but in severe anæmias it may be necessary to count in all the squares. To avoid counting the corpuscles twice, those which touch a line bounding a square should *only be counted on the top and left-hand lines*; those on the right or bottom lines will be counted as the left and top lines of other squares (*Fig.* 336).

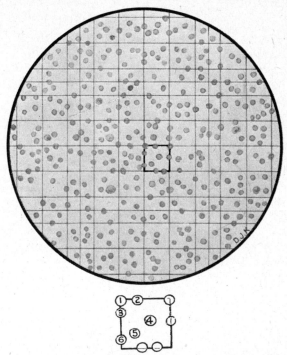

Fig. 336.—The hæmacytometer counting chamber. The mode of counting will be seen in the square which has been outlined in black (cf. inset). The cells on the upper and left-hand lines are counted but not those on the right and lower lines.

Calculation.—Each small square has a cubic capacity of $\frac{1}{4000}$ c.mm., so that if the dilution is known, the number of corpuscles per cubic millimetre can be easily calculated. For simplicity, the *total number of red corpuscles counted in five large squares (eighty small squares)* × 10,000 = *R.B.C. per c.mm. if the dilution is* 1 *in* 200.

Example : 600 cells counted in five large squares ; dilution 1–200.
R.B.C. per c.mm. = 600 × 10,000 = 6,000,000
Calculation in full :

$$\text{R.B.C. per c.mm.} = \frac{600 \text{ (R.B.C.)}}{80 \text{ (small squares)}} \times 200 \text{ (dilution)} \times 4000$$

(cubic capacity of squares) = 6,000,000.

If the dilution is 1 in 100 the number of corpuscles counted must be multiplied by 5000. If it is desirable to count a large number of cells, ten or fifteen large squares may be counted and the result divided by two or three respectively.

WHITE CORPUSCLES.—The method of counting the white cells is similar to that for the red cells. A smaller pipette is used, graduated to 0.5 and 1 on the stem and 11 above the bulb (*see Fig.* 335). The blood is thus diluted to 1–20 or 1–10. A special diluting fluid (2 per cent acetic acid containing a trace of methyl green) is used which dissolves the red corpuscles and stains the white cells. The total number of white corpuscles is relatively small, and it is necessary to count all the squares.

Calculation : *Example.*—

$$\frac{24 \text{ (no. of corpuscles)}}{256 \text{ (small squares)}} \times 20 \text{ (dilution)} \times 4000 \text{ (cubic capacity of}$$

squares) = 7500.

Simplification : Count cells in all 256 squares and multiply by 312, e.g.—

$$24 = 312 \times 7488$$

If a dilution of 1–10 is used the number of cells counted should be multiplied by 156.

Differential Count.—The blood-film is stained with Leishman and 200 leucocytes are enumerated (*see also* pp. 216 and 437). The number of each type of cell is expressed as a percentage.

PLATELETS.—As there is a tendency for these bodies to clump on contact with a glass surface, ideally all glassware should be waxed. The following gives a reasonably accurate result. Prepare a solution of brilliant cresyl blue in citrate to the colour of mixed Fehling's solution. Place a drop on the patient's finger and prick through it. Let 2 or 3 drops of the blood and citrate mixture drop into a small wax crucible containing more cresyl blue and citrate. Mix with a waxed pipette, and transfer a suitable drop to a glazed Thoma counting chamber. Allow to stand 15 minutes while the platelets settle, and count the number of red cells and platelets in several sets of small squares. By this a ratio of platelets to red cells is obtained, and, by reference to the total red cells counted in the normal manner, the absolute figure per cubic millimetre. The normal range is 200,000–400,000 per c.mm. The most marked reduction is in purpura hæmorrhagica, and a large decrease is noted after splenectomy.

Estimation of Hæmoglobin.—The *Haldane hæmoglobinometer* (*Fig.* 337) is the most suitable for ordinary purposes. The blood is taken up to the graduated mark on a special pipette. The outside of the tube is wiped, and the blood blown into a graduated tube (B) at the bottom of which a little distilled water is placed (up to the mark 10). Shake gently to mix the blood with the water. Now bubble coal gas through the blood mixture with a fine glass tube attached to the gas by rubber tubing. This converts the oxyhæmoglobin into carboxyhæmoglobin. Having completed this process, add distilled water drop by drop, mixing after each addition, until the colour of the solution matches the standard, and read off. Always match in daylight if possible. The standard consists of a tube (A) which contains a jelly, coloured with a solution of carboxyhæmoglobin. The standard is an arbitrary

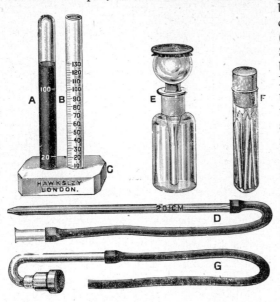

Fig. 337.—Haldane's hæmoglobinometer. A, Glass tube containing blood solution of standard tint ; B, Graduated tube ; C, Rubber stand for tubes A and B; D, Capillary pipette and suction tube—wires for cleaning the pipette are supplied ; E, Bottle with pipette stopper ; F, Glass tube holding six lancets ; G, Tube and cap for fixing over ordinary gas-burners.

one representing " 100 per cent " of hæmoglobin.

The *Dare Hæmoglobinometer* is somewhat expensive, but if available gives rapid and fairly satisfactory results in amateur hands. The undiluted blood is sandwiched between small plates of glass and porcelain, illuminated by an electric light, and compared with a wedge of coloured glass, which can be revolved until the colours match.

OTHER SPECIAL INVESTIGATIONS

The Clotting Time.—The time taken for blood to clot, namely, about 1 to 2 minutes (Dale and Laidlaw's method—variations according to other methods) is greatly prolonged in *hæmophilia*, which serves to distinguish this from other hæmorrhagic diseases.

The Bleeding Time.—This is the length of time the blood continues to flow when the finger or the lobe of the ear is pricked. In certain forms of *purpura* it may be prolonged, *especially during the phases in which the patient is actually bleeding*. It is normally about 4 minutes (Janet Vaughan), but may be 5 to 10 minutes or longer when the blood-platelet count is low. The bleeding time, therefore, should also be ascertained in diseases characterized by hæmorrhage.

Fragility of the Red Corpuscles.—The resistance of the red corpuscles to the hæmolytic effects of saline solutions of different strengths is a useful criterion of their fragility. *Increased fragility is a peculiar characteristic of acholuric familial jaundice.* Normal corpuscles hæmolyse in salines of strengths between 0·45 and 0·3, but excessively fragile corpuscles may hæmolyse in a solution of 0·6 per cent or even greater strength.

Sedimentation Rate.—If blood, rendered non-coagulable, is allowed to stand in special tubes kept strictly vertical, the corpuscles settle from the plasma at a fairly constant rate, varying somewhat in men and women. Several methods are in use to determine this rate of sedimentation : Wintrobe's is described. Collect 5 c.c. of blood in a tube containing a mixture of 6 mg. of ammonium oxalate and 4 mg. of potassium oxalate. (This anti-coagulant prevents cell shrinkage.) Fill the hæmatocrit (*Fig.* 338) with blood and stand in a vertical position. Read off the level to which the cells have fallen in an hour. The hæmatocrit is then centrifuged, and the volume of packed red cells determined by reading the new level of cells. For this read from the bottom upwards. By means of correlating these two results with a special chart, correction may be made for anæmia. By this method the normal sedimentation rate for men is 0–9 mm. and for women 0–20 mm. A great increase in the rapidity of the sedimentation rate is observed in many infections, in nephritis, pregnancy, carcinoma, and other conditions. The test is therefore of *little diagnostic value*, but has its place in prognosis. For example, the rapid sedimentation rate of active pulmonary tuberculosis may become slower as the patient responds to treatment. Similarly the test may have a prognostic value in nephritis, when the rate may remain persistently high in cases which are progressive or showing no signs of recovery. A rapid sedimentation rate is considered as evidence of activity in rheumatoid arthritis and is taken as one indication for gold therapy.

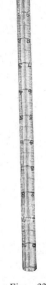

Fig. 338.— Wintrobe's hæmatocrit for measuring sedimentation rate of red blood-corpuscles.

Sternal Puncture.—A small quantity of bone-marrow is aspirated by inserting a large needle into the sternum. Smears are made from the marrow, stained, and a differential count of cells performed. The procedure may be of value in the diagnosis of some obscure cases of anæmia, and in leukæmia with an atypical peripheral blood-picture.

Prothrombin Time.—The level of the prothrombin in the blood is tested by noting the time taken for plasma to clot when mixed with thrombokinase and calcium chloride. The test is not yet standardized and times differ according to the method used. The estimation *is* of value in certain cases with hæmorrhagic tendencies due to a low prothrombin level in the blood. Examples are obstructive jaundice and hæmorrhagic disease of the newborn.

Blood Culture.—An attempt to grow organisms from the blood must be made in all cases of suspected septicæmia. Even when the clinical signs leave no doubt of the existence of a blood-stream infection, it is essential to know the nature of the organism. If the only organism reported as present is the *Staphylococcus albus*, the possibility of a skin contamination should be excluded by repeating the investigation. In low-grade septicæmia the organisms may not be constantly present in the blood—e.g., in subacute infective endocarditis—and repeated cultures are necessary. The blood should be taken, if possible, whilst the temperature is rising.

Agglutination Reactions.—In certain diseases, the patient's serum is capable of agglutinating or massing together an emulsion of the causal organ. This fact is of great value in the diagnosis of enteric and other infections. It becomes particularly important if fever is present with few or no other abnormal physical signs (*see* FEVER, Chap. X). In most persons, antibodies remain in health below a certain limit. Some of these agglutination limits are set forth below.—

1 in 10—*B. paratyphosum* A, H, and O ; *B. dysenteriæ* (Sonne).

1 in 25—*B. typhosum* H ; *B. paratyphosum* B,H, and C,H, ; *B. enteritidis* (Gaertner) ; *Br. melitensis and abortus* ; *B. dysenteriæ* (Shiga).

1 in 50—*B. typhosum* O, ; and various food poisoning organisms.

Usually if the titre is higher than these average figures, active antibody formation may be suspected from which activity of the disease may be deduced. It is, however, essential to make allowance for occasional wider variations in the normal titre, especially in Flexner dysentery. This serves to emphasize the importance of repeated agglutinin tests so that the results may be compared. A rising titre is far more valuable evidence of active infection than a single estimate, however high the titre may be. It should be pointed out, also, that some persons normally have a very low titre and that in them the rise of agglutinins may still remain below the average normal and yet signify activity. Conversely, inoculations against enteric fever may increase the titre so much that single estimate is quite unreliable. After prophylactic inoculation, the titre of H agglutinins may remain at levels of several hundred and that of O agglutinins at about 25, for many years.

Search for Parasites.—Search for parasites should be made in cases of intermittent or irregular fever when the patient has been abroad. Malarial parasites are the most important found, but others such as trypanosomes or Leishman-Donovan bodies may occasionally be found in patients in general hospitals in this country. (*See* EXAMINATION FOR TROPICAL PARASITES, p. 437.)

CHEMICAL EXAMINATION OF THE URINE

Before testing for abnormal constituents, the urine should be inspected. The quantity, colour, odour, and specific gravity should be noted, and the reaction to litmus tested. If the urine is shaken a froth may appear, which if it lasts for more than two minutes may suggest the presence of protein or bile-salts, but may be caused by rarer constituents.

Turbid urines are often found, commonly due to urates, phosphates, bacteria, blood-, or pus-cells (*see also* Chapter V). *Urates* disappear on heating. *Phosphates* disappear when heated with a few drops of strong acetic acid. *Bacteria, blood-cells, and pus* require filtration or centrifuging for their removal. If the urine is not cleared by heat or the addition of acetic acid, it should be filtered, and, if still cloudy, kieselguhr should be added and the urine filtered again, before applying tests for albumin.

Albuminuria (proteinuria—for most practical purposes it is not necessary to distinguish between albumin and globulin).—

Heat Coagulation Test.—Half fill a test-tube with urine. Boil the top portion. Turbidity occurs from phosphates, but disappears with the addition of a few drops of strong acetic acid. Any remaining turbidity is due to proteins, and is well shown up by the clear layers of urine below the boiled portion (*Fig.* 339).

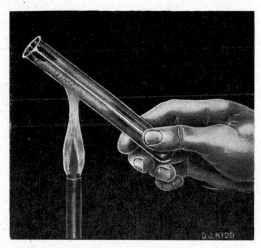

Fig. 339.—A postive reaction in testing urine for albumin.

Nitric Acid Test.—This will sometimes show traces of protein not demonstrable by boiling. Fill the test-tube one third full with urine. Slowly pour a few c.c. strong nitric acid down the side of the sloped tube. A cloud of ' albumin ' results at the junction of the acid and urine.

Salicylsulphonic Acid Test.—To a test-tube one-third filled with urine add 2 to 3 c.c. 10 per cent salicylsulphonic acid. Turbidity occurs from proteins and proteoses, but the latter disappear on boiling. The *test is a very delicate one*, detecting very small amounts of coagulable protein.

Quantitative Estimation of Albumin.—In cases of nephritis a daily estimation of the albumin in the urine is of value in determining the progress of the disease. For this an *Esbach's albuminometer* (*Fig.* 340) is generally employed. The urine is poured into the tube up to the mark U. The Esbach reagent (picric and citric acid) is added to the mark R. The tube is corked, and inverted several times to mix thoroughly. A white precipitate of protein results and is allowed to stand for twenty-four hours. The scale is graduated in figures representing grammes of albumin per litre, and the percentage is therefore obtained by dividing the result by 10. The longer the precipitate stands the less will be the percentage recorded, so it is necessary to allow a uniform time for each estimation.

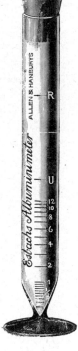

Fig. 340.—Esbach's albuminometer.

If the amount of albumin is very great or the specific gravity is over 1015, the urine should be diluted with an equal quantity of water and the necessary adjustment made in calculating the percentage of albumin.

Small amounts of albumin cannot be recorded by Esbach's method, and it is sufficient to record the amount in such terms as faint trace, trace, or cloud of albumin. An estimation of the quantity of albumin may be obtained more rapidly by the addition of salicylsulphonic acid and comparison of the resultant turbidity with standard tubes representing various percentages of albumin.

Estimation of Urea in Urine.—Most methods of estimating urea depend upon the liberation of nitrogen from the urea by a solution of hypobromite. Several types of apparatus are in use, but the illustration of *Little's nitrometer* (*Fig.* 341) shows one of simple pattern, suitable for use in the clinic room. Little gives the following description of its use :—

Directions for Use.—

1. Distilled water, coloured with a drop or two of red ink, should be poured down the upright tube to the level of first graduation.

2. Pour into empty bulb about 5 c.c. of fresh hypobromite solution.

3. Introduce carefully the rubber stopper.

4. Fill the syringe with the urine to be tested, then screw the regulating nut down to file mark on piston which indicates 1 c.c.

5. Insert the nozzle of the syringe deeply into opening of stopper.

6. Note the level of the liquid on the upright graduated tube.

7. Slowly inject the urine and rotate slightly, grasping the instrument by the top arch.

8. When the effervescence has ceased, read off the level of the fluid in the upright graduated tube. The excess over the former reading (less 1 c.c.) represents the volume of nitrogen evolved from 1 c.c. of urine.

9. Refer to accompanying Table (p. 429) for percentage of urea.

Each capsule of bromine (2 c.c.) added to half an ounce of a 40 per cent solution of caustic soda yields that amount of sodium hypobromite solution which may be used at about 5–10 c.c. at a time for each estimation.

LITTLE'S NITROMETER TABLE

Nitrogen in c.c.	In Grammes per 100 c.c.	In Grains per fl. oz.
0·5	0·14	0·61
1·0	0·28	1·23
1·5	0·42	1·85
2·0	0·56	2·47
2·5	0·70	3·10
3·0	0·84	3·71
3·5	0·98	4·32
4·0	1·13	4·94
4·5	1·27	5·56
5·0	1·41	6·18
5·5	1·55	6·80
6·0	1·69	7·41
6·5	1·83	8·03
7·0	1·97	8·65
7·5	2·11	9·27
8·0	2·25	9·88
8·5	2·40	10·50
9·0	2·54	11·12
9·5	2·68	11·74
10·0	2·82	12·35
10·5	2·96	12·97
11·0	3·10	13·59
11·5	3·24	14·21
12·0	3·39	14·83
12·5	3·53	15·45
13·0	3·67	16·06
13·5	3·81	16·68
14·0	3·95	17·30
14·5	4·09	17·92
15·0	4·23	18·53
15·5	4·37	19·15
16·0	4·52	19·77
16·5	4·66	20·39
17·0	4·80	21·01
17·5	4·94	21·63
18·0	5·08	22·24
18·5	5·22	22·86
19·0	5·36	23·48
19·5	5·50	24·10
20·0	5·65	24·71

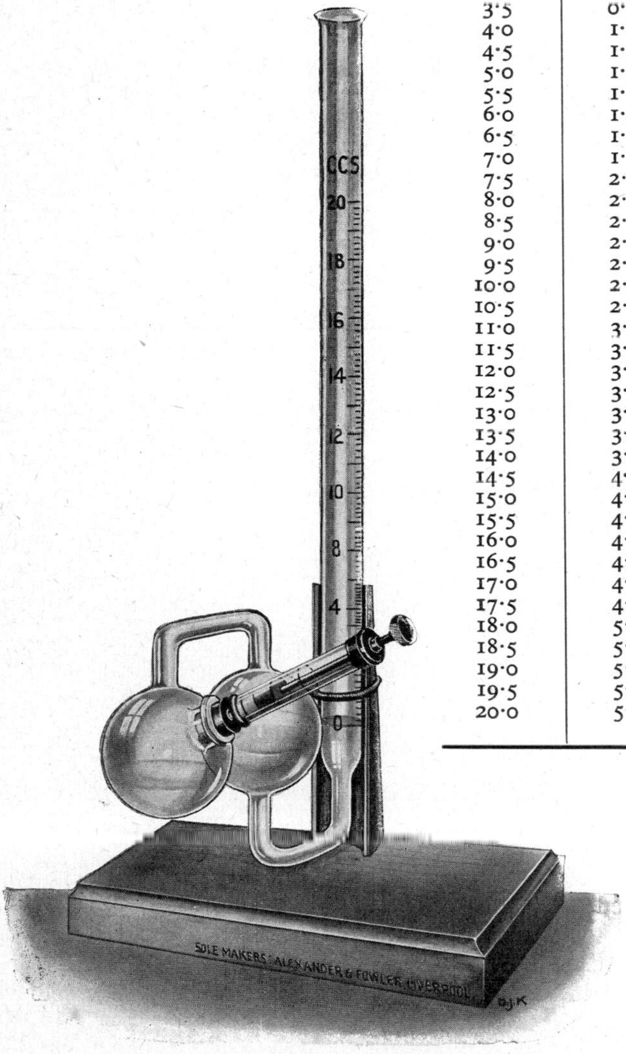

Fig. 341.—Little's nitrometer.

Proteinuria (Bence-Jones protein).—This peculiar protein body is found in the urine in large amounts in certain cases of multiple myelomatosis.

To demonstrate its presence the urine is acidified slightly with acetic acid in a test-tube, to which a thermometer is attached with the aid of elastic bands on the outside of the tube. The whole is placed in a water bath and the temperature raised gradually and kept uniform by stirring, using the tube and thermometer for the purpose. The Bence-Jones protein is precipitated between temperatures of $40°$ and $60°$ C., first at the lower temperature as a uniform turbidity and later at $60°$ C. as a flocculent precipitate. As the temperature approaches $100°$ C. the precipitate almost completely disappears—and reappears on cooling.

Glycosuria (sugar in urine).—

Fehling's Test.—Mix a few c.c. of urine with an equal quantity of Fehling's solution (the latter is usually dispensed in two solutions, one containing sodium potassium tartrate, the other copper sulphate). Boil the mixture for three minutes. A yellow or red *precipitate* generally denotes the presence of sugar (including lactose in lactating women). A greenish or even yellowish *discoloration of the urine without a precipitate* occurs from several reducing agents, especially uric acid, creatinine, salicylic acid derivatives, chloral hydrate, chloroform, and from minute traces of sugar.

Benedict's Test.—The reagent used in this test has the advantage that it is not reduced by uric acid, glycuronic acid, and creatinine, which may cause normal urine to reduce Fehling's solution.

To 5 c.c. of Benedict's solution add 8 drops of urine and boil for 2 minutes. Sugar is present in appreciable amounts if the fluid becomes brick-red, yellow, or brown and on standing a deposit of similar colour will form.

Sometimes the fluid merely becomes green and turbid, but this is *not* to be taken as evidence of sugar unless a *deposit* forms on standing, which may occur with very small quantities of sugar.

A rough estimation of the amount of sugar may thus be made from the colour and amount of the deposit, providing 8 drops of urine only are used.

Quantitative Estimation of Sugar : Benedict's Method.—If the urine is of high specific gravity indicating a high sugar content (after first testing qualitatively with Fehling), it should be diluted 1–10 before proceeding to the estimation. If a weak Fehling reaction and a low specific gravity is found, the undiluted urine is used.

Technique :—

1. Measure 25 c.c. of Benedict's reagent into a porcelain evaporating dish about 30 cm. in diameter. Add about 5 g. of anhydrous sodium carbonate.

2. Fill a 25-c.c. burette with the urine, place it in a stand suspended over the evaporating dish, which has been placed on a tripod.

3. Heat the contents of the evaporating dish until they boil vigorously, and, while constantly stirring, rapidly run in the urine from the burette until a heavy white precipitate is produced and the blue colour of the solution diminishes. From this point the urine is run in more slowly, with constant *vigorous boiling*, until the last trace of blue colour disappears ; this is the end point of the titration. If the volume of fluid in the evaporating dish is reduced considerably by evaporation, the volume can be restored by the addition of distilled water.

4. *Calculation* : 25 c.c. of Benedict's reagent are reduced exactly by 50 mg. of glucose. Therefore the amount of urine used to complete the reduction contained 50 mg. of sugar. The formula for calculating the percentage of sugar is as follows :—

For undiluted urine : $\dfrac{0.050}{X} \times 100 = $ g. per cent of sugar.

For urine diluted 1–10 : multiply by 1000 instead of 100.

X = c.c. of urine required to reduce 25 c.c. of the reagent.

Example : 2.5 c.c. of undiluted urine are used. Then sugar content is :— $\dfrac{0.05}{2.5} \times 100 = 2$ g. per cent glucose.

To convert the result into grains per fluid ounce, multiply by 4.375.

Ketonuria.—

Ferric Chloride Test for Diacetic Acid (Gerhardt's Reaction).—To a few c.c. of urine add about a quarter its volume of ferric chloride solution. Filter if a precipitate forms. In the presence of diacetic acid a claret colour develops. A similar reaction may be given by salicylic acid derivatives, gallates, and antipyrin, but more elaborate technique is required for differentiation.

Rothera's Nitroprusside Reaction for Diacetic acid and Acetone.—Take several c.c. of urine. Add solid ammonium sulphate to saturation point, then a few drops of freshly prepared sodium nitroprusside solution, mix, and finally pour a few c.c. strong ammonia down the slope of the test-tube. The presence of diacetic acid and acetone is shown by the development of a purple colour which deepens on standing, the intensity of the colour depending on the amount present. The test is much more delicate than the ferric chloride reaction.

Bilinuria.—Bile in urine may be discovered by tests dependent upon the presence of bile-pigments or bile-salts.

Iodine Test.—This reaction depends upon the presence of bile-pigments. One c.c. of tincture of iodine is *slowly* poured into a few c.c. of urine. A positive reaction is the development of a greenish-blue colour at the level of the iodine.

Gmelin's Test.—If urine containing bile is passed through filter-paper, the deposit formed on the paper will yield a series of brilliant colours radiating from the point where a drop of nitric acid is placed—yellow, red, violet, and green. A test for bile-pigments.

Hay's Test.—A test for bile-salts. The urine should be put in a small beaker and powdered sulphur sprinkled gently on its surface. Some of the sulphur sinks when bile is present, but floats in normal urine.

Urobilinuria.—First add a few drops of tincture of iodine to 5 c.c. of urine. This converts urobilinogen into urobilin. Then add 5 c.c. of a saturated alcoholic solution of zinc acetate. Shake the mixture and filter. A greenish fluorescence results if urobilin is present in excess. A *very faint* reaction may occur in normal urine.

Urobilinogen in Urine.—Add 2 drops of a 3 per cent solution of Ehrlich's reagent (paradimethylaminobenzaldehyde in 50 per cent hydrochloric acid) to 5 c.c. of urine. In the presence of an excess of urobilinogen, a deep-red colour develops.

Hæmaturia.—Blood is most satisfactorily detected by microscopical examination of the urine. The following chemical tests are also commonly employed.

Direct Guaiacum Test.—To 10 c.c. of urine add 2 or 3 drops of fresh tincture of guaiacum. The resulting cloudiness is cleared by addition of sufficient alcohol. Then add 10 drops of hydrogen peroxide or ozonic ether. A blue colour results from the presence of blood or certain other substances, notably pus.

The test is most valuable as a negative one, for *if no blue colour results blood is absent in any quantity*.

Extraction Guaiacum Test.—If the above reaction is positive, a further test is necessary to distinguish blood from other substances giving the same result.

Take 20 c.c. of urine. Add 3 c.c. strong acetic acid and boil the mixture. *Cool* and extract by shaking up with 5 c.c. of ether. Pipette the ethereal extract into another test-tube and add 3 drops of tincture of guaiacum and 5 drops of hydrogen peroxide. A blue colour denotes the presence of blood if the possibility of iodides in the urine can be excluded.

Hæmoglobinuria.—The urine has not the bright-red appearance of hæmaturia. It is often port-wine-coloured, and varies from a red to a dark brown. On standing there is a heavy brownish deposit which, under the microscope, shows no intact red cells. The usual chemical tests for blood are positive, so that microscopy is necessary to eliminate hæmaturia.

Vitamin C in Urine.—The test is dependent upon the power of ascorbic acid (vitamin C) to discharge the colour of the indicator, dichlorophenolindophenol. Normally the excretion of ascorbic acid is over 13 mg. in 24 hours, and figures less than this may indicate subnutrition. It is more satisfactory, however, to estimate the urinary content after administration of a test dose. Persons with a sufficiency immediately respond by an increase of urinary excretion. Those suffering from subnutrition or scurvy show a delayed response depending upon the time taken for the tissues to become saturated. Test outfits suitable for the clinic room may be obtained.

OTHER SPECIAL INVESTIGATIONS

Renal Function Tests.—In purely medical diseases of the kidney, especially in the different types of nephritis, the special investigations of most value are those throwing light on the functional capacity of the kidneys. Three of considerable importance may be mentioned.

1. *The Urea Concentration Test.*—In this test, 15 grammes of urea are given to the patient by mouth, and the amount excreted in the urine is estimated hourly during the succeeding three hours. The normal kidney possesses the power of concentrating urea so that between 2 and 4 per cent should be passed in one or more of the analysed specimens. If the concentration is less than 2 per cent in all specimens, some renal insufficiency may be presumed unless diuresis is very marked. Usually not more than 120 c.c. should be passed in the first hour, nor more than 100 c.c. in the second and third hours. If the diuresis is greater than this, the test should be repeated. The urea concentration test often shows up early defects in renal adequacy.

2. *The Urea Clearance Test.*—This test attempts to assess the renal function by measuring the quantity of blood cleared of urea by the kidneys in a given time. The patient, who should be in bed, is first given a glass of water. The bladder is emptied completely, and the specimen discarded. Exactly one hour and two hours later (by stop watch) the bladder is again emptied, and the volume of each specimen noted. Blood is taken for urea estimation just before the first hour's collection of urine. According to whether the urinary volume is more or less than 2 c.c. per minute, the formula for 'maximum or standard' clearance is applied, and the result expressed as a percentage of normal. The two hourly specimens are taken as a check upon each other and should agree to within 10 per cent. The test is invalidated by carelessness in collection, or incomplete evacuation of the bladder. Normal renal function is indicated by a result of over 70 per cent of average normal clearance. Moderate impairment gives figures from 40 to 20 per cent, and uræmia is present when the urea clearance falls below 5 per cent.

3. *Estimation of Non-Protein Nitrogen (N.P.N.) or Blood-Urea.*— In more serious cases of renal insufficiency there may be retention of nitrogenous products, especially urea, in the blood. This is particularly so in some types of chronic renal disease, and sometimes in acute nephritis and in renal changes secondary to obstruction to the urinary flow, e.g., in enlargement of the prostate. In uræmia the N.P.N. or blood-urea may attain very high values. The normal N.P.N. or blood-urea content is about 30 mg. per cent, but may be as high as 40 mg. per cent without pathological significance. In renal disease, especially with uræmia, figures from fifty to several hundred milligrammes may be reached, but do not always bear a direct relationship to the severity of the clinical condition.

28

In surgical diseases of the urinary tract these three methods of assessing kidney function are also employed, but other methods of great value are available (X rays, cystoscopy, and ureteric catheterization).

GLUCOSE TOLERANCE TEST

Fifty or a hundred grammes of glucose are given to the patient in a flavoured watery solution. Samples of blood and urine are taken immediately before, and at intervals of half an hour afterwards, usually for two and a half hours. In a normal tolerance test the blood-sugar rises rapidly from its fasting level of 100 mg. per cent (average) to 170-180 mg. per cent, at which point the storage mechanisms prevent further rise. The peak of the curve is generally reached half an hour after the ingestion of the glucose, and thereafter falls to normal in another one to one and a half hours. Considerable variation in the time taken to return to fasting values is shown by different individuals. Normally no sugar appears in the urine during this test. (*Fig.* 342.)

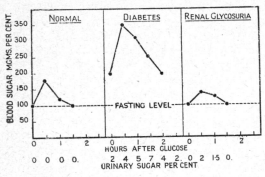

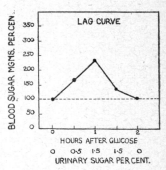

Fig. 342.—Glucose tolerance test. Examples of responses.   *Fig.* 343.—Glucose test in lag glycosuria.

The fasting level of blood-sugar is the same in capillary (arterial) or venous blood. After the ingestion of glucose, however, the capillary blood-sugar is somewhat higher than the venous.

In the *diabetic*, the fasting blood-sugar is high (200–300 mg. per cent in cases of average severity), there is a great rise after ingestion of sugar (300–500 mg. per cent), and a very slow return to the fasting level.

In most cases sugar is found in each specimen of the urine unless the ' leak point ' is high, i.e., if the kidney will not secrete sugar until the blood-sugar rises to more than 200 mg. per cent.

In *renal glycosuria* the leak point is low. After ingestion of glucose, sugar soon appears in the urine although the blood-sugar may never rise above normal values.

In *lag glycosuria* the fasting blood-sugar is normal, but after ingestion of glucose it rises rapidly to above 180 mg. per cent, returning however to normal in $1\frac{1}{2}$–2 hrs. (*Fig.* 343). Sugar appears in the urine. It is due to a delay in the action of the sugar storage mechanism. Clinically it is symptomless.

STAINING FOR BACTERIA

The following brief description includes the more common stains which the student or practitioner will require. Methods requiring elaborate technique have been omitted.

Before the application of the stain a careful preparation of the material must be made. This should be spread on a glass slide in sufficient amount for the bacteria to be shown up, but too thick a layer should be avoided. The preparation should be fixed by gently heating above a Bunsen flame (never in it).

Löffler's Methylene Blue.—This is a general stain which can be used for all cells and bacteria. It is useful in a routine examination of sputum, throat swabs, etc.

Technique.—Stain the preparation for three minutes. Then wash in water. Organisms and cellular nuclei stain deep blue, cytoplasm a pale blue.

Gram's Stain.—Gram's stain is probably the most commonly used of all bacterial stains. It is used to demonstrate bacteria in sputum, blood, purulent exudates, urine, cerebrospinal fluid, and so forth. Its principal value is the fact that it divides bacteria into two classes : (1) Those which take on a bluish colour with gentian violet and retain this colour after decolorizing the film with alcohol (Gram-positive) ; (2) Those which do not retain the blue colour (Gram-negative) but require to be shown up by an acid counterstain.

Technique.—

1. Stain with aniline gentian violet (or carbol gentian violet) for 1 to 2 minutes.

2. Drain off the gentian violet and replace with Gram's iodine. Allow this to act for 1 minute.

3. Without washing, pour off the iodine and decolorize the film with spirit until the violet colour is dispersed. (Avoid over-decolorization by controlling under the microscope if in doubt.)

4. Wash the film with water.

5. Counterstain with dilute carbol-fuchsin (1–10) for 10 to 20 seconds.

6. Wash with water and dry with blotting or filter paper.

Ziehl-Neelsen's Carbol-fuchsin Stain.—This method is used for demonstrating tubercle bacilli. In the case of sputum and cerebrospinal fluid it may be applied directly to a dried preparation from these, though the cerebrospinal fluid should be centrifuged in order to concentrate the bacteria. When the bacilli are likely to be obscured by other constituents of the preparation, e.g., in fæces and urine, special methods of dissolving these other constituents are employed, e.g., the antiformin method.

Technique.—

1. Heat about 5 c.c. of filtered Ziehl-Neelsen carbol-fuchsin in a test-tube until nearly boiling.

2. Flood the film with the hot solution and allow to act for 5 to 10 minutes (avoid allowing the stain to dry on the slide).

3. Wash with water.

4. With the aid of a pair of forceps immerse the whole of the slide in a 25 per cent solution of sulphuric acid in alcohol. The red colour changes to a yellowish brown. Remove the slide after one minute and wash with water ; the film becomes reddish-pink again. This process should be repeated several times until finally the film assumes a faint pink after washing.

5. Wash thoroughly with water.

6. Counterstain with Löffler's methylene blue for 30 seconds.

7. Wash, blot, and dry.

The tubercle bacilli stain red, the remainder of the preparation blue.

Neisser's Stain.—This stain is used to demonstrate diphtheria bacilli.

Technique.—

1. Flood the film with Neisser's stain (acid methylene blue) and allow to act for 30 seconds.

2. Wash with water.

3. Counterstain with Bismarck brown or chrysoidin for 15 to 20 seconds.

4. Wash with water and dry.

This stains the bodies of the bacilli brown, and the metachromatic granules blue.

Emrys Roberts's Method.—

1. Stain with Neisser for 30 seconds.

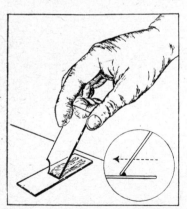

Fig. 344.—Preparing a blood-film. If the corner of the slide is cut off the smear will occupy only a portion of the other slide, and its edges can therefore be examined easily. This is of value, as the leucocytes are more numerous at the edges.

2. Wash.

3. Stain with Lugol's iodine for 1 minute.

4. Wash and dry.

The polar bodies of the bacilli stain blue, and stroma light brown.

Giemsa's Stain.—This method is employed for staining blood-films, especially when searching for parasites such as the malarial parasite, trypanosomes, and spirochætes.

Technique (rapid method).—

1. Fix the film in methyl alcohol for 3 minutes.

2. Flood with a mixture of 1 part stain and 2 parts distilled water. Allow to act for 5 minutes.

3. Wash with distilled water and allow to act for about $\frac{1}{2}$ minute.

4. Blot and allow to dry in the air.

Leishman's Stain.—Used chiefly as a blood stain.

Technique.—Make a blood-film as indicated in the illustration (*Fig.* 344). The film should be even and not too thick. Allow to dry in the air. Place slide on staining rack and flood with Leishman's stain. Allow to act for 5 minutes. Dilute with equal volume of distilled water and mix well with pipette ; the mixture should remain on for a further period of 10 minutes. Wash film in distilled water and allow it to remain for further 30 seconds covered with water. Drain and dry in air, or between absorbent paper. The staining can be controlled by examining the wet preparation under the microscope.

EXAMINATION FOR TROPICAL PARASITES

By A. R. D. ADAMS, M.D., D.T.M.

Stool Examination (*Fig.* 345).—The proper examination of fæces for protozoal and helminthic intestinal parasites requires some skill and much practice. The material to be examined must be reasonably fresh, and in those cases where the vegetative or unencysted forms of protozoa alone are to be found, the examination must be made within an hour or so of the passage of the specimen. The vegetative protozoal forms die and disintegrate very rapidly, but the cysts last for a day or two. A loose stool is likely to contain the unencysted vegetative forms, while a formed stool contains only the cystic forms of protozoa. A simple method of searching a stool for such parasites is the emulsification of a loopful in a drop of water or saline on a slide. This is then covered with a glass slip and examined with the 2/3 in. microscope objective, the light being cut down with the iris diaphragm. The vegetative and cystic forms of the intestinal protozoa, and helminth ova, can be found by this method ; more detail can then be seen by using the higher objectives. While helminth ova can readily be identified by their size, shape, and structure, employing this technique, the protozoal cysts have to be stained to show their morphology. A simple method of staining is the emulsification of a loopful of stool in a drop of 3 per cent aqueous iodine solution*. It will be found that the nuclei of the cysts are stained by the iodine and their number and structure are thus revealed, enabling an identification of the species to be made. A word of warning about the employment of an iodine-stained film initially is advisable : this apparent short cut may result in missing the cysts entirely, iodine staining making them much more difficult to find.

Concentration methods for protozoal cysts are of dubious clinical value ; one used for certain helminth ova, more especially hookworm ova, will greatly increase the chances of finding the ova when scanty in number. Certain eggs float in a saturated brine solution, and if about a gramme of fæces is emulsified in a few cubic centimetres of such a solution in a wide-mouthed tube, and the tube is then carefully filled brim-full

---

* Iodide .1 part ; Potassium iodide, 2 parts ; Distilled water, 100 parts.

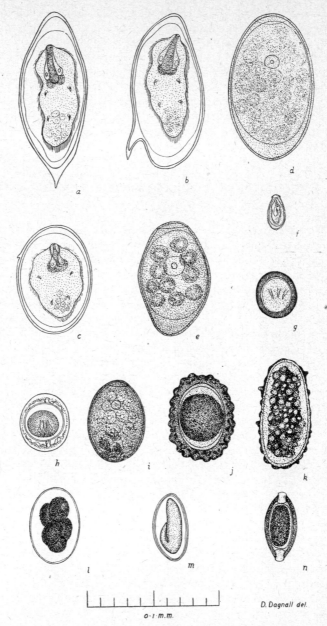

D. Dagnall del.

o · 1 · m.m.

Fig. 345.—HELMINTH EGGS.—Drawn to show relative sizes and appearances. Found in fæces unless otherwise noted.

a, Schistosoma hæmatobium (urine, rarely fæces) ; *b,* Schistosoma mansoni ; *c,* Schistosoma japonicum ; *d,* Fasciolopsis buskii ; *e,* Paragonimus westermanii (sputum) ; *f,* Clonorchis sinensis ; *g,* Tænia spp. ; *h,* Hymenolepis nana ; *i,* Diphyllobothrium latum ; *j,* Ascaris lumbricoides ; *k,* Unfertilized Ascaris ; *l,* Hookworm—Ancylostoma duodenale and Necator americanus ; *m,* Enterobius vermicularis (perianal skin) ; *n,* Trichuris trichiura.

with the salt solution, the eggs float to the top. They can be picked off by touching a slide on the meniscus and examining the collected material microscopically after covering with a cover-slip. This technique is of no value in recovering such eggs as those of *Ascaris* or *Tænia*.

Blood Examination (*Fig.* 346).—The examination of blood for *malaria* parasites calls first for the preparation and proper staining of well-made films. Thin films can conveniently and rapidly be stained with Leishman's stain ; after staining, the Leishman should merely be flushed off. But little washing is advisable, as it removes the blue dye. The parasites are in the red cells, and, when numerous, their recognition is not of great difficulty. When scanty, however, they may be excessively hard to find, and here the thick film is of great value in skilled hands. Thick films are made by putting two or three drops of blood in the middle of a slide and then rubbing evenly together with a needle over an area to a thickness such that the hands of a watch can be seen through the film. This film, after thorough drying, must be de-hæmoglobinized before staining and examination, or it will be opaque. It can be inverted in water, then dried and stained with Leishman's stain ; it can be stained with Giemsa's stain ; or, preferably, it can be stained by Field's technique*, which gives much superior results. The recognition of the deformed parasites after such treatment requires skill and much practice, but, when these are acquired, parasites can be found where too scanty to be seen in thin films of the same blood.

Other parasites which may occur in the blood are the trypanosomes of *African sleeping sickness* and of *Chagas's disease*, the spirochætes of the *relapsing fevers*, *Leptospira icterohæmorrhagiæ* causing *Weil's disease*, *Spirillum minus* the cause of *rat-bite fever*, and certain larval filarial worms referred to as *microfilariæ*. All these parasites may be detected by putting a drop of fresh blood on a slide and examining microscopically under a cover-slip as a wet preparation with a suitable objective, using either the ordinary illumination or, preferably, a dark-ground condenser. They may also be seen in thick or thin films stained as for malaria parasites : microfilariæ are best seen in thick films stained with Mayer's hæmalum.

---

* **Field's Technique for Staining Thick Blood-films.—**

Stain A.—

Methylene blue	.. ..	0·8 g.
Azur I	..	0·5 ,,
Disodium hydrogen phosphate (anhydrous)		5·0
Potassium dihydrogen phosphate (anhydrous)	..	6·25 ,,
Distilled water	..	500 c.c.

Stain B.—

Eosin	..	1·0 g.
Disodium hydrogen phosphate (anhydrous)	..	5·0 ,,
Potassium dihydrogen phosphate (anhydrous)	..	6·25 ,,
Distilled water	..	500 c.c.

Method.—Dry thick film in air or at 37° C. Dip for 3 seconds in Stain A. Rinse for 5 seconds in water. Dip for 3 seconds in Stain B. Rinse in water. Drain and allow to dry in air. Examine with 1/12 in. oil-immersion objective.

To find the Leishman-Donovan bodies responsible for visceral *leishmaniasis*, which are parasitic in endothelial cells, microscopical examination of blood is wholly inadequate and virtually useless. The blood can be cultured in suitable media and may well give a positive culture, but the organisms at best are excessively scanty in it; they must be recovered from the spleen, liver, or bone-marrow to be seen and recognized in appreciable numbers. In cutaneous leishmaniasis the bodies can be found in large numbers in the endothelial cells in the *walls* of the lesions; they will not be recognizable in the pus discharged from the ulcers, and they do not invade the body as a whole.

Fig. 346.—MALARIA PARASITES.—Nos. 1 to 26—thin films, Leishman's stain ; Nos. 27 to 29—thick films, Field's stain. Smears made from peripheral blood unless otherwise noted. (× 600.)

Plasmodium falciparum (malignant tertian malaria) (Nos. 1 to 8.) 1, Ring. 2, Ring with two chromatin dots. 3, Double infection of red cell. Marginal or accolé forms. 4, Ring in deeply stained cell showing coarse stippling (Stephen's and Christopher's dots). 5, Male sexual form. Gametocyte or crescent. Note purplish cytoplasm and scattered pigment. 6, Female sexual form. Gametocyte or crescent. Note slaty-blue cytoplasm and compact pigment. 7, Half-grown asexual form from spleen smear of fatal case. 8, Fully-grown asexual form (schizont) from spleen smear. 9, Macrophage containing ingested malarial pigment.

Plasmodiam malariæ (quartan). (Nos. 10 to 15.) 10, Ring. 11, 12, Trophozoites. Note compactness of cytoplasm and heavy pigment. No. 12 shows an equatorial form. 13, Schizont. Typical rosette form consisting of a central mass of pigment surrounded by 8 merozoites. 14, Male gametocyte. Shows diffusion of nucleus and scattered pigment. 15, Female gametocyte. Shows compactness of nucleus and pigment.

16, Blood-platelet superimposed on red cell. Often mistaken for a malarial parasite.

Plasmodium vivax (simple or benign tertian). (Nos. 17 to 21.) 17, Ring. 18, Trophozoite. Note amœboid cytoplasm and paleness of red cell, which is enlarged and stippled with fine red dots (Schüffner's dots). 19, Schizont. Red cell enlarged, pale, and stippled with Schüffner's dots. 20, Male gametocyte. 21, Female gametocyte. The gametocytes differ from those of quartan in being enclosed in enlarged, stippled cells, and in having finer pigment.

Plasmodium ovale (tertian). (Nos. 22 to 26.) 22, Ring. 23, Trophozoite. Differs from the trophozoite of *P. vivax* in being more solid, and is often found in an oval red cell with fimbriated edges. The stippling is heavier than in *P. vivax.* 24, Schizont. The number of merozoites (12), is less than in *P. vivax*, which has 16 to 24. 25, Male gametocyte. 26, Female gametocyte.

27, *P. falciparum* : thick film. Shows several rings lying at various angles, a gametocyte, and some blue-staining bodies, reticulocytes.

28, *P. malariæ* : thick film. Shows two trophozoites and a schizont. Included in the field are blood-platelets, a punctate basophil, and a lymphocyte.

29, *P. vivax* : thick film. Shows three trophozoites. Note apparent breaking-up of cytoplasm, a typical feature. The outline of the infected red cells can be traced by the Schüffner's dots. Included are a neutrophil polymorphonuclear leucocyte, platelets, and a reticulocyte.

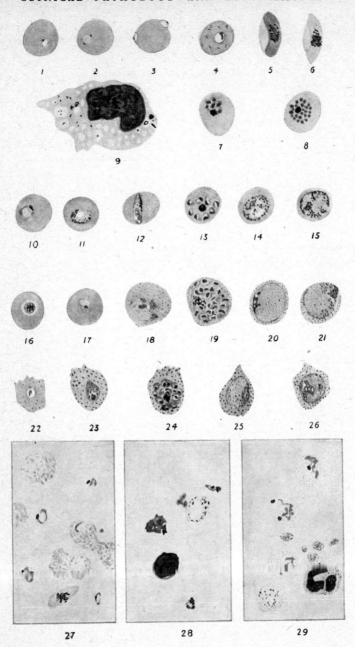

D. Dagnall del.

Fig. 346.—For description see facing page.

TABLE OF BIOCHEMICAL STANDARDS

Blood.— *Mg. per 100 c.c.*

N.P.N.		25–35
Urea		15–40
Uric acid		2–3·5
Ammonia N		0·1–0·2
Glucose		80–120
Cholesterol (serum)		150–190
Cholesterol (whole blood)		140–180
Bilirubin		0·3–0·8
Chlorides (as NaCl)		450–500
Phosphates (P)		3–4
Calcium (serum)		9–11
Sodium		170–225

Urine.—(Results of 24-hour specimen ; mixed diet ; volume 1500 c.c.)

Reaction	pH 6·0 (mean)
Ammonia	about 0·7 g.
Diastase	5–30 units (average 10)
Sodium chloride	16·5 g. (1·1 per cent)
Total N	10–17 g.
Urea	20–35 g.

Cerebrospinal Fluid.— *Mg. per cent*

Proteins (total coagulable)	20–30
Glucose	45–100
Chlorides (as NaCl)	700–760
Urea	10–40
Phosphates	1·5–2

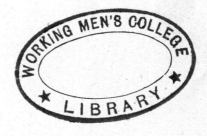

443

INDEX

PRINTED IN GREAT BRITAIN BY JOHN WRIGHT AND SONS LTD., BRISTOL

11 DEC 1956

17 DEC 1956

7 FEB 1957

2 5 FEB 1959

8 JAN 1973

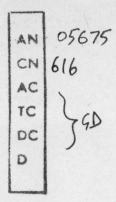

AN	05675
CN	616
AC	} SD
TC	
DC	
D	